NMS Q&A
Family Medicine

3rd EDITION

NMS Q&A
Family Medicine

3rd EDITION

David R. Rudy, MD, MPH
Clinical Professor of Family Medicine
The Ohio State University
Professor, Chairman, Retired
Department of Family and Preventive Medicine
The Chicago Medical School

Wolters Kluwer | Lippincott Williams & Wilkins
Health
Philadelphia • Baltimore • New York • London
Buenos Aires • Hong Kong • Sydney • Tokyo

Acquisitions Editor: Susan Rhyner
Product Manager: Stacey Sebring
Marketing Manager: Joy Fischer-Williams
Vendor Manager: Alicia Jackson
Designer: Holly McLaughlin
Compositor: Aptara, Inc.

351 West Camden Street
Baltimore, MD 21201

Two Commerce Square, 2001 Market Street
Philadelphia, PA 19103

Printed in China

Library of Congress Cataloging-in-Publication Data

Rudy, David R.
    Family medicine / David R. Rudy.—3rd ed.
        p. ; cm.—(NMS Q&A)
    NMS Q&A family medicine
    Includes bibliographical references and index.
    ISBN 978-1-60831-577-2 (alk. paper)
 1. Family medicine—Examinations, questions, etc.   I. Title.
 II. Title: NMS Q&A family medicine.   III. Series: NMS Q&A.
    [DNLM: 1. Family Practice—Examination Questions. WB 18.2]
    RC58.R83   2011
    616—dc22
                                            2011016385

To purchase additional copies of this book, call our customer service department at **(800) 638–3030** or fax orders to **(301) 223–2320.** International customers should call **(301) 223–2300.**

Visit Lippincott Williams & Wilkins on the Internet: http://www.LWW.com. Lippincott Williams & Wilkins customer service representatives are available from 8:30 am to 6:00 pm, EST.

1 2 3 4 5 6 7 8 9 10

This work is dedicated to my wife, Rose Mary S. Rudy, PhD; our children Douglas David Rudy (IT executive), Steven William Rudy (aerospace engineer), Katharine Rudy Hoffer, RN, MA and Hunter Ashley Elam, PhD and to our seven grandchildren. Finally, I dedicate this work to the memories of my parents, Robert Sale Rudy, CPA, late retired CFO of the White Castle Corporation and Lois May Arthur Rudy; and to my late older, mentoring twin brothers, John Franklin (MWE) and James Arthur Rudy (MME), Master level engineers.

Foreword to the First Edition

Family medicine was the first specialty to require recertification to ensure that family physicians remain current in advances in medicine. We are continually challenging ourselves with questions of the type presented in this book. These questions help us remain abreast of new information and prepare for written examinations, whether they be the in-training exams given in the medical clerkships, to family practice residents, or the certification and recertification exams taken by physicians in practice.

The questions in this book focus on practical issues also presented in *Family Medicine: The House Officer Series*. The answers not only give the preferred course of action but also discuss why other options are incorrect.

New information is added, supplementing that provided in *Family Medicine: The House Officer Series*. These questions and the discussions of the answers give the reader insight into the problem-solving process in primary care, which often differs from that in the consulting specialties.

Dr. Rudy has, through *Family Medicine: The House Officer Series* and *NMS Q&A Family Medicine*, provided the reader with an excellent overview of our discipline by reflecting the variety of problems encountered in practice. It is this variety that keeps us perpetually challenged. These books let us keep pace with modern advances and help us sustain the excitement and satisfaction of primary care.

Robert E. Rakel, MD

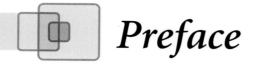

Preface

The third edition of *Family Medicine Q&A,* in the respected NMS series, is more student friendly and more amenable to reference in that there is a complete index. The main objective of the third edition remains the provision of study material for students in preparation for USMLE Steps 2 and 3 and Family Medicine clerkships. Every item from the second edition was revisited; obsolete material was deleted and material still relevant was presented anew from different pedagogical angles. New questions are more likely to have originated from material taken from the latest Scientific Assembly of the American Academy of Family Medicine and from late issues of the American Family Physician. A few questions remain virtually verbatim from the second edition because they bear repetition, unchanged in form from the second edition. As with the first and second editions, the exacting standards of Lippincott Williams & Wilkins ensure quality worthy of the NMS. I consider it an honor to have brought the project to its third edition and hope that students and residents will continue to benefit in their preparation for their futures.

David R. Rudy, MD, MPH

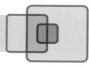

Acknowledgments

For the contributions to medical education I hope will be conveyed through book, I acknowledge the academic leadership of Family Medicine and their untiring dedication to continued growth and keeping pace with the ever-expanding fund of knowledge. Furthermore, I greatly appreciate the professionalism as well as literary friendship and close working relationship with my freelance editor, Julie Scardiglia. I also thank Sirkka Howes, managing editor at LWW, for all her support to this project. Finally, I wish the best for Charley Mitchell, my first contact at Williams & Wilkins and publisher for LWW at the time of the initiation of this edition.

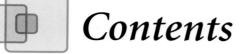

Contents

SECTION XII ALLERGIES

SECTION XIII PREVENTIVE HEALTH CARE

SECTION XIV BEHAVIOR AND PSYCHOLOGY IN PRIMARY CARE

SECTION XV MISCELLANEOUS AREAS OF CLINICAL PRACTICE

Urgent Care

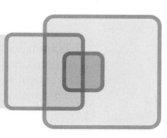

chapter 1

Urgent Care in Family Practice

Examination questions: *Unless instructed otherwise, choose the ONE lettered answer or completion that is BEST in each case.*

1 A 72-year-old male had the onset, within the last 60 minutes, of right hemiparesis and expressive aphasia. Which of the following is the most important variable to monitor on this patient while a decision is being made regarding whether to employ thrombolytic therapy?

(A) WBC
(B) Hemoglobin
(C) Blood sugar
(D) Serum electrolytes
(E) Oxygenation status

2 A morbidly obese 19-year-old male fell 3 days ago on the ice with his legs going "out from under," sitting down hard. He complains of increasing pain in the lumbar region with radiation down the left lateral posterior thigh. On examination, he manifests positive straight leg raising test at 45 degrees on the left and 60 degrees on the right; both maneuvers result in shock with shooting pains into the lower extremities. Knee-jerk reflexes are 2+ bilateral; ankle-jerk reflexes are 2+ left and consistently 0–1 on the right. Heel

walking is normally demonstrated. Toe walking is weak on the right. Which of the following is the most urgent finding thus far in forming an immediate differential diagnosis in this patient?

(A) The pattern of radiation of the pain
(B) Asymmetry in the deep tendon reflexes of the lower extremities
(C) Bilateral presentation of signs and symptoms
(D) Weakness of the Achilles apparatus
(E) Severity of the pain

3 Regarding Question 2, which of the following is most critical in supplementing the history taken thus far?

(A) Presence or absence of numbness in the lower extremities
(B) Presence or absence of visceral symptomatology
(C) Investigation of possible drug-seeking behavior
(D) Ability to bend forward in lifting
(E) Whether or not the accident was work-site connected

4 Regarding the patient in Questions 2 and 3, the patient admits that he has had trouble holding his urine without spilling into his clothing or on the floor en route to the bathroom; which of the following is most necessary to complete the physical examination?

(A) Check for plantar reflex response
(B) Complete neurological examination
(C) Visual-field examination
(D) Checking the perineum and inner thighs for touch, sharp and dull pain perception and conducting a digital rectal examination
(E) Test for proprioception in the lower extremities

5 What is the average maximum time period from the onset of symptoms and signs for the diagnosis and treatment of the patient in questions 2 through 4 in order to achieve the best therapeutic result?

(A) Hours
(B) 48 hours
(C) 72 hours
(D) 5 days
(E) Days

6 A 60-year-old male—newly diagnosed Type II diabetic—complains of unremitting and increasingly severe low back pain for the past 48 hours. He has been unable to find a comfortable position, that is, whether he is sitting, standing, flexed at the hips supine or on his side. There is radiation down the left lateral thigh. He denies urinary symptoms of any sort. His vital signs are normal except for a temperature of 100.8°F. Examination shows no abdominal mass or tenderness, and there is no costovertebral angle or other back tenderness. There is no saddle numbness or sensory loss. Deep tendon reflexes of the lower extremities are brisk and symmetrical. Straight-leg-raising test is unworkable due to the patient writhing in pain when in the supine position. Complete blood count (CBC) shows a leukocytosis of 18,000 with 80 neutrophils and a slight shift toward immature forms. The urinalysis is unremarkable. Which of the following is the most important next step in evaluating this patient?

(A) 100 mg meperidine intravenously for empiric evaluation of his response
(B) Urology consultation for a possible obstructing urolith accounting for normal urinalysis
(C) Computed tomography (CT) of the lumbosacral spine
(D) Stat blood cultures to be drawn
(E) Start intravenous levofloxacin

7 Of the following, which is the most urgent of the possible diagnoses of the patient in Question 6?

(A) Acute pyelonephritis
(B) Metastatic malignancy in the spinal cord or column

(C) Vertebral body pathologic fracture due to osteoporosis
(D) Epidural abscess
(E) Acute cholecystitis

8 A 63-year-old Caucasian male, with a history of frequent headaches during his adult years, was leaving his yacht club after docking his boat and, en route to his car, noted the onset, over less than a minute, of a severe headache; he had no history whatsoever of headaches in the past. His friend drove him to the family doctor's office within 15 minutes of the onset. The patient, who walked into the office accompanied by his friend, was by that time having difficulty remembering what he was trying to say when he would start a sentence. However, there was no aphasia noted, neither motor nor expressive. In ordering the patient to be delivered forthwith to the nearest emergency department (ED), which of the following is the most logical of urgent diagnostic studies to be obtained?

(A) CT scan of the head without contrast
(B) Lumbar puncture
(C) CT scan of the head with contrast
(D) Magnetic resonance imaging (MRI) of the brain
(E) Stat CBC and differential

9 A 25-year-old woman suffers a direct blow to the head from the elbow of a teammate in a volleyball game. She manifests a few minutes of confusion after which she is oriented to person, place and time and notes tenderness and swelling on the right frontal eminence of her head where the blow occurred. She is playing in her hometown and lives with her husband. Which of the following constitutes the most reasonable approach if she consults her family physician in a private office setting?

(A) Reassurance and arrangements for the patient to call the office or the nearest ED if symptoms recur
(B) Ordering an emergency MRI of the head
(C) Instructing her husband in checking the patient's pupil sizes and reactivity plus her state of alertness frequently over the next 48 hours
(D) Ordering routine skull x-rays and discharging if negative, after instructing in observational care over the next 48 hours
(E) Ordering an emergency CT scan of the head with contrast

10 If the husband of the patient in Question 9 calls later that day, after hours, to express concern over the patient's alertness, which of the following dispositions is the correct one?

(A) Order stat plain films of the skull at the nearest hospital ED.

(B) Order stat CT scan of the head without contrast at the ED.

(C) Order stat MRI at the ED.

(D) Call the neurosurgeon on call at the hospital at which the physician has staff privileges.

(E) Arrange to meet the patient at the office for a repeat examination.

11 The obstetrics department at 3 AM calls the ED doctor to the floor because of respiratory suppression in a 35-year-old G2/P2 white female during her care for tocolysis (the on-call obstetrician is in the middle of an emergency Cesarean section). On which of the following tocolytic medications is she most likely to be?

(A) Indomethacin

(B) Nifedipine

(C) Magnesium sulfate → *resp ↓*

(D) Terbutaline

(E) Ritodrine

12 A young male complains of the rapid onset of left testicular pain over a 2-hour period. Which of the following is the least compatible with the diagnosis of testicular torsion?

(A) Compromise of circulation to the testicle denoted by ultrasound

(B) Irregular palpable testicular mass

(C) Testicle is positioned in a transverse position and found significantly higher than the right testicle

(D) The left-sided cremasteric reflex is absent

(E) Excruciatingly painful involved testicle

13 A 25-year-old female has been treated with fluoxetine (Prozac) for depression, monthly hydrochlorothiazide for 1 week before her menses for premenstrual syndrome and omeprazole (Prilosec) for gastroesophageal reflux. On the third day of her monthly fluoxetine, she began to complain of muscle spasms about the neck and shoulders. She then grabbed a friend's tramadol for her "wry neck." Within 2 hours of her first dose of tramadol, her muscle spasms became worse, and she began to complain of chills, goose bumps and mental agitation. In the nearby ED, she manifests hyperreflexia. Which of the following is the most likely cause of these symptoms and signs?

(A) Bacteremia

(B) Overt indulgence in cocaine

(C) Drug interaction *SSRI + tramadol*

(D) Thyrotoxicosis

(E) Carcinoid syndrome

14 A 57-year-old ex-smoker has been followed for chronic obstructive pulmonary disease (COPD). His dyspnea has become worse over the past week. Queries to discern whether the patient exhibits orthopnea lead nowhere, because the patient has always slept sitting up since his early adulthood. The neck veins are unremarkable. Which of the following findings would best support specifically the possibility that the patient is suffering from congestive heart failure (CHF)?

(A) Sinus tachycardia

(B) "P pulmonale" in Lead II on electrocardiogram

(C) Afternoon fatigue

(D) Elevated beta-natriuretic protein (BNP)

(E) Peripheral edema

15 Which of the following is the likely diagnosis of a deformed and laterally displaced nose in which examination reveals a dark red swelling on the side of the blow incurred a short time ago in an athletic contest?

(A) Orbital fracture

(B) Zygoma fracture

(C) Basal skull fracture *raccoon*

(D) Septal hematoma → *ipsi side swelling*

(E) Simple nasal fracture

16 An 18-year-old woman falls onto her outstretched hand and complains of wrist pain. The distal radius and distal ulna are not tender or deformed, but there is tenderness to palpation of the anatomic snuffbox and of the scaphoid tubercle. Plain x-rays of the hand are read by the radiologist as negative. What is the most sensible disposition today?

(A) Wrap the wrist and hand in a 4-in. ACE bandage, and see the patient back in 1 week.

(B) Apply a thumb spica and wrap in ACE bandages for 2 weeks, at which time the x-rays are repeated.

(C) Advise passive range of motion for 1 week and reexamine.

(D) Advise active range of motion and re-examine in 1 week.

(E) Place the forearm and wrist in a sling and re-examine in 1 week.

17 A middle-aged man is brought to an urgent-care center, giving a vague and unintelligible story. He is unkempt and unclean. He is disoriented in time, gives only a first name and does not answer when asked his age. His blood alcohol level is approximately half the legally allowed limit for driving an automobile. He is confused but seemingly unconcerned. He manifests nystagmus, both horizontal and vertical. On physical examination, you note a few spider angiomata over the anterior chest and purple dilated flank veins on the abdominal. Which of the following must be treated while the confusional state is being managed?

(A) Acute schizophrenia
(B) Wernicke's encephalopathy
(C) Alzheimer's disease
(D) Acute alcohol intoxication
(E) Bipolar disease in manic phase

18 A 70-year-old man is hospitalized with pneumonia, having been a 2-pack-per-day cigarette smoker for 50 years. He was placed on oxygen for abnormally low arterial oxygen content. On the third day of hospitalization, he was transferred to the intensive care unit. That afternoon, he was found to be confused, disoriented and having vivid visual hallucinations of spiders crawling inside his teacup. Which of the following is the best treatment to manage the cognitive dysfunction?

(A) Benztropine (Cogentin)
(B) Diazepam (Valium)
(C) Fluoxetine (Prozac)
(D) Haloperidol (Haldol)
(E) Modafinil (Provigil)

Examination Answers

1. The answer is E. Oxygenation status is more important in limiting neurological damage within the first few hours than the other factors presented.

2. The answer is C. Bilateral presentation of signs and symptoms. The presence of bilateral symptoms and/or signs of radiculopathy pose the question of central disc herniation if present in the acute setting. This patient manifests left-sided radiation of the pain, bilateral, albeit asymmetrically positive, straight-leg-raising tests and decreased Achilles tendon reflex on the right.

3. The answer is B. Presence or absence of visceral symptomatology. The presence of bowel or bladder control symptoms would pose further evidence of central herniation. Sensory loss is reasonably well-tolerated in nerve root compression syndromes; while drug seeking is important in all aspects of patient care, particularly frequent in back pain, diagnosis of this issues is not urgent. Limitation of the ability to bend to lift is common in back syndromes and important in prognostication after diagnosis and in setting activity restrictions but is not of critical value to acute diagnosis. Work connectedness is relevant to worker's compensation claims but is not of critical importance medically.

4. The answer is D. Check the perineum and inner thighs for touch, sharp and dull sensation. The urgency of timely diagnosis in this case is the possibility of acute cauda equina syndrome (CES). Alertness to that condition should have been stimulated by the history and physical findings of bilateral (and not necessarily symmetrical) symptoms and/or signs suggesting radiculopathy, that is, left lateral thigh radiation and right-sided reflex change as well as straight-leg-raising test positive on both sides. Other combinations may include sensory changes or motor deficits pointing to different sides. If the condition is not diagnosed in a timely fashion, the patient is at great risk of various degrees and combinations of paraparesis, bowel and bladder control, and sexual impotence in the male and the equivalent in the female.

5. The answer is B. 48 hours. Notice that the question seeks the average ideal time. For this purpose, the onset of CES is defined as when the bowel and bladder dysfunction begin. Incomplete CES (CESI) is defined as consisting of irritative bladder symptoms and confers a better prognosis than urinary retention (CESR). Two-thirds of cases will do well if diagnosed and treated by emergency laminectomy or other posterior decompression within 48 hours of the onset of bladder symptoms, whereas only

one-third will do well if treated later than 48 hours from that onset. The earlier group is more likely to be in the CESI stage, and the later-treated group is more likely to be CESR. Patients are not likely to self-refer to a neurosurgeon, and due to the rarity of the condition, it is quite likely to be overlooked in the primary care setting.

6. The answer is C. CT of the lumbosacral spine. A patient with unremitting low back pain with or without evidence of infection must be evaluated for urgent conditions in the spinal area before other diagnoses are considered.

7. The answer is D. Epidural abscess. This is a rare and critical condition but one that is more likely to be seen in primary care than in an orthopedic or neurosurgical practice. Spinal epidural abscess (SEA) must be diagnosed within a short time after onset (ranging from 3 to 5 days) to avoid the development of paraplegia. If emergency laminectomy followed by antibiotics are instituted before neurologic symptoms and signs occur, neurological disaster may be avoided, with the latter consisting most frequently of paraplegia. Risk factors include diabetes, alcoholism and recent spinal tap. Patients may or may not manifest radicular symptoms due to encroachment on neural foramina. Leukocytosis occurs in only about 2/3 of cases and bacteremia in about 60%. There may be an overlap of CES and SEA in that abscesses may encroach on the cauda. Pyelonephritis would manifest urine abnormalities (unless secondary to a totally obstructing urolith) but would have a lateralizing presentation and associated CVA tenderness. Malignant metastases may pose a surgical emergency as well but the reward is less significant for metastatic disease than for a timely diagnosis of SEA. Delay in the diagnosis of pyelonephritis is more forgiving as well as unlikely because of its more common occurrence. Vertebral body fracture due to osteoporosis is quite painful but requires no special urgency for diagnosis, and it runs a benign course in the vast majority of cases. Cholecystitis, on occasion, may refer only to the lower thoracic back instead of having the classic band-like referral around the right flank. This case is taken from a medicolegal file in which the patient was sent out of an ED despite the unremitting pain, low fever and leukocytosis after receiving meperidine IV with instructions to see his primary care physician if the pain did not remit within the next 2 days. Before he could see his regular doctor, he awoke in the middle of the night to void urine and fell down, becoming rapidly paraplegic. If diagnosed timely with a CT–myelogram scan or MRI, both of which are 90% sensitive, surgical treatment will guarantee a result free of neurological complications. "Timely" appears to be defined as treatment taking place when there is back pain only (Stage 1) or pain with radiculopathy (Stage 2). If motor weakness (Stage 3) or paralysis sets on, intervention should take place within 24 to 36 hours; the longer the delay beyond 24 hours, the worse the ultimate result.

8. The answer is A. CT scan of the head without contrast. An acute event in the head as described is quite likely to be hemorrhagic; the "worst headache I've ever had" is a subarachnoid hemorrhage until proven otherwise. Contrast is not needed to see hemorrhage of or around the brain.

9. The answer is C. Instruct her husband in checking the patient's pupil sizes and reactivity plus her state of alertness frequently over the next 48 hours.

10. The answer is B. CT scan of the head without contrast. The chief concern at this time would be to rule out a temporal-bone skull fracture transecting the middle meningeal artery, resulting in epidural hemorrhage. This is an arterial hemorrhage, and the classic clinical presentation is head trauma with or without attendant concussion followed by a "lucid interval" of minutes to 24 to 48 hours, after which the patient becomes obtunded (decreasing level of consciousness). It constitutes a neurosurgical emergency. CT need not—and should not—be carried out with contrast since the presence of blood is clearly shown without contrast. CT is superior to MRI in showing hemorrhage within or on the brain. Reexamination is unlikely to produce a reassuring result and would cost valuable time. Calling the neurosurgeon might be appropriate after the order for the CT scan, but the latter would take precedence in urgency since it would have to be accomplished in any event.

11. The answer is C. Magnesium sulfate is the tocolytic medication most likely to be associated with respiratory depression. Nifedipine and indomethacin, while used as tocolytics, do not cause respiratory depression. Terbutaline and ritodrine cause respiratory distress due to pulmonary edema but do not suppress respiration.

12. The answer is B. Irregular testicular mass. Testicular torsion is a surgical emergency requiring correction within 6 hours to avoid the loss of spermatogenesis. Testicular torsion occurs in adolescent boys older than 12 years. The cremasteric reflex is virtually absent. 99mTc or color Doppler ultrasonography is 95% "accurate" (implying 95% sensitivity and 95% specificity). However, specificity is clinically <95%, because damage may ensue with <360 degrees of torsion, thus allowing some arterial circulation. Emergency surgery should not be withheld if the clinical picture is otherwise compatible with the diagnosis. Although the testicle is classically found to ride higher than the contralateral organ, it retains its natural

shape. An irregular mass is most likely caused by epididymitis or, if present over time and painless, possibly cancer.

13. The answer is C. Patients who are on SSRIs along with serotonin-increasing drugs such as tramadol, meperidine, monoamine oxidase inhibitors (MAOIs), sibutramine, sumatriptan, lithium, St John's wort and Ginkgo may result in serotonin syndrome. Findings include mental status changes, agitation, myoclonus, hyperreflexia, diaphoresis, goose bumps and shivering, tremor, diarrhea, ataxia, and fever. This can be life threatening. Further, SSRIs can increase the levels or pharmacological effects of warfarin and of the tricyclic antidepressants. Although the other choices are each somewhat plausible in certain details, the drug interaction described is by far the most likely under the circumstances portrayed in the vignette.

14. The answer is D. BNP secreted in the ventricles is a sensitive indicator of CHF and may be helpful in differentiating cardiac dyspnea from other causes of dyspnea such as COPD, reactive airway disease and air hunger from acute blood loss. Although there is a gray zone of uncertainty in evaluating the significance of BNP, a level <100 pg/mL excludes CHF and a level >400 pg/mL confers a 95% chance of CHF.

15. The answer is D. Septal hematoma. This must be diagnosed and drained as soon as possible to avoid infection and a saddle nose deformity. The reduction of the fracture can wait to be dealt with electively over the following few days. Of course, the other diagnoses mentioned should be ruled out since they may have occurred concomitantly. Basal skull fractures classically manifest raccoon eyes and spinal fluid rhinorrhea; orbital and zygoma fractures manifest palpable deformity and appropriate tenderness to palpation; simple, uncomplicated fractures of the nose, while they may bleed, do not manifest submucosal hematoma in the nose.

16. The answer is B. Apply a thumb spica and wrap in ACE bandages for 2 weeks, at which time the x-rays are repeated. This is to rule out a fracture of the scaphoid (navicular, semilunar), showing only by an emerging fracture line, which may have been missed in the acute films. The scaphoid has arterial supply only from the distal end of the bone. Thus, if the fracture is not carefully immobilized for an adequate period of time, the result is aseptic necrosis of the proximal end and chronic pain in the wrist.

17. The answer is B. Wernicke's encephalopathy. Alcohol withdrawal leading to delirium tremens, in the absence of adequate nutrition, occurs with a drop in blood alcohol level from the range at which it has been for significant periods of time, even when there may be significant levels remaining. The direct cause of Wernicke's is vitamin B1 (thiamine) deficiency. The patient manifests inattention to himself/herself as well as diplopia due to extraocular muscle paralysis, most notably in the lateral rectus or recti, gaze disturbance (horizontal and vertical nystagmus—weakness of lateral recti), confident confusion. Immediate treatment with thiamine is necessary.

18. The answer is D, haloperidol. The patient described has manifested delirium. As opposed to dementia, delirium has an onset that is rapid; it may be precipitated by acute illness, particularly in people over 65; more specific precipitating factors include hypoxia and various medications.

Haloperidol is dosed intravenously and increased every 30 minutes until the signs and symptoms improve. Anticholinergics such as benztropine (Cogentin, choice A) are contraindicated in dementia and delirium and in older people in general since they may precipitate confusion. As a sedating drug—its primary effect—diazepam is contraindicated in all confusional states for the same reasons. Fluoxetine (Prozac) is an antidepressant of the SSRI family, and modafinil is a central stimulant used for daytime relief in narcoleptic states.

Reference

Family Medicine Board Review sponsored by the American Academy of Family Practice, 2009. May 3–9, 2009.

SECTION II

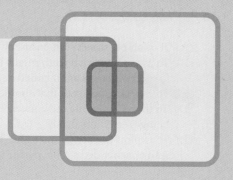

Oto-ophthalmolaryngology

chapter 2

The Oral Cavity in Primary Care

Examination questions: Unless instructed otherwise, choose the ONE lettered answer or completion that is BEST in each case.

1 A 33-year-old man complains of "canker sores," present for about a week. Physical examination shows a 4-mm ulcerated area on the left side of the oral buccal mucosa. You prescribe fluocinonide in the adhesive ointment Orabase, which he may apply as needed with no limit on the frequency of applications. You advise him that the painful stage should last 7 to 10 days, and he should be healed within 3 weeks. Six weeks later, he returns and says the ulcer is still present and just as irritating. Each of the following may be associated with persistent aphthous ulcers except

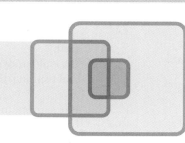

- ✗(A) Erythema multiforme
- (B) Scleroderma & oral ulcers
- ✗(C) Drug allergies
- (D) Pemphigus
- ✗ (E) Herpes simplex

2 A 36-year-old male comes to his family doctor with irritating sores in his mouth, which have been present on and off for 6 weeks. Examination reveals a white plaque or membrane on the base of the right tonsillar pillar. There are no enlarged or tender lymph nodes. The membrane is easily rubbed off, leaving an erythematous base. Which of the following is the most likely diagnosis of the finding?

- (A) Leukoplakia
- (B) Aphthous ulcer
- (C) Candidiasis
- (D) Infectious mononucleosis
- (E) Streptococcal pharyngitis

3 Your 45-year-old pipe-smoking male patient recently decided (and succeeded) to quit smoking and is now motivated to be alert to oral cancer. Which of the following is most likely to be a sign of mouth cancer?

- (A) Nonhealing sore in the mouth
- (B) Leukoplakia
- (C) White pseudo-membrane that is removed with difficulty
- (D) Erythroplakia
- (E) Persistent earache or sore throat.

4 Which of the following is the best reason to consult the patient's personal dentist prior to initiating radiation therapy to the head and neck area?

(A) To plan posttreatment cosmetic repair
(B) To ascertain which teeth might be candidates for radiotherapy as an added benefit
(C) To examine for teeth that should be extracted
(D) To thoroughly rule out cancers besides what is being treated primarily
(E) To exploit the dental insurance before cycling into another deductible period

5 A new mother brings in her 2-month-old daughter for routine well-baby care. She was born vaginally at 40 weeks of gestation and has had an uneventful course to date. The mother asks about dental care. Which of the following statements is true regarding routine pediatric dental care and prevention of caries?

(A) Dental care need not be initiated until the secondary teeth have all erupted.
(B) Because the family lives in a community that has fluoridation of the water system, caries will not be a problem.
(C) As long as the child is trained to avoid sugars, caries can be evaded.
(D) Starting between 6 and 12 months of age, the child is at risk of developing caries.
(E) Prevention of caries is a moot point in dealing with deciduous teeth.

6 The mother of a 3-month-old child asks which of the following food substances is the least likely to cause cavities in her child's teeth. You answer would be

(A) Cow's milk   *lactose is protective*
(B) Enfamil
(C) Soy formula with sucrose
(D) Similac
(E) On-demand mother's milk

7 At what age of the child should one expect the eruption of the last of the deciduous dentition?

(A) 18 months
(B) 2.5 years
(C) 3.5 years
(D) 4 years
(E) 6 years

8 At what age should the first permanent teeth erupt?

(A) 4 to 6 years
(B) 6 to 7 years
(C) 9 to 10 years
(D) 12 to 13 years
(E) 17 to 22 years

9 What is the standard concentration of fluoride in treated public water supply?

(A) 0.6 parts per million (ppm)
(B) 1 ppm
(C) 2 ppm
(D) 2 mg/kg/day
(E) 5 mg/kg/day

10 The foregoing notwithstanding, at what age should a child be started on fluoride treatments?

(A) Birth
(B) 3 months
(C) 6 months
(D) 1 year
(E) 2 years

11 Which of the following statements about *home* dental care of children is true?

(A) The parents should take the child to the dentist for the first time by the age of 26 months, about the age of eruption of the last of the deciduous teeth.
(B) If a child under the age of 18 months is irritable and teething, the child may have a low-grade fever.
(C) Bottle propping is acceptable as long as the bottle does not contain sugary liquids.
(D) Dental caries in parents may lead to dental caries in their children.
(E) The earliest sign of caries in children is a brown or black concavity in a tooth.

12 A 75-year-old man complains for 3 weeks of irritation of the tongue. An examination shows fiery redness of the entire dorsum of the tongue. The causes of this condition include all but *which* of the following?

(A) Pernicious anemia
(B) Riboflavin deficiency
(C) Iron deficiency
(D) Excessive smoking
(E) Rubeola

13 A 22-year-old woman complains of an increasingly severe sore throat over the last 4 days, worse in the evening, without evolution to coryza or cough. The appearance of the throat is that of diffuse redness; anterior cervical lymph nodes are tender. Which of the following organisms is virtually the sole possible bacterial cause of this condition?

(A) Streptococcus pneumoniae
(B) Streptococcus pyogenes
(C) Staphylococcus aureus
(D) Moraxella catarrhalis
(E) Hemophilus influenzae

14 A 35-year-old male patient comes to you for a second opinion, having been to his dentist by whom he was advised to undergo extraction of his remaining three unerupted third molars ("wisdom teeth"). One month ago, he had undergone incision and drainage of an abscess formed around his left lower third molar, which had only partially erupted, showing two cusps above the gum line. In your response, which of the following do you indicate is the most significant sequela of failure of eruption and consequent impaction of third molars?

(A) Malocclusion
(B) Cosmetic implications
(C) Inability to masticate with the molars
(D) Formation of dentigerous cysts
(E) Abscess formation

15 A 17-year-old girl is brought to you for the complaint of a sore throat. You note the presence of petechiae of the mucosa overlying the hard palate. Cervical lymph nodes are notably enlarged and palpable but not tender. Which of the following *nonbacterial* diseases could explain the foregoing?

(A) Herpes simplex I
(B) Infectious mononucleosis
(C) Herpes simplex II
(D) Influenza A virus
(E) Rhinovirus

16 A male teenager and his family complain of his having severe mouth soreness for the last 10 days. Examination discloses a fetid odor and fibrous pseudomembranes on many gingival crests. Which of the following diagnoses best fits this situation?

(A) Acute necrotizing gingivitis
(B) Periodontal abscess
(C) Dentigerous cyst
(D) Herpes labialis
(E) Molar impaction

17 A 55-year-old man was found sleeping in an alley and smelling of alcohol. He complained of swelling of the anterior neck and was brought to the emergency department of your hospital. Physical examination shows edema and erythema of the area of the anterior neck as it merges with the floor of the mouth. Percussion of the teeth reveals a tender area surrounding a lower partially erupted third molar. What is this form of oral cavity infection called?

(A) Caseous scrofula
(B) Cavity formation with secondary lymph nodes
(C) Coronary insufficiency
(D) Ludwig angina
(E) Mucosal epidermolysis

Examination Answers

1. The answer is B. Scleroderma is one condition among the choices given that is not associated with persistent aphthous stomatitis. Erythema multiforme, drug allergies, pemphigus, pemphigoid, herpes simplex and bullous lichen planus, Behcet's disease (a condition of the small vessels associated with aphthous ulcers of the oral and pharyngeal mucosa and genitalia, severe uveitis, retinal vasculitis and optic nerve atrophy), squamous cell carcinoma and inflammatory bowel disease may each be associated with aphthous stomatitis (i.e. canker sores).

2. The answer is C. Candidiasis is the diagnosis of the white membrane that is easily removable, leaving a red base that is nonulcerated, not to be confused with an exudate, the latter being more of a viscous fluid. Leukoplakia is not removable without a minor surgical procedure. Aphthous ulcers are ulcerated, and any exudate that is removed leaves a whitish base. Infectious mono is often characterized by an exudate that is more yellowish than white and, being an exudate, does not come off in leaflets as does a membrane; mono nearly always manifests nontender cervical adenopathy. Streptococcal exudate is grayish white and more fluid than membrane and is usually associated with tender cervical adenopathy, albeit not necessarily markedly enlarged.

3. The answer is D. Erythroplakia is the most likely to indicate an oral cancer. 70% of cases of erythroplakia are cancerous or precancerous. While leukoplakia is better known historically as a precancerous sign, only about 25% of leukoplakia falls into that category. Although each of the other symptoms or findings may be precancerous, they are highly nonspecific, usually having benign causes. In the case of persistent earache, it would occur as referral of the throat pain via the eustachian tube.

4. The answer is C. To examine for teeth that should be extracted is the best reason for consulting a patient's personal physician before initiating radiation therapy to the head and neck area. Recent extraction sites heal poorly and slowly if radiation therapy occurs during the healing phase. If indicated, extractions take place before the onset of radiotherapy; three weeks must be allowed for healing before radiotherapy begins. In addition, all bisphosphonates, albeit rarely, may cause osteonecrosis, and the most common site affected is the jaw, particularly in the situation of dental extraction.

5. The answer is D. Children are at risk of development of caries from the age of their first (primary) dentition. The central maxillary incisors erupt when the child is between the ages of 6 and 12 months. At about 1 year, the first molars erupt; at 2 years, the second or posterior molars erupt. Fluoridation of water or systemic fluoridation by medication reduces the chances of caries formation by 50%. Avoidance of sugar is important but not a guarantor against tooth decay. Soy-based formulas have a tendency to contain sucrose, which is an obvious risk factor for caries formation.

6. The answer is A. Cow's milk (which is also the basis of Enfamil and Similac) and mother's milk are the least likely among baby foods to predispose babies to caries formation. The lactose of cow's milk may actually be protective. Indigenously present sugars, such as fructose, are less cariogenic than introduced sugars such as sucrose. Premature birth (low birth weight) and low socioeconomic status are strong risk factors for caries formation. Bottle propping, particularly when the feed contains sweetening, predisposes to cavities. Propping, a substitute for attention, presumably results in unnecessarily prolonged exposure to the cariogenic substance. Having carious deciduous teeth constitutes a risk factor for having caries in permanent dentition.

7. The answer is B. The last teeth should have erupted by the age of 30 months. The peak times of eruption for the individual teeth are as follows (note that they erupt in mesiolateral order, front to back): Maxillary and mandibular medial incisors, 6 to 12 months; mandibular and maxillary lateral incisors, 11 to 13.2 months; mandibular and maxillary cuspids ("canines"), 15.6 to 16 months; mandibular and maxillary first molars, 19.5 to 19.6 months; mandibular and maxillary second molars, 26.5 to 28 months.

8. The answer is B. The first permanent teeth to erupt would be the mandibular premolars at 6 to 6.3 years. These are followed by central and lateral mandibular incisors at 7.2 years; maxillary incisors, 8.5 years; mandibular cuspids (canines), 9.7 years; maxillary cuspids, 11.6 years; maxillary premolars, 10 to 10.7; mandibular premolars, 10.7 to 11.5 years; first molars, 6 to 7 years; second molars, 10.7 to 11.5 years; and third molars (wisdom teeth) 20 to 20.5 years.

9. The answer is B. The standard for fluoride supplementation in public water supplies is 1 ppm; 0.6 ppm is the point below which prescriptive supplementation should be initiated. A major overdose would be 2.2 mg/kg/day; however, 2.2 mg of sodium fluoride daily is the recommended dosage to obtain 1 mg of fluoride in communities without supplementation in their water supply at or above 0.03 ppm for children in the age range of 6 to 16 years. In a single dose, 5 mg/kg constitutes a critical toxic dose.

10. The answer is C. Six months is the age at which children should be receiving fluoride. This would be in the form of a supplement if the household water is not fluoridated commercially, publicly or in well water at a concentration of >6 ppm. Supplement should be either topical or oral or both. The child should not receive fluoride supplementation if it is breastfeeding and in any event not until the age of 6 months. Overdose can cause hypocalcemia, convulsions, tetany and cardiac dysrhythmias.

11. The answer is D. Bacteria that cause dental caries (i.e., mutans streptococci in the great majority) can be transferred among members of a household, including from mother to newborn child. Children should be taken to the dentist by the age of 1 year. Teething is not a cause of fever in infants. Bottle propping is unacceptable according to dental opinion, for many reasons: First, because of the temptation to overfeed improper foods; second, there may eventually be mechanical effects on the dentition. The typical yellow to brown to black discoloration is not the first appearance of caries. They are preceded by white spots or lines.

12. The answer is E. Rubeola or "hard measles," although classically producing the buccal Koplik spot, does not cause glossitis. All the other listed conditions may be associated with glossitis.

13. The answer is B. Beta-hemolytic streptococcus is virtually the only bacterial cause of bacterial pharyngitis. Streptococcal pharyngitis causes increasingly severe symptoms throughout the day, whereas viral pharyngitis, as the harbinger of a viral upper respiratory infection, is worst in the morning upon awakening. Although there is no single reliable symptom or sign of streptococcal infection in the throat, the combination of the chronicity and progression of symptoms in this case, along with tenderness of the anterior cervical nodes and the cellulitic appearance of the throat, point to such an infection. *S. pneumoniae*, the most common cause of bacterial pneumonia, is not an oral pathogen, neither are Staphylococci (except in unusual circumstances), *M. catarrhalis*, or *H. influenzae*.

14. The answer is D. Dentigerous cysts. The third molars are commonly only partially erupted in the adult. For this reason, they are the foci of frequent abscesses that are due, of course, to the beta-hemolytic *S. pyogenes*. Further, when third molars or wisdom teeth remain totally unerupted, they may form dentigerous cysts (expansions of the original cocoon of the molar roots); these may grow slowly over time, taking on the characteristics of benign tumors, dislodging other teeth, and eroding the maxillary or mandibular arch. Malocclusion is not a significant occurrence in this condition. There are no cosmetic implications with unerupted third molars. Chewing is seldom a problem except in the partially erupted molar that has abscess formation.

15. The answer is B. Infectious mononucleosis and streptococcal pharyngitis each may cause petechiae over the hard palate, though the question regards a nonbacterial cause only. Furthermore, adenopathy due to Bets strep is virtually always tender whereas that due to infectious mono is virtually never tender. In children, herpangina (not mentioned among the choices) causes palatal petechiae and occurs mostly in preschool-age children, generally up to 4 years of age. It may occur, however, as late in childhood as 16 years. In the present case, the existence of impressive lymphadenopathy without tenderness is typical of mononucleosis.

16. The answer is A. Periodontitis progresses to gingivitis, which, if untreated and severe, leads to acute necrotizing gingivitis or trench mouth. Periodontal abscess consists of a focal lesion under pressure, which is quite painful. Dentigerous cysts are not visible on oral examination. Molar impaction is the primary lesion from which dentigerous cysts form, nearly always involving a third molar that has not erupted and that impinges on surrounding structures, particularly after cyst formation (see the discussion of Question 13).

17. The answer is D. Ludwig angina is cellulitis of the submandibular space by extension from the sublingual area. It usually results from an infection of a dental site, such as that from an infected extraction site, root canal therapy or abscessed third molar. Scrofula is tuberculous involvement of cervical nodes and, as such, consists of obvious adenopathy. Coronary insufficiency may cause anginal pains that radiate into the neck, but nearly always this occurs unilaterally and is not associated with local findings. Mucosal epidermolysis occurs on the mucosa, not the skin.

References

Douglass JM, Douglass AB, Silk HI. A practical guide to infant oral health. *Am Fam Phys* 2004; 70(11):2113–2119.

M.D. Anderson, University of Texas. www.mdanderson.org/patient-and-cancer-information

Tryon AF, Streckfus CF. Problems of the oral cavity. In: Rudy DR, Kurowski K, eds. *Family Medicine: House Officer Series.* Baltimore: Williams & Wilkins; 1997:27–42.

US Preventive Services Task Force. Prevention of dental caries in preschool children: recommendations and rationale. *Am Fam Phys* 2004; 70(8):1529–1532.

Ward, Daniel, DDS, Clinical Associate Professor, The Ohio State University: Personal communication.

chapter 3

Otolaryngology in Primary Care

Examination questions: Unless instructed otherwise, choose the ONE lettered answer or completion that is BEST in each case.

1 A 35-year-old male smoker for 18 pack years complains of hoarseness and cough for 10 days. He denies weight loss and other constitutional symptoms. His friends have noted frequent throat clearings. Which of the following is the <u>least</u> likely cause of the dysphonia?

(A) Atopic allergy
(B) Carcinoma of the larynx
(C) Reaction to tobacco smoke
(D) Pharyngolaryngeal reflex
(E) Viral URI

2 A 55-year-old man with 35 pack years smoking history has had hoarseness for 3 months, and recently, there has been inspiratory stridor. Which of the following diagnostic measures is the most sensitive first step in diagnostic evaluation to determine the cause of the dysphonia?

(A) Laryngoscopy
(B) Magnetic resonance imaging (MRI)
(C) Computed tomography (CT) scan of the larynx
(D) Diagnostic therapeutic trial of proton pump inhibitors.
(E) Serum T_4, T_3, and thyroid stimulating hormone (TSH) levels

3 A 17-year-old atopic male sales manager makes an appointment for complaint of a prolonged course of cold. Until the last year, his allergic rhinitis has seldom required antihistamine therapy during his peak season of mid-August until the first cool weather. He noted the onset of coryza 2 1/2 weeks ago during the 4th month of August and that his rhinorrhea has persisted, producing a tenacious discharge, sometimes blood streaked, from the right naris. When he leans forward, he feels a pain in his right facial region and sometimes a sense of shifting fluid in the right cheek

anteriorly. On examination, he manifests tenderness of the right nasal rim of the orbit. Which of the following would be a logical therapeutic plan?

(A) Refer for allergy evaluation
(B) Obtain otolaryngology consultation
(C) Prescribe a course of levofloxin
(D) Administer a 500-mg ceftriaxone injection
(E) Prescribe amoxicillin 500 mg thrice per day

4 The atopic patient in Question 3, immediately after filling his prescription, joined his friends on a canoeing trip into the wilds of the great north woods of Canada. On the 3rd day, he accidentally drops his pill bottle overboard. After the group had reached a distance 5 days from motorized transportation, the 17-year-old man with known ethmoid and maxillary sinusitis notes the onset of diplopia and inability to direct his right eye gaze within the normal range. His friends notice the right eye has become chemotic (shows excessive edema of the conjunctivae). In addition, the man complains of blurred vision on the right. Which of the following is his likely complication?

(A) Brain abscess
(B) Osteomyelitis of the frontal bone
(C) Mucocele of the ethmoid
(D) Cavernous sinus thrombosis
(E) Orbital cellulitis

5 A 4-year-old girl has had five middle ear infections in each of the past 3 years, and now, on March 15, she is brought to you with an acute attack of earache on the right side; the Weber test lateralizing to the left ear and red, immobile eardrum with pus fluid level on the right. Last September, you gave both influenza and pneumococcal vaccines and prescribed amoxicillin daily between December 1 and March 1. You plan a course of amoxicillin/clavulanate (Augmentin). Assuming a satisfactory response, what should be your next therapeutic move?

1st (A) Prescribe inhaled glucocorticoids
2nd (B) Arrange consultation for placement of ventilation tubes
3rd (C) Consult otolaryngology for possible adenoidectomy
(D) Consult otolaryngology for possible tonsillectomy
(E) Skin test for desensitization

6 A 24-year-old male is in the examining room to complain of stuffy nose in the aftermath of a viral cold of 5-day duration. He relates that he has taken a proprietary nasal spray for self-treatment of this symptom for the past 3 days and has noted that the stuffiness has become bilateral and has now interfered seriously with his sleep. Which of the following is an accepted rational approach to the treatment of this condition?

(A) Moist warm air nasal inhalation and inhaled glucocorticoids while the topical medication is withdrawn
(B) Prescribing more potent vasoconstrictors in a topical preparation
(C) Prescription of longer acting nasal decongestants
(D) Discontinue the nose drops and skin test for desensitization to treat atopic allergies
(E) Topical application of a basophile stabilizing agent such as cromolyn

7 An African American child has an earache with onset the previous night and an associated fever, temperature 38.3°C (101°F). The mother is concerned over the fact that he has had five bouts of middle ear infection over the past year, three of which have occurred in the past 6 months. It is the month of February. Which of the following is the most likely underlying risk factor in the recurrence of the child's condition?

(A) Atopic constitution
(B) African American ancestry
(C) Exposure to cold winds
(D) Tonsillar hypertrophy or tonsillitis
(E) Anterior attached frenulum

8 A 2-year-old child is brought to you for apparent dyspnea 4 days that followed coryza and fever (39.5°C, 103.1°F). The fever is abating in the past 24 hours, but the child is now coughing. Respiratory rate is 50/minute. The lung fields manifest prolonged *expiratory phase* as well as diffuse crackles during the expiratory phase. Which of the following statements is true regarding this condition?

(A) It is caused by influenza A/B
(B) The chances of follicular tonsillitis are increased
(C) There is a scant chance of future respiratory sequelae

(D) The possibility of coincident otitis media is higher than with other upper respiratory infections
(E) It is caused by an adenovirus

9 A mother brings to you her 4-year-old child complaining of right-sided earache for 12 hours following three days of coryza, giving way to cough over the past 2 days. The external ear is not tender nor is the tempero-mandibular joint. The eardrum is retracted, fiery red, slightly bulging, and reveals a pus/fluid level. What are the three top-ranking bacterial organisms in the causation of this condition, in descending order of frequency?

(A) *Streptococcus pyogenes, Staphylococcus aureus, Klebsiella pneumoniae*
(B) *Moraxella catarrhalis, Streptococcus pyogenes, Staphylococcus aureus*
(C) *Moraxella catarrhalis, Pseudomonas species, Haemophilus influenzae*
(D) *Haemophilus influenzae, Streptococcus pyogenes, Staphylococcus aureus*
(E) *Streptococcus pneumoniae, Haemophilus influenzae, Moraxella catarrhalis*

10 In the preceding vignette, which of the following approximates the proportion of organisms involved in otitis media, which would be expected to be resistant to penicillin and ampicillin?

(A) 10% to 20%
(B) 20% to 30%
(C) 30% to 40%
(D) 40% to 50%
(E) 50% to 75%

11 A 26-year-old woman complains of gradually developing hearing loss on the left side. Her left tympanic membrane appears to be discolored red as compared to the right. Which of the following must be present to make the diagnosis of otitis media?

(A) Air conduction better than bone conduction in the involved ear
(B) Fever >101°F
(C) Fiery red tympanic membrane
(D) Local tenderness of the tragus
(E) Conductive hearing loss in the involved ear

12 A 5-year-old girl is brought by her mother for a routine physical examination to meet health standards requirements before entry into the first grade in school. She appears to have no complaints. On the examination, you are reminded that you treated her for otitis tympanic membrane, which manifests a purplish color. When you mention this to the mother, she expresses concern and asks whether further treatment is required. Which of the following is your most appropriate answer?

(A) Yes. Otitis media should be entirely cleared by 10 days after treatment.

(B) Yes. Otitis media should be entirely cleared by 3 weeks after treatment.

(C) No. Treatment failure of otitis media is not established until 6 weeks have passed.

(D) No. Treatment failure of otitis media is not established until 16 weeks have passed.

(E) No. An adequate course of an appropriate antibiotic is all that one needs to ascertain in prognosticating on the course of otitis media.

13 A 24-year-old man with type I diabetes mellitus comes to you with complaint of severe pain in the right ear with onset over the previous 24 hours. On examination, you find the ear to be extremely tender upon light touch of the tragus and slight manipulation of the auricle. You diagnose external otitis and consider the possibility of malignant otitis externa. Which of the following defines that condition?

(A) Conductive hearing loss

(B) *Pseudomonas* species

(C) Associated diabetes mellitus

(D) Osteomyelitis of the bony canal or mastoid   *Pseudomonas*

(E) Requirement of intravenous antibiotics

14 A 35-year-old female who works on a noisy assembly line received a routine audiogram at her place of employment, which showed a hearing loss on the left. She was vaguely aware of increasingly turning her right ear toward conversation and in talking on the telephone. She denies pain, recent upper respiratory infection, and atopic constitution or allergic symptoms. Both eardrums move briskly when the patient performs a modified Valsalva maneuver (forced expiration against a closed nasopharyngeal cavity). The tympanic membrane exhibits a color more erythematous on the left than the right eardrum. The Weber test shows bone conduction better on the left than on the right. Which of the following is the most likely diagnosis?

(A) Mild otitis media of the left ear

(B) Otosclerosis of the left ear — *conductive loss 3 (inherited)*

(C) Noise-induced sensorineural hearing loss on the left

(D) Meniere's disease on the left

(E) Labyrinthitis

15 An 18-year-old male patient complains of sore throat that began 5 days ago. There has been no preceding or accompanying coryza or cough, and the pain has been worse toward the day's end. On examination, you see a diffusely red posterior palate and the

anterior lymph nodes are enlarged and tender. Assuming a bacterial cause, which of the following is the most likely causation?

(A) *Neisseria meningitidis*

(B) *Staphylococcus aureus*

(C) *Moraxella catarrhalis*

(D) Beta-hemolytic *Streptococcus pyogenes*

(E) *Klebsiella pneumoniae*

16 A 45-year-old male, a right-handed, devout game hunter, complains that his wife notes he often turns his right ear to her to understand her in conversation. Which of the following is the most likely pattern to be found on a multiple-frequency audiogram?

(A) Flat audiogram across multiple frequencies in both ears

(B) Low-frequency hearing loss in the left ear

(C) Early complaint of difficulty hearing at a conversational level

(D) Deep involvement of the 4,000 cps in the left ear

(E) Crisp response to a hearing aid

17 A 42-year-old male patient is sent to you for follow-up from your junior partner's care 2 days ago with a diagnosis of left otitis media for which he was prescribed amoxicillin and told to see the sought treatment, and he answers that he complained of hearing loss, gradually increasing over several months before he felt it necessary to seek a medical opinion. He denies previous coryza and vertigo. He does not shoot guns and works in an office as a public accountant. He notes tinnitus has gradually become prominent on the left. He says that the gradually increasing symptoms are unremitting and not occurring in paroxysms. You examine him and find that his tympanic membrane is mobile, but the color of the left eardrum is red streaked as compared to the right. The Weber test indicates sensorineural loss on the left (i.e., lateralizes to the right). Which of the following is the most likely cause of his symptoms?

(A) Meniere's disease   *episodic*

(B) Mild otitis media of the left ear   *conduction*

(C) Acoustic neuroma

(D) Impacted cerumen, left ear   *conduction*

(E) Acoustic trauma to the left ear   *slowly : hx will tell*

18 Your 38-year-old patient, a Mexican-American man, who runs his own landscaping business, comes to you for a routine physical examination, interested in knowing the status of his lipids and blood sugar. On routine otoscopy, you notice that the anatomy of the left ear in the region of the tympanic membrane is unrecognizable. The patient then says that he has had a perforated eardrum for several years. Weber and

Rinne' tests indicate conductive hearing loss on the left side. Which of the following is the diagnosis?

(A) Otosclerosis
(B) Malignant external otitis
(C) Cholesteatoma → result of non healing busted TM
(D) Meniere's disease
(E) Bullous myringitis

19 A 55-year-old woman comes to you for vertigo of recent and violent onset. She denies hearing loss and tinnitus. Which of the following characteristics reveals this as of peripheral origin (labyrinth) as opposed to central origin?

(A) Immediate onset of nystagmus and vertigo with the Hallpike maneuver
(B) Violent symptoms after a latent period upon motion of the head affecting the semicircular canals
(C) Causes include basilar artery insufficiency
(D) Associated nystagmus exhibits pendular motion
(E) This entity is associated with a conductive hearing loss.

20 A 3-year-old girl presents with foul smelling postnasal drip, temperature of 102°F, and perceptible swelling of the face. Which of the following is the most important reason to diagnose and treat this condition in timely fashion?

(A) It presents with a malodorous discharge
(B) To avert febrile seizure
(C) It may be caused by lactamase-producing organisms
(D) Orbital cellulitis is a feared complication {Ethmoid sinusitis}
(E) Treatment must be carried out for 3 weeks

21 A 12-year-old female patient is diagnosed as having streptococcal pharyngitis. To prevent rheumatic fever in this child, how soon must the treatment begin to eradicate the *Streptococcus*?

(A) 48 hours
(B) Five days
(C) Nine days   7-9 days
(D) Fifteen days
(E) Twenty days

22 A 22-year-old male medical student complains of severe sore throat for 3 days and says that he has been unable to ingest solid foods for the past 2 days. He appears moderately ill and in pain, with his head held in a "sniffing"-type position, lips slightly parted, grimacing while swallowing saliva. His speech is muffled and sounds as though the patient is trying to talk with a hot potato in his mouth. There is no stridor. His temperature is 101°F (38.3°C). His cervical lymph nodes are visibly and palpably enlarged but not tender to palpation; tonsils are present and show an exudate whose color is a mixture of white and yellowish against an erythematous and edematous background. There are palatal petechiae. The rim of the epiglottis is visible above the base of the tongue and appears normal in color and size. Survey for other adenopathy yields nothing of note, and abdominal examination is negative for masses and organomegaly. A rapid streptococcal screen is negative. Therefore, you order a stat spot test for infectious mononucleosis, which is also negative. Despite the latter findings, due to the patient's state of illness, you elect to treat him with penicillin V, potassium 250 mg qid for 10 days. He returns in 4 days complaining that he is not improved and in fact is "miserable"; he appears just as uncomfortable as during the last visit and the cervical adenopathy has not abated discernibly. Which of the following is the most logical measure you should take at this time?

(A) Change the antibiotic to ampicillin 500 mg tid for the balance of 10 days and instruct him to return in 48 to 72 hours
(B) Repeat the Monospot test
(C) Change the antibiotic to a newer macrolide (e.g., azithromycin) for the balance of 10 days
(D) Check human immunodeficiency virus (HIV) status and assume cytomegalovirus (CMV) is the cause of seronegative mononucleosis
(E) Hospitalize and consult an infectious disease specialist

23 A 35-year-old woman complains of cough that has become debilitating, although not very productive. The onset of her illness was 2 days before and was gradual, with low-grade fever, malaise, headache, and cough that was at first mild. On inspection, she does not appear seriously ill; she manifests tender red nodules on her anterior lower legs. Otologic examination reveals an abnormality of the left eardrum. The patient denies hearing loss, and the eardrum moves *bullous myringitis* when the patient performs a modified Valsalva maneuver, but the Weber subtly lateralizes to the left side. Which of the following is the most logical empiric therapeutic approach to this patient?

(A) Prescribe penicillin V-K 250 mg 4 times daily for 10 days
(B) Prescribe a codeine-containing antitussive medication
(C) Prescribe clarithromycin, 500 mg extended release, two tablets daily for 3 weeks
(D) Prescribe amoxicillin 875 mg 3 times a day for 10 days
(E) Prescribe an expectorant and reassure the patient

Macrolide → mycoplasma
Tetracycline

24 A 42-year-old Caucasian woman has been followed for episodic sensorineural hearing loss. The attacks are accompanied by tinnitus and vertigo. Her physician has been treating with every accepted medical treatment for the condition. Each of the following treatment modalities would be beneficial except for which one?

(A) Salt restricted diet
(B) Smoking cessation
(C) Elimination of xanthines from her diet *(choco/caffein)*
(D) Referral for possible endolymphatic shunt
(E) Institute meclizine by prescription

Menière's Dz → refractory to medical management

Examination Answers

1. The answer is B. The least likely cause of 10 days of hoarseness and cough, even in a heavy smoker, is carcinoma. This is because of the short chronicity and the presence of cough. These two factors favor an irritative phenomenon. The latter includes all the other choices, including irritation due to inhaled smoke. Although cancer is a possibility in a smoker, there is no time urgency in the present case.

2. The answer is A. Laryngoscopy is the easiest, least expensive, and most sensitive of all the choices given for diagnosis of long-standing hoarseness. The differential diagnosis of new onset hoarseness of some chronicity includes carcinoma, granulomas, leukoplakia, nodules, and polyps. One arbitrary cut point for chronicity of hoarseness as a criterion for decision to obtain laryngoscopy is 2 weeks. An MRI or CT scan at some point may be indicated, for example, in determining the extent of spread contiguously or distantly. A diagnostic therapeutic trial of proton pump inhibitors may be useful after mass lesions have been ruled out (by biopsy if necessary). Although hypothyroidism can be a cause of dysphonia, serum T_4, T_3, and TSH levels too would be useful after ruling out mass lesions.

3. The answer is E. Prescribe amoxicillin 500 mg 3 times per day. This patient has typical right ethmoid sinusitis (tenderness of the right orbital rim) as well as right maxillary sinusitis (based on the history of shifting fluid in the cheek area). Ethmoiditis seldom occurs without concurrent maxillary sinusitis. Levofloxicin and ceftriaxone are too radical for this sinusitis that had not been treated for at least 3 years, hence not expected to involve exotic or resistant organisms. They should be held in reserve. The sinusitis is likely a complication of allergic rhinitis, for which summer "cold" is a code word. Uncomplicated, it responds to antihistamines throughout the season of allergic symptoms, unlike viral colds, in which antihistamines remediate symptoms for no more than 3 to 4 days. Allergists seldom have anything to offer during the acute phase of complications. ENT consultation would be grossly premature.

4. The answer is D. This complication of ethmoid sinusitis is cavernous sinus thrombosis. At first glance, it may be easily confused with orbital cellulitis, also a complication of ethmoid sinusitis. The difference in clinical presentation is that orbital cellulitis manifests proptosis of the involved eye and edema of the eyelids, as opposed to chemosis and ophthalmoplegia. Both conditions are medical emergencies and require rapid intervention with

intravenous antibiotics (the outdoorsman in the vignette must phone in for life flight out of the bush). Mucocele is relatively benign by comparison and requires only aspiration and evacuation by an otolaryngologist. Brain abscess can be a complication of sinusitis and would present with neurologic symptoms and signs. Osteomyelitis of the frontal bone is a complication of frontal sinusitis and presents with swelling of the frontal bone.

5. The answer is A. Prescribe inhaled glucocorticoids to attempt to prevent recurrences of otitis media. Choices B and C, ventilation tubes and referral for adenoidectomy, would be the second and third choices in that order, if the foregoing measures do not result in a decreased frequency of middle ear infections.

6. The answer is A. Mist or warm moist towels for nasal inhalation combined with inhaled glucocorticoids for a brief period following withdrawal of the inhaled vasoconstriction is an accepted rational approach to the treatment of *rhinitis medicamentosa*. Other approaches are short-term systemic glucocorticoids. Prescription of longer lasting topical decongestants is not a solution to this problem, which has been brought on by the overuse of such medications. When prescribed, topical decongestants should be used only intermittently, most likely on one side of the nose only and at the time of sleep onset. Although this condition may be more prevalent in atopic individuals, allergy is not the proximate cause and the condition is not served by skin testing at this point in the course.

7. The answer is A. Atopic constitution is an underlying factor in recurrence of otitis media; in fact, probably, the most prevalent one in this disorder. Native American, but not African American race, would be a factor. Contrary to earlier teaching, tonsillar hypertrophy and/or tonsillitis is/are not factor(s), although adenoidal hypertrophy is the second most prevalent underlying risk factor. Congenital palatal deformity renders one susceptible to recurrent otitis media. Anterior attached frenulum, or "tongue tied" state, is not a risk factor for recurrent otitis media. As the most common precipitating insult is viral URI, superimposed on one of the foregoing risks, exposure to a population with increased incidence of viral URI is also an underlying risk factor.

8. The answer is D. The child has a respiratory infection and bronchiolitis caused by a respiratory syncytial virus (RSV), a member of the family Paromyxiviridae, species *pneumovirus*. RSV carries a 30% to 60% risk of otitis media as a sequela, as compared with about 10% of cases of respiratory infections caused by the plurality of common colds, rhinoviruses (about 25% of common colds). Expiratory rales or "crackles" are unique to bronchiolitis in children. It is found that children who had bronchiolitis caused by RSV are at increased risk for asthma in the future.

9. The answer is E. *S. pneumoniae, H. influenzae, M. catarrhalis* are the three most frequent bacterial causes of otitis media. *S. pyogenes*, the cause of "strep" pharyngitis and tonsillitis, is the agent of otitis media in just 5%, according to a typical study finding by DelBoccaro *et al.*, J. Pediatr 1992; 120(1): 81–84.

10. The answer is B. Twenty to thirty percent approximates the proportion of organisms involved in otitis media, which would be expected to be resistant to penicillin and ampicillin. One-third of the 19% of otitides mediae caused by *H. influenzae* (some 6% of the total) are highly lactamase producing, whereas 80% to 90% of the 22% of cases caused by *M. catarrhalis* (some 20% of the total) are "low-grade" producers.

11. The answer is E. Hearing loss in the involved ear, which is conductive in character, is a *sine qua non* for otitis media (assuming it is a hearing ear). Thus, the Weber test should lateralize to the symptomatic ear, and bone conduction would be better than air conduction in the ear with conductive loss. A common mistake is to overinterpret perceived color change in the eardrum without checking whether there is a conductive hearing loss before making the diagnosis. Color changes attendant to otitis media vary from fiery red through purple and the creamy hue of pus. Apparent color change may be the stable state of an eardrum that is overlain with vascular ectasia.

12. The answer is D. No, further treatment is not indicated at this time. Although most children will show nearly normal middle ear findings by 3 to 4 weeks (or even less) after treatment is instituted (or often even without treatment), otolaryngologists will not define a case as failure to respond based on persistent effusion until 16 weeks have passed. The "correct antibiotic" is never known until an empirically good result is observed after a sufficient time has elapsed, but presumptive success may be assumed if there is early disappearance of fever and pain, that is, within 4 days or sooner. However, persistence of fluid into the 6th week, for example, if the patient is otherwise asymptomatic, does not signal therapeutic failure.

13. The answer is D. Osteomyelitis of the bony canal or mastoid is present by definition in malignant otitis externa. The characteristics listed in the distracters are all true except that conductive hearing loss, although often present in external otitis secondary to debris blocking the canal, is not necessary for the diagnosis and not necessar-

ily present in either uncomplicated or malignant external otitis. *Pseudomonas* species remains the most common pathogen. Associated diabetes mellitus is the most common underlying condition rendering the patient susceptible, and there is virtually always a requirement of intravenous antibiotics.

14. The answer is B. The patient has otosclerosis. In otosclerosis, a conductive loss occurs in the face of completely normal physical examination, including mobile tympanic membrane. Any perceived color change of the eardrum on the affected side is a "red herring." Otitis media cannot exist without a conductive hearing loss. In all other forms of conductive hearing loss, either the external canal is occluded on examination or the tympanic membrane is immobile or nearly so, due to exudate, purulent or serous, or nonfunctional due to perforation. A noise-induced hearing loss is a sensorineural loss, not a conductive loss, that is, the Weber test with tuning fork set in vibration in the midline of the skull, is heard better in the symptomatic ear in conduction loss while a sensorineural loss results in bone conduction heard better in the asymptomatic ear. Meniere's disease also causes a sensorineural loss and classically is associated with prominent tinnitus and vertigo. Labyrinthitis causes vertigo without hearing loss. In otosclerosis, a conductive loss is the first clinical manifestation. It is a curable cause of hearing loss through surgery to free the adhesive new bone formation that prevents vibration of the stapes' footplate within the oval window. Otosclerosis is inherited as an incompletely penetrant Mendelian dominant trait that affects Caucasians more than other groups. Its progress is accelerated by pregnancy.

15. The answer is D. Beta-hemolytic *Streptococcus* is virtually the only cause of bacterial pharyngitis; any other bacterial causes are relatively rare. *Corynebacterium diphtheriae* and *Neisseria gonorrhoeae* make up about 5% of bacterial pharyngitis, according to some texts (in primary care, those incidences are far lower). Epiglottitis is caused by *H. influenzae*. Although it is often said that no one historical or physical finding can differentiate streptococcal from viral pharyngitis, the constellation shown in this vignette is significant and helpful. These are first and continuing dominant symptom is sore throat; symptoms are worse toward the end of the day (while viral sore throat usually worst in the morning); coryza and cough are generally absent and tender adenopathy favors beta-hemolytic strep.

16. The answer is D. The patient has hearing loss due to chronic exposure to noise, affecting the left ear selectively in a right-handed rifle shooter. The left ear is positioned closer to the muzzle blast when the right eye is on sight. On an audiogram, the vertical axis represents decibels (db) of hearing *loss* ranging from "−10" (10 db better

TABLE 3–1   Audiogram Showing the Noise-Induced V Shape

db	500 Hz	1 kHz	2 kHz	3 kHz	4 kHz	5 kHz	6 kHz	7 kHz	8 kHz
0									
10		x	x				x	x	x
20				x		x			
30									
40					x				

than "normal" at the top to up to 60 db loss going downward on the chart). The horizontal axis shows the sound frequencies in the hearing range in cps or Hertz moving upward in frequency from left to right (connecting the points of hearing threshold normal hearing would be a flat line across the top of the graph). The 4,000 cps is the first and most severely affected frequency (deepest loss on a tonal audiogram) involved in noise-induced hearing loss. As the 4,000 cps (4 kHz) frequency is more deeply affected, the adjacent frequencies become involved (e.g., 3,000 and 5,000 cps), producing on the audiogram the noise-induced "V." See Table 3–1. A flat audiogram showing depression of threshold uniformly across the frequencies is more characteristic of a conductive hearing loss than of a sensorineural loss. Early involvement of conversational frequencies is not a strong characteristic of noise-induced loss, as most conversation occurs at lower frequencies. However, when conversation is effected, higher voices such as females' are the first problems to be noted. As a sensorineural hearing loss, noise-induced loss is not as amenable to a hearing aid as are conductive losses, although developing technology has resulted in great improvement in this deficit.

17. The answer is C. Acoustic neuroma is the most likely cause of the symptoms. Acoustic neuroma is a slowly growing benign growth, the most common of cerebellopontine angle tumors, comprising 78% of that category. Gradual expansion may involve other cranial nerves as well, for example, the trigeminal and visual dysfunction can result through space occupation. Acoustic neuromas present with hearing loss, sensorineural to be sure, in little more than 50% of cases, the remainder presenting with tinnitus, vertigo (9%), or unsteadiness. Females are involved more than males in a ratio of 3:2. When bilateral, acoustic neuroma may be a manifestation of Von Recklinghausen's disease. Both otitis media and cerumen impaction cause conductive hearing loss. Acoustic trauma causes sensory hearing loss but comes on more slowly and is associated with clearly identified causes by history. Although Meniere's disease may present as isolated hearing loss without vertigo (and acoustic neuroma with vertigo and tinnitus, much like Meniere's disease), the course or Meniere's disease is always episodic rather than steadily progressive. The perceived color change does not fit with other findings in this case and thus must be attributed to

an unrelated cause, for example, a vascular variation on the tympanic membrane.

18. The answer is C. Cholesteatoma. Owing to chronic otitis media, this complication is nearly always the result of a nonhealing perforated tympanic membrane. The interaction of the ectodermal and entodermal elements of the eardrum combine to form an expanding "benign" mass that occupies space and may destroy the ossicular chain, impinge on the facial nerve, and lead to complications such as meningitis. Treatment is usually surgical. Neither otosclerosis nor Meniere's disease manifests any visible abnormalities on examination. Although this condition may resemble chronic external otitis in that the latter would show debris in the canal, the area of the tympanic membrane would be expected to be nonvisualized due to the debris. Bullous myringitis is easily seen as a deformity of a recognizable eardrum.

19. The answer is B. Vertigo of peripheral (vestibular) origin is characterized by violent symptoms after a latent period of 15 to 60 seconds, after motion of the head affecting the semicircular canals, for example, the Hallpike maneuver, in which the patient is told to lie back to the supine position while the examiner holds the patient's head and turns it simultaneously 90 degrees and the patient told to stare onto a blank wall. Symptoms of vertigo and the sign of horizontal nystagmus after a latent period of 30 to 60 seconds upon motion of the head affecting the semicircular canals is characteristic of peripherally based vertigo. This syndrome may be caused by vestibular neuronitis, benign positional vertigo, and Meniere's disease, among others, although Meniere's usually is associated with hearing loss and tinnitus – and would be expected to recur). The nystagmus due to a peripheral cause manifests fast and slow phases in nystagmus and tends to be relieved by fixation of gaze upon a fixed point. Nystagmus and symptoms that occur immediately upon completing the maneuver indicate centrally based vertigo. That nystagmus is pendular in that the eye movements are most rapid at the midpoint of the movement and the movement is symmetrical.

20. The answer is D. The patient has ethmoid sinusitis (ethmoiditis). The most important reason to diagnose and treat this condition within a day or two is the feared complication, orbital cellulitis. The other statements are all true as well except that in cases diagnosed early, treatment may be completed within 10 days instead of a mandatory 3 weeks.

21. The answer is C. Beta Strep must be treated within 7 to 9 days to be certain of prevention of rheumatic fever in children infected with Group A beta-hemolytic *S. pyogenes*. The first attack of rheumatic fever occurs between the ages of 5 and 15 years. Secondary attacks may occur up until 25 years.

22. The answer is B. Repeat the Monospot test. The clinical picture is classic for infectious mononucleosis, given the description and severity of symptoms in the absence of lymph node tenderness. The immunologic screens and certainly the heterophile agglutination test are known to require 5 to 7 days of illness before they become positive and in some cases as long as 4 weeks. Nevertheless, the decision to treat as streptococcal disease was justified, given the degree of illness, even though the streptococcal screen was negative. Rapid screening tests are only 80% to 87% sensitive. Not mentioned is that this patient, if he has infectious mononucleosis, would have greater than a 90% chance of developing a maculopapular or sometimes a petechial rash if ampicillin was instituted, compared with 15% in infectious mononucleosis cases not treated with ampicillin. Generalized adenopathy, although expected logically, given the pathophysiology of infectious mononucleosis, is often not appreciable. The cervical adenopathy is frequently notable posteriorly rather than anteriorly as is found in streptococcal disease, but this is not a dependable distinction. With infectious mononucleosis, there is a 50% chance of splenomegaly. For that reason, patients must be cautioned to avoid sports for at least 6 weeks. CMV infection is the most common cause of "seronegative" mononucleosis (wherein the heterophile antibodies, the basis of the Monospot test, never rise). Both CMV and toxoplasmosis may present similarly to infectious mononucleosis but are less likely to manifest exudative pharyngitis. CMV can be cultured, but if strongly suspected and the culture is negative, then HIV should be tested for as the possible underlying basis for susceptibility to CMV.

23. The answer is C. Change to a macrolide. Given the subacute onset of febrile disease (in influenza, fever is present from the first hours), the hacking, troubling cough, the headache, and the bullous myringitis, a good clinical empiric approach is expectant treatment for mycoplasmal disease. This is the classic cause of the definitive atypical pneumonia (although mycoplasma disease causes pneumonia in only 5% to 10% of patients who have the infection). Mycoplasma responds to tetracyclines and to the macrolides, including clarithromycin – not to the penicillins. Expectorants and antitussives are needed as supportive therapy but are not truly therapeutic. Bullous myringitis is defined as a bleb on the eardrum formed by fluid dissecting the ectodermal and entodermal elements of the tympanic membrane, without necessarily eustachian tube dysfunction being present. Owing to the awkwardness of eardrum mobility, it might be expected to be a mild conductive hearing loss.

24. The answer is E. The patient has classic Meniere's disease, which has proved to be refractory to medical management. The standard treatment consists of dietary salt restriction, elimination of xanthines (caffeine and chocolate), and smoking cessation for prevention and prescription of diuretics as well as judicious use of valium during attacks. Meclizine, helpful in most vertiginous states, does not appear to be effective in Meniere's disease. Although Meniere's disease is usually self-limited, it can cause severe disability, and this case patient has had the benefit of all the foregoing measures. The patient may be a candidate for surgical relief, the most common approach being endolymphatic shunt. If the procedure must be repeated, the most definitive operation is vestibular nerve section.

References

Ear Surgery Information Center. www.earsurgery.org/site/ages/conditions/menieres-syndrome.php.

Ear Surgery Information Center. www.earsurgery.org/site/pages/conditions/menieres-syndrome.php.

Handel O, Halperin D. Necrotizing (malignant) external otitis. *Am Fam Physician*. 2003; 68:309–312.

Neff M. AAP, AAFP, AAO-HNS Release Guideline on Diagnosis and Management of Otitis Media with Effusion. *Am Fam Physician*. 2004; 69:2929–2931.

Rudy DR. Problems of the ears, throat and sinuses. In: Rudy DR, Kurowski K, eds. *Family Medicine, House Officers Series*. Baltimore: Williams & Wilkins; 1997:1–26.

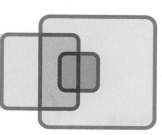

chapter 4

Pain and Headache Management

Examination questions: *Unless instructed otherwise, choose the ONE lettered answer or completion that is BEST in each case.*

1 Each of the following is a solid indication for neuroimaging in a patient with headache except:

(A) Onset of headaches over the age of 50 years
(B) Seizures associated
(C) Prolonged aura
(D) Nausea and vomiting *common c̄ migraines*
(E) Headache worsening with movement

2 Triptans, selective serotonin receptor agonists (SSRAs), have made a huge impact on treatment of migraine and to some extent cluster headaches. Of the many contraindications to their usage, which of the following is not a contraindication to taking a triptan?

(A) Presence of ischemic heart disease
(B) Taking within 24 hours of another triptan
(C) Concomitant use with nonsteroidal antiinflammatory drugs (NSAIDs) → *↑ efficacy*
(D) Taking in concert with ergotamine
(E) Taking during a prolonged aura

3 All of the following are commonly found in cluster headache except for which one?

(A) Alcohol ingestion
(B) Tearing and rhinorrhea
(C) Visual aura
(D) Abrupt onset
(E) Eyelid edema, ptosis

4 A 26-year-old woman in her second trimester of pregnancy complains of a recurrence of right hemicranial headache that has been present for 24 hours and is associated with photophobia and nausea as occurred on numerous previous occasions. Which of the following is acceptable and safe for relief of her headache?

(A) Gabapentin (Neurontin) → *safe in preggos*
(B) Valproic acid *NTD*

(C) Vitamin B2
(D) Lisinopril (Prinivil)
(E) Candesartan (Atacand)

5 A patient enters your practice with complaint of recent onset of acute headache. Which of the following would be the least indicative of serious pathology underlying the cause of the headache?

(A) Occipitonuchal distribution
(B) Age 50 years
(C) Headache waking the patient from sleep
(D) History of taking ibuprofen daily for arthritis
(E) Increasing frequency of the headaches over time

6 A 35-year-old woman complains of headaches that are throbbing and frontal or occipital in distribution. These have been occurring for most of her adult life but have become more severe over the last several days, lasting the whole day, several times per week. They require her to take over-the-counter ibuprofen once or twice weekly and usually respond thereto. Although the headaches remit during sleep, they recur during the day. Neurological history (including inquiry regarding visual and other neurological symptoms accompanying the headaches) and examination are negative. Funduscopy is negative for hemorrhages, exudates, and papilledema. Blood pressure is 116/75. Which of the following is most likely as the diagnosis of the headaches?

(A) Tension headache
(B) Cluster headache
(C) Migraine headache
(D) Intracranial hemorrhage
(E) Sinusitis

7 A 45-year-old man complains of daily unilateral headaches associated with rhinorrhea and tearing for the past several weeks. Vascular examination is normal. There are no visual or musculoskeletal symptoms. Which of the following is the most likely diagnosis?

(A) Migraine headache
(B) Temporal arteritis
(C) Cluster headache ◊persistent !
(D) Hemicrania continua autonomic Sx , persistent
(E) Sinusitis

8 A 42-year-old woman complains of recent onset of facial pain in the areas of the left cheek, left jaw, and the ante-auricular area on the left side. There has been no rash and this is the first time the patient has experienced these symptoms. The pain is lancinating, and it is precipitated by touching the skin of the affected areas, by chewing, and sometimes by talking. Which of the following is possibly associated with this syndrome?

trigeminal neuralgia

(A) Dental abscess
(B) Temporomandibular joint arthritis
(C) Vascular compression of the gasserian ganglion
(D) Maxillary sinusitis
(E) Herpes zoster (HZ)

9 A patient presents exactly as the person in Question 8 except that she complains also of disturbed vision and recent onset of urinary retention. Which of the following is the most likely cause of this patient's symptoms?

trigeminal neuralgia   optic neuritis

(A) Vascular impingement on the gasserian ganglion
(B) Posterior fossa epidermoid cyst
(C) Multiple sclerosis
(D) Sepsis
(E) Amyotrophic lateral sclerosis

10 Your female patient, an elementary school teacher, complains of paroxysms of right occipital pain. Examination is negative except for local tenderness over the right side of the occipital scalp at the ridge, and tapping the area produces a shocklike pain in the area of the headache. What is this pain called?

(A) Tension headache
(B) Occipital neuralgia —◊ Tinel's sign
(C) Migraine variant
(D) Cluster headache
(E) Giant cell arteritis

11 Which of the following patients with HZ (or shingles) is *least* likely to suffer from postherpetic neuralgia?

(A) A 25-year-old woman with abdominal zoster, one dermatome involved   & facial zoster
(B) A 76-year-old man with abdominal dermatomal involvement
(C) A 25-year-old man with HZ involvement of the ophthalmic branch of the trigeminal nerve

(D) A 45-year-old person with sacral involvement
(E) A 55-year-old person with sciatic branch involvement

12 You are examining a 66-year-old man who was brought to you by a friend; the man states that less than an hour earlier, he was walking from his yacht club to his car and abruptly developed a very severe headache in his occipital area and upper neck. He had never before experienced a headache. There is no reported drug use, and he denies taking any prescription medication. Vital signs are normal, except for blood pressure, which is 150/90. The patient's head shows no ecchymosis, and stethoscopy reveals no bruits. For the eyes, the pupils are equal and reactive. Fundi appear normal; extraocular movements are normal. There is resistance to flexing and rotation in the neck. Neurologically, the patient is sleepy but arousable. He can respond to questions, but they must frequently be repeated. He can move all extremities, and sensation to touch is intact in all extremities. Deep tendon reflexes are normally reactive and symmetrical. Which of the following would you order first to evaluate this patient?

(A) A computed tomography (CT) scan of head without contrast
(B) A CT scan of head with contrast
(C) A magnetic resonance image (MRI) of the brain
(D) A cerebrospinal fluid examination
(E) An erythrocyte sedimentation rate

13 A 71-year-old man complains of right-sided headache, coming on only within the last several months. Last week, he noted that, when he was chewing enthusiastically, his jaw on the right side began to be stiff and painful. Examination reveals tenderness of the right temporal artery. Dental examination is negative. A complete blood count is within normal limits, except that the sedimentation rate is 65 mm/hour. Which of the following is the most likely diagnosis?

(A) Migraine headache
(B) Subarachnoid hemorrhage (SAH)
(C) Cluster headache
(D) Giant cell arteritis   Temporal
(E) Dental infection in the right mandibular arch

14 Each of the following is associated with the condition portrayed in the 71-year-old man in Question 13 except for one. Which one is not associated with that condition?

(A) Pain in the hip and shoulder   polymyalgia rheumatica
(B) Unilateral visual loss
(C) Jaw muscle pain during mastication

(D) A photosensitive macular rash over the facial cheeks

(E) Fever

15 A 30-year-old woman complains of headaches that have often occurred during her menstrual periods. Recently, she has begun hearing her own pulsation in her right ear. She weighs 120 lb (54.4 kg) and is 5 ft, 4 in. (1.63 m) tall; she has no blood pressure or lipid abnormalities. You place your stethoscope over her optic orbits and hear no abnormal sounds. When you move the scope to the mastoid areas, you hear on the right a bruit timed with her peripheral pulse. What is the most likely explanation of these findings?

(A) Atherosclerotic stenosis of the right external carotid artery

(B) Arteriovenous malformation

(C) Migraine headache

(D) Cluster headache

(E) Temporal arteritis

16 A 28-year-old woman complains of a 10-year history of headaches. These headaches are fronto-occipital in location and are noted often at the end of workdays; they are more likely when sleep has been poor or short and they are generally relieved by sleep. They have always been quickly relieved by the use of NSAIDs. She does note an increase in her headaches when she is under stress or *anticipates* stress. Which of the following characteristics is most commonly associated with this type of headache?

(A) There is an aura about 30 minutes before onset of the headache.

(B) There is nausea and emesis.

(C) There is a gradual, often not precisely noticed, start and end to the headaches.   tension /vascular HA

(D) They are more common in men.

(E) They are frequently brought on by oral contraceptive usage.

17 A 45-year-old man began 2 weeks ago to have headaches on a daily basis. They last 1 to 2 hours and are associated with erythema of the face and rhinorrhea. The man says that he had a string of similar headaches about a year ago. He suffered a concussion 2 years ago and had headaches for several months afterward, but he has had none since until the recurrent headaches a year ago. Which of the following does this patient have?

(A) Allergic rhinitis

(B) Classic migraine

(C) Cluster headache   daily, short lived, remission

(D) Tension, vascular headache

(E) Post-traumatic headache

Examination Answers

1. The answer is D. Vomiting with nausea is not a solid indication for neuroimaging during management of a migraine headache. Although some have said that vomiting with or without nausea is an indication for neuroimaging, actually nausea and vomiting associated with migraine is relatively common and not of great concern except when there is no history of these symptoms being associated with headaches or if there be anything "different" about the headache that presents with nausea or vomiting. Certain indications for neuroimaging with migraine include seizures, prolonged aura, onset of headaches over the age of 50 years, headache worsening with movement, symptoms of systemic illness (e.g., fever), and any neurological signs that were not present at baseline.

2. The answer is C. Concomitant use with NSAIDs with triptans is not contraindicated. Actually, NSAIDs increase the efficacy of triptans. Ischemic heart disease that is active (e.g., symptomatic angina) is unsafe because of triptans' vasoconstrictive effects that would aggravate the pathology in play; ergotamine, itself a vasoconstrictor, is unsafe with a triptan due to the danger of exaggerating the vasoconstrictive effects; a prolonged aura, that is, continuation of the vasoconstrictive phase of the migraine process, could result in prolonged cerebral ischemia and precipitate a stroke.

3. The answer is C. Each of the characteristics or paired factors given is associated with cluster headaches except visual or other neurologic aura. Alcohol ingestion may precipitate attacks; tearing and rhinorrhea are part of the classic presentation of cluster headache as are eyelid edema and ptosis; cluster headache has an abrupt onset and short period of duration, generally a maximum of 3 hours.

4. The answer is A. Gabapentin is safe in pregnancy. Lisinopril and all other angiotensin-converting enzyme (ACE) inhibitors can cause fetal and neonatal morbidity and death if they are taken during the second and third trimesters, but not the first trimester of pregnancy; the same applies to ACE receptor-blocking agents such as candesartan. Valproate in pregnancy can be teratogenic, resulting especially in neural tube defects. Vitamin B2 is also said to be contraindicated in pregnancy. Acceptable drugs for migraine relief in pregnancy include fluoxetine, propranolol, amitriptyline, gabapentin, and topiramate.

5. The answer is D. Daily use of medication commonly results in rebound headache. Conversely, daily use of analgesics often fails to respond to preventive therapy. All analgesics may result in this phenomenon, including the triptans. Although occipital and uncial distribution of headache is common in tension-type (sometimes called vascular) headaches, rapid onset may be a sign of an intracranial vascular phenomenon or cervical spine syndromes. Headache that awakens the patient in the night is unlikely to have a benign cause unless there are associated migraine features or in the case of cluster headache. Increasing frequency of headaches, especially when worse in the mornings or associated with nausea, must be evaluated for intracranial pathology.

6. The answer is A. The description is typical of tension headache, albeit changing in intensity over the recent past. In a patient such as this, the first step after the neurologic history and examination is to investigate for increased tension in her life. Sources of such tension might be recent relative sleep deprivation, onset of anxiety or depression, onset of a systemic condition such as a chronic infection, a metabolic abnormality or anemia, or other life changes. Cluster headache is strictly unilateral and occurs daily or several times per day, albeit lasting less than 4 hours. Migraine headaches do not usually occur in the frequency given in this vignette and are classically unilateral. Intracranial hemorrhage is unlikely, given the overall chronicity. Ninety percent of patients who complain of "sinus headache" have identifiable forms of headache.

7. The answer is D. Hemicrania continua is associated with autonomic symptoms such as rhinorrhea and tearing. So are cluster headaches; however, cluster headaches are not persistent and do not last throughout the day. Temporal arteritis is associated with tenderness of the temporal artery. Migraine is classically hemicranial as well but is not daily in frequency. It appears that all types of vascular headaches are treated with the same battery of medications, with the exception that migraine and cluster headaches are treated specifically with the triptan group in addition.

8. The answer is C. This patient has typical trigeminal neuralgia ("tic douloureux"). Causes have become better understood within the past few years, and in fact, a majority of these cases are now thought to be caused by anatomic aberrations, including posterior fossa tumors, meningioma, schwannoma, epidermoid cyst, and basilar artery aneurysm. Another surgically approachable cause is arterial or venous pressure on the gasserian (trigeminal) ganglion. Other invasive approaches include methods of destruction of the ganglion or the root, such as radio frequency, glycerol, or balloon compression, all three of which may result in corneal anesthesia. The surgery is dramatically successful. Regardless, the initial treatment should be conservative, to which 70% of patients will respond. CT scan and MRI are often negative in the foregoing syndromes; therefore, exploration has become more common for making the diagnosis. The first drug of choice is carbamazepine (Tegretol). Other drugs used are phenytoin, baclofen, lamotrigine (Lamictal), gabapentin (Neurontin), topiramate (Topamax), and clonazepam (Klonopin). Neither temporomandibular joint syndrome nor maxillary sinusitis has sensory stimulatory precipitation. HZ acutely causes a typical rash. Postherpetic (zoster) pain is precipitated by sensory stimulation, but this patient had no preceding rash.

9. The answer is C. Multiple sclerosis can be a cause of trigeminal neuralgia. The common pathological pathway of trigeminal neuralgia includes demyelination of the nerve root near the ganglion, which may be on a mechanical basis as described in Question 5 or by the mechanism involved in multiple sclerosis. Sepsis could not explain the symptoms described without having more than one focus. Amyotrophic lateral sclerosis is entirely a motor degenerative neurologic disease. Mechanical causes of compression of the ganglion would not explain the urinary and the ophthalmologic symptoms.

10. The answer is B. Occipital neuralgia is caused by compression of the greater occipital nerve, by underlying entities such as posterior head trauma or compression of the occipital nerves by muscle tension (a possible cause in a "burned out" elementary school teacher). Tapping to stimulate electric shocklike pain is here called the Tinel's sign, just as it is in relationship to carpal tunnel syndrome. Such muscle tension can be secondary to osteoarthritis of the cervical spine, and on occasion, the cause cannot be found. Tension headache is not characterized by local tenderness or other neuralgic traits, although some patients complain of generalized scalp tenderness; migraine and cluster headaches are not neuralgic in character. Giant cell arteritis does not produce nerve tenderness.

11. The answer is A. Postherpetic neuralgia occurs increasingly with the age of the patient, rising from 9% in younger people to as high as 70% in patients older than 75 years. The other significant risk factor is acute HZ involvement of the ophthalmic branch of the trigeminal nerve. Sacral involvement may result in bladder dysfunction but no particular risk for postherpetic neuralgia. Incidence in all settings is reduced by acute (within 72 hours of onset) treatment with antiviral agents such as acyclovir and famciclovir.

12. The answer is A. A CT scan of head without contrast should be taken. Sudden severe headache, sometimes called "the worst headache I've ever had," should be assumed to be due to SAH until proven otherwise. A CT scan of the head without contrast is 90% sensitive in detecting SAH. Using a contrast agent or MRI confers no greater sensitivity; these procedures require more time and are more expensive. Cerebrospinal fluid examination is not necessary if blood is visible in the ventricles on the CT scan. Such procedures should be resorted to in the event of a negative CT study, when SAH is still suspected, to avoid brainstem herniation. Sedimentation rate elevation is sensitive for temporal arteritis, which occurs in the age group of this patient. SAH is a neurosurgical emergency.

13. The answer is D. Giant cell arteritis is the cause of temporal arteritis, which this patient has. The disease is a medical urgency because it can be the cause of blindness, based on occlusion of the ophthalmic artery. The jaw pain is the ischemic pain of claudication. The diagnosis is confirmed by biopsy of the temporal artery. Giant cell disease can affect many other parts of the arterial vascularity, which accounts for various presentations other than the headache of temporal arteritis. The disease responds dramatically to systemic glucocorticoids, and these do not have to be continued indefinitely.

14. The answer is D. A photosensitive, macular rash over the facial cheeks is *not* known to be associated with temporal arteritis. Temporal arteritis may lead to the symptoms of polymyalgia rheumatica (or the symptoms of both may develop simultaneously). Unilateral vision loss is present in only about 7% of patients at the time of presentation, but it will develop in about 44% of patients if they are not treated. Temporal arteritis is characterized by a strikingly elevated sedimentation rate. Temporal arteritis must be considered as a potential source of fever in those patients who are older than 50 years.

15. The answer is B. There is an intracranial arteriovenous malformation. Arteriovenous malformation may present with headache, seizures, or focal neurologic symptom or hemorrhage, but the latter is the most common, constituting the clinical presentation in 30% to 60% of cases. Headaches are the presenting complaint in 5% to 25% of the cases, and seizures in 20% to 40%. Bruits may be heard over a mastoid bone or an optical orbit. Carotid atheromatous stenosis causes pulsations audible to the patient on occasion but are not often heard by the stethoscope. Carotid atheromas would most likely occur in people with risk factors such as hypertension, dyslipidemia, or diabetes, and nearly always in individuals in their fifth or sixth decades or older. Migraine headaches often recur during various stages of the menstrual cycle, but the bruit would have to be explained otherwise. The same is said regarding cluster headaches, and these do not recur with such wide ranges of periods between attacks. See

Questions 11 and 12 for the clinical setting of temporal arteritis. Although it might briefly be considered, again the bruit would have to be otherwise explained.

16. The answer is C. These are prototypical tension or vascular headaches. Onsets are gradual, are often not precisely noted, and subside gradually. The presence of aura, as well as exacerbation perimenstrually, perimenopausally, during pregnancy, and with oral contraceptives, is characteristic of migraine headaches. Migraine headaches are frequently associated with nausea and emesis, unlike tension or cluster headaches. Both migraine and tension headaches are more common in women.

17. The answer is C. The patient has typical cluster headaches. The defining pattern is the daily recurring but short-lived headache, the associated facial flushing and rhinorrhea, and the "remission" of a year between clusters. Retro-orbital headache is also a characteristic of cluster headaches. These headaches traditionally affect men eight times as frequently as women and come on between the ages of 30 and 50 years. That said, recent reports indicate the gender gap has been closing markedly in recent years. Allergic rhinitis causes rhinorrhea but is not well noted for headache. (Many people with self-proclaimed sinus headaches may actually have cluster headaches.) Migraine headaches last longer but do not recur in clusters. The patient's history suggests that he once had traumatic headaches following a concussion, but they would not recur after a year's absence. Tension headaches are known for gradual beginnings and endings rather than the sudden starts and stops depicted in the vignette.

References

Beck E, Sioeber WJ, Frejo R. Management of cluster headaches. *Am Fam Physician*. 2005; 71:717–724, 728.

Family Medicine Board Review 2009. May 3–9, 2009.

Kurowski K. Headache. In: Rudy DR, Kurowski K, eds. *Family Medicine: House Officer Series*. Baltimore: Williams & Wilkins; 1997:43–56.

Maitzels M. The patient with daily headaches. *Am Fam Physician*. 2004; 70:2299–2306.

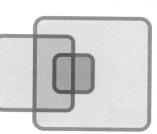

chapter 5

The Eye in Primary Care

Examination questions: *Unless instructed otherwise, choose the ONE lettered answer or completion that is BEST in each case.*

1 A 60-year-old Caucasian male complains of decreased visual acuity, noted when he reads. The complaint applies more or less equally to both eyes. His peripheral vision is intact to the usual office testing. He sees movement at 100 degrees laterally and 90 degrees inferiorly in both eyes. Nasal and superior fields are intact as well, limited only by the nose and brow respectively. He counts fingers from center in all directions. Fundoscopy reveals clusters of yellowish round, small lesions rather close to the center of the retinal fields in both eyes. What are the lesions?

(A) Drusen *age related macular degeneration*
(B) Cotton wool exudates
(C) Microaneurysms
(D) Flame hemorrhages
(E) Point of arterioles where they cross venules

2 Your patient is a 60-year-old Caucasian male of Scandinavian descent who has noticed transient blind areas when gazing into the direction of the sun. His confrontation visual fields appear to reveal a significant area of blindness in each eye, the left showing the scotoma above center and the right eye below center. Intraocular pressure is low normal in both eyes. An ophthalmologist consultant corroborates the foregoing and diagnoses cataracts. Which of the following is the strongest possibility for the surgeon to encounter at the time of a lens implant?

(A) Detached retina
(B) Anterior synechiae of the lens capsule to the iris
(C) Flame hemorrhages
(D) Fragility of the zonules holding the lens capsule
(E) Fragility of the cornea

3 A 71-year-old white woman complains of a visual disturbance over the last 2 days. She read in a family health journal about retinal detachment and fears she may have that problem. Which of the following symptoms would lead you to have her evaluated for that condition?

(A) Sudden loss of central vision in one eye
(B) Homonymous right-side visual field loss
(C) Peripheral visual loss in one eye with progression toward the central visual field over several hours
(D) Diplopia after a head contusion
(E) Irritation and tearing of the right eye over a period of 24 hours

4 A 55-year-old African-American man complains of the sensation of "a curtain" dropping over the peripheral visual field of his left eye. He complains of headache as well but no eye pain or photophobia. The patient has worn glasses for farsightedness. He denies history of intraocular hemorrhage, inflammatory conditions of the eye, eye infections, or eye surgery. He denies any increased incidence of "floaters" over the past weeks or months. Upon obtaining further history, you find the patient has a known history of hypertension that has been treated in the past; however, treatment lapsed about a year ago when the patient moved to his present location from another city. You examine him and find a blood pressure of 220/110. Pupils are equal, round, and reactive to light and accommodation. His fundi show hemorrhages typical of uncontrolled hypertension, but there is no papilledema. Which of the following is the best plan of action for today?

serous retinal detach (A) Start aggressive treatment to control blood pressure and call for an ophthalmologic opinion.
(B) Perform a slit-lamp examination.
(C) Hospitalize and start intravenous mannitol at 1 to 2 g/kg.
(D) Obtain a magnetic resonance image of the head with and without contrast medium.
(E) Obtain a carotid artery duplex Doppler study.

5 A 25-year-old mother of two children complains of pain in the right eye immediately after the fifth fingernail of her 6-month-old baby swiped across her eye during bottle feeding 4 hours ago. On physical examination, she exhibits striking photophobia. Which of the following is the key aspect of diagnosis of this condition?

(A) Disturbance in visual acuity
(B) Presence of diplopia
(C) Presence of limbal flush
(D) Matting of the eyelids
(E) Presence of green color upon examination of the cornea when a cobalt blue light is shone after application of fluorescein

corneal abrasion

6 You have diagnosed an 18-year-old man who plays on the high school varsity basketball team and incurred an injury to the left eye when another player poked his finger into the eye an hour ago. Fluorescein staining of the cornea is positive. Which of the following is the mainstay of treatment of this condition?

healing is rapid

(A) Topical and oral analgesics with a follow-up in 24 hours
(B) Antibiotic ointment followed by double patching and taping to prevent relative movement of the eye during the healing process
(C) Mydriatic drops followed by patching with follow-up in 24 hours
(D) Meiotic drops followed by patching with follow-up in 24 hours
(E) Immediate referral to an ophthalmologist

7 A 2-year-old boy is brought to your office by his parents for the first time, after a day care attendant expressed concern because the boy's eyes do not appear to be in parallel position. He and the mother are concerned that the child has "cockeyes": One eye falls consistently to the outside of the direction of his gaze. As a permanent condition, this is most often caused by which of the following visual defects?

(A) Myopia
(B) Amblyopia
(C) Hyperopia
(D) Astigmatism
(E) Exotropia

8 A 3-week-old female infant is brought to you by her mother, who is concerned by the child's left eye; it shows crusting and matting of a conjunctival discharge. The pupils are equal and reactive to light and there appears to be no photophobia. What is the most likely cause of this finding and what must be done, if anything, to remediate the condition?

(A) Bacterial conjunctivitis—use ophthalmic antibiotic drops
(B) Viral conjunctivitis—use ophthalmic antibiotic drops
(C) Iritis—use patching and instill an ophthalmic glucocorticoid preparation
(D) Obstructed lacrimal duct—use observation and consider probing the lacrimal duct

(E) Foreign body—perform double eversion of the eyelid and removal of same

9 At what age can the foregoing condition be expected to resolve physiologically?

(A) 3 to 4 weeks
(B) 4 to 5 weeks
(C) 3 to 5 months
(D) 9 to 11 months
(E) 2 to 3 years

10 A 52-year-old white woman calls your office and asks for an appointment the same day because she has had rapid onset of pain in her right eye. You see her within the hour and notice injection of her right eye and that she is unable to open her eye easily in the bright light of your examining room. She complains of pain that is 8 on a scale of 10, and the pain is felt in the eye as opposed to the anterior aspects of the eye as in foreign body or corneal injury. You have her visual acuity measured while she wears her glasses that correct for myopia. Her right eye, normally correctable to 20/25, is now 20/50 at distance. On examination in the light, the right pupil is dilated as compared with the left. In the dark, however, the right eye pupil dilates no further while the left eye pupil dilates and becomes larger than the right pupil. Which of the following does the patient have until proven otherwise?

nonreactive

(A) Acute iritis
(B) Allergic conjunctivitis
(C) Chronic simple glaucoma
(D) Acute (angle closure) glaucoma   *fixed pupil*
(E) Retinal detachment

11 A 35-year-old white man complains of the onset of photophobia over 2 days and blurred near vision of the left eye. He is not aware of getting a foreign body in his eye and the irritation of which he complains is unlike that of a foreign body sensation. Review of his medical history reveals that he has been diagnosed with psoriasis and has been under treatment for the past 2 years. On examination, the pupils are unequal; the left eye is meiotic (constricted) as compared with the right eye. The left eye has been tearing, and the patient has difficulty opening the eye widely when a light is shone into it. His corneae show no fluorescein uptake and no foreign body is found on the double upper-lid inversion. Which of the following diagnoses is the most probable explanation of this patient's eye complaints?

(A) Acute angle closure glaucoma
(B) Unseen foreign body in the left eye
(C) Retinal detachment of the left eye
(D) Bacterial conjunctivitis
(E) Anterior uveitis   *autoimmune predilection*

12 A 58-year-old woman complains of <u>dryness</u> of her <u>eyes</u> for the past several months and that, when she has had occasion to cry, her tear production is sparse. Over the last 2 years, she has had a spate of recurrent <u>dental caries</u>. Within the last 2 weeks, she has noted soreness of an enlargement behind her left ear and that her mouth is dry most of the time. Which of the following is most likely to be associated with her condition?

(A) Atherosclerosis
(B) Multiple endocrine neoplasia type I
(C) Hashimoto thyroiditis
(D) Diabetes type II
(E) Colorectal cancer   *Sjögrens*

13 You have instituted screening for glaucoma in certain routine preventive complete physical examinations. Which of the following is a <u>risk factor</u> for primary <u>open angle glaucoma</u>?

(A) Age >35 years in the absence of other risk factors
(B) Female sex
(C) Mexican or indigenous American race
(D) Excess exposure to sunlight
(E) African-American race *begin at age 35*

14 A 55-year-old white male patient enters your practice for the first time and has scheduled a complete history and physical examination. Specifically, he asks to be checked for chronic glaucoma, as he works with a person who informs him that he must take drops in his eyes daily for glaucoma. You do a measurement of intraocular tension and find it to be 16 mm Hg OS and 15 mm Hg OD (normal ≤25 mm Hg). However, on completing the general examination, you make a finding that tells you that you have not definitely ruled out open angle (chronic) glaucoma in the left eye. Which of the following is that finding?

Cup : disc > 30%

(A) Optic cup in the left eye is 40% the diameter of the optic disc.
(B) The patient exhibits a change in distant visual acuity with correction from 20/20 to 20/50.
(C) There is erythema of the left eye conjunctiva.
(D) There is papilledema of the left eye.
(E) There is a mydriatic pupil in the left eye.

15 A 20-year-old student is being brought to you directly from the scene of a bar fight in which he received a fist blow to his left eye orbit. He manifests an impressive periorbital hematoma ("black eye"), but no hyphema is seen. The pupils are equal and round and reactive equally to light. He complains of <u>diplopia when he directs his gaze to the right</u>, and you find that his left eye cannot follow your penlight more than 15 degrees past the midline toward the right. Which of the following is the likely cause of this complaint and finding?

(A) Direct blow to the eyeball
(B) Rupture of the eyeball
(C) Fracture of the orbital rim *EOM entrapped*
(D) Traumatic iritis
(E) VI nerve palsy precipitated by trauma in a diabetic patient

16 You have diagnosed chronic (open angle) <u>glaucoma</u> by a Schiotz tonometer and wish to do an in-office check of the patient's peripheral vision to make an informed referral for consultation of an ophthalmologist. When having the patient count fingers to ascertain visual fields, at what <u>angle</u> from the central visual axis should you hold your fingers?

(A) 15 degrees
(B) 25 degrees
(C) 30 degrees
(D) 45 degrees
(E) 60 degrees

Examination Answers

1. The answer is A. The clusters of little yellow dots are drusen. They have great pathological significance in that they signal the presence of non-exudative (age-related) macular degeneration, the most common cause of permanent blindness in the elderly. Cotton wool exudates resemble just that larger than drusen and white as opposed to yellow and they signify diabetic retinopathy. Microaneurysms are blood colored and the same or smaller than cotton wool exudates and are pathognomonic of diabetes. Flame hemorrhages are well named for their appearance and signify advanced staging of hypertension. The points of crossings of arterioles and venules are notching caused by traction on the venules by the thicker-walled arterioles as they deform with sclerotic change.

2. The answer is D. Fragility of the zonules holding the lens capsule, that is, the guy wires that suspend the lens capsule containing the lens. This occurs with the condition called the pseudo-exfoliation syndrome or simply exfoliation syndrome. It consists of proteinaceous material that escapes from the iris and appears to clog up the canals of Schlemm impeding reabsorption of the aqueous fluid in the anterior chamber. That is not the entire explanation of the pathophysiology, however, because the glaucoma with which it is associated is of low pressure (thus, the vignette). It occurs predominantly in people of Scandinavian descent. The largest database on the condition comes from Iceland. During lens implantation on patients with this condition, special rings may have to be inserted into the capsule after the old lens is extracted to distribute the tension more evenly among zonules if some have begun the rupturing process during the procedure. One message to the primary care physician is that not all destructive glaucoma is characterized by high intraocular pressure.

3. The answer is C. Peripheral loss of vision in a curtain type of blockage, as opposed to central loss, is typical of retinal detachment. Central visual loss occurs in optic neuritis or macular degeneration. Homonymous scotomas are always due to central lesions. Those that involve the right field of both visual fields would occur through a lesion of the left optic radiation or the left visual projection area of the occipital cortex. Diplopia is a result of pathology other than retinal function. Tearing is caused by irritation of anterior structures such as corneae, conjunctivae, or sclerae and also may be a response to pain and irritation associated with iritis and acute glaucoma, among other problems.

4. The answer is A. Given the history, it is likely that the patient has had a serous type of retinal detachment. This is brought about by effusion of serum behind the retina, secondary to uncontrolled disease states such as hypertension or uveitis. Treatment consists of medical control of the underlying disease (e.g., labetalol, perhaps combined with a thiazide diuretic in an Africa-American) and usually results in complete recovery of vision. However, most primary care physicians would make early judicious inquiry of an ophthalmologist as they begin to control the hypertension (as in this case). A second type of detachment is tractional retinal detachment and is due to intraocular fibrotic processes caused by previous hemorrhage. Treatment consists of surgical disengagement of the scar tissue from the retina by a trained ophthalmologist. The third type is the most common and is called rhegmatogenous detachment, related to initial detachment of the vitreous from the retina. One-fourth of the population will experience this condition between the ages of 61 and 70 years. At this stage, the symptoms are mild, consisting of an increased frequency of vitreous floaters. However, 15% of people with vitreous detachment progress to develop a retinal flap or tear or a hole. Besides the risk factor of age, rhegmatogenous retinal detachment occurs more often in myopic individuals and in those who have undergone cataract removal. The word *rhegmatogenous* is derived from the Greek word for rupture.

Slit-lamp examinations are not normally expected of primary care physicians. Intravenous mannitol is an accepted therapeutic modality for acute angle closure glaucoma. Acute glaucoma is characterized by intraocular pain and ipsilateral mid-position fixed pupil. A magnetic resonance image of the head would be indicated for suspicion of vascular accident or neoplastic disease, neither of which is suggested by the findings given. A carotid artery duplex Doppler study would be indicated for suspicion of visual disturbance that is due to carotid artery insufficiency. The latter may cause amaurosis fugax, that is, ipsilateral transient total blindness (or partial visual cuts, such as unilateral quadrantanopsia), caused by embolism of small flakes of coagulum or ruptured plaque from an atherosclerotic site of carotid artery stenosis. This patient did not exhibit that constellation of symptoms.

5. The answer is E. The patient has either a corneal abrasion or corneal laceration. Either lesion shows a green color in the area of abrasion, keratitis, or laceration of the cornea with cobalt blue light after instillation of fluorescein. The shape of the defect will determine whether one is dealing with a laceration or an abrasion. If the injury is associated with an embedded corneal foreign body, the defect will outline the speck. The aforementioned patient might well have a laceration or an abrasion, but it is unlikely that there would be a foreign body. Keratitis, depending on the cause, results in an array of pinpoint fluorescein positive areas, ulceration in patches, or a dendritic pattern. In any event, the course would not be so rapid in onset and would not be associated with trauma. Acute visual disturbance, decreased visual acuity, occurs with many problems of the eye, such as acute glaucoma, marked changes in blood sugar in diabetes, conjunctivitis with profuse exudate, or corneal injury. Limbal flush, which is a thin, red halo surrounding the limbus of the cornea, is reputed to be a hallmark of angle closure glaucoma. Matting of the eyelids, which is crusting of the lids to the point that they tend to stick together upon opening, is a sign of the profusion of exudate. Matting occurs especially in conjunctivitis, more so in bacterial as compared with viral causation.

6. The answer is A. Management of corneal abrasion has been greatly simplified. Essentially, supportive and symptomatic care consisting of topical and oral analgesics is all that is necessary and efficacious. Follow-up in 24 hours by the treating physician is prudent. Healing takes place rapidly and often is virtually complete within 24 hours and certainly so in 3 to 4 days. Patching as management of corneal injury has been eclipsed in light of meta-analyses that show that patching neither promotes more rapid healing nor relieves pain. Antibiotics, whether ointment or drops, are probably irrelevant, although they are often used. Bacterial infection is rare as a complication of corneal abrasion or laceration, as long as the injury is not deforming or ablative. Neither therapeutic mydriasis nor meiosis has a place in the treatment of corneal injury. Mydriasis was once used on the basis of relief of ciliary muscle spasm (there sometimes being ciliary spasm, hence a meiotic pupil as occurs in iritis) and resultant pain. Referral to an ophthalmologist is seldom necessary because of the benign natural course of this condition. However, if healing has not occurred within 4 days, then such referral is warranted and indicated. Many corneal abrasions are secondary to contact lens use. In those cases, if they recur, contact lenses should be discontinued.

7. The answer is A. Myopia is most often the result of a congenitally elongated eyeball. This leads early to unsuccessful attempts to relax accommodation for distance, resulting in relaxation of convergence to a degree that goes beyond parallel and thus is divergent. The resultant divergence is called exotropia. Thus, exotropia is a synonym for divergent gaze, not a cause thereof; the choice of letter E is therefore wrong. Basically, the eyeball that is abnormally long in relation to the focal distance capability of the lens and cornea must relax accommodation of the ciliary apparatus even for reading; in the extreme, this is unsuccessful even for reading. Accommodation and convergence are enervated together and act synchronously. In some cases, gaze malalignment occurs only

when fusion of gaze is broken up ("lazy eye") and thus shows no visible strabismus under usual circumstances. In such cases, the cover–uncover test is performed. The patient is instructed to fix the gaze on a point beyond 20 ft, or 6 m (i.e., "infinity"). Then an obstructing cover is placed over one eye, serving to break up the fusion or point fixation. Upon removal of the cover, in a person with lazy eye, the previously covered eye is seen to return to the original gaze from either a lateral position (exophoria, which is the subclinical phase of exotropia) or medially (esophoria, which is the subclinical phase of esotropia). Eventually, the diplopia that occurs is no longer tolerated by the brain, and the weaker eye's vision is suppressed. This condition is called suppression amblyopia and such cortical blindness may become permanent. Amblyopia is central blindness as defined herein, but the described case does not illustrate that condition. Hyperopia, farsightedness, is caused by an abnormally shortened eyeball at birth. The age range of 3 to 5 years for correction through surgery or eye exercises is chosen so that the child can be mature enough to cooperate in the therapy and the procedure would be early enough for the condition to still be reversible. Astigmatism is a refractory error produced when the cornea, which accounts for 65% to 75% of the refraction of light to the eyes, is set in a less than perfect spherical surface.

8. The answer is D. An obstructed lacrimal duct (physiological) is a common cause of conjunctival discharge after the first month of life. Treatment generally is nonspecific and supportive as the condition is self-limited. Occasionally, the lacrimal duct and sac become infected. In either case, the pressure on the lacrimal sac expresses fluid from the ipsilateral punctum or through the nose and thereby affects the opening of a congenital obstruction.

9. The answer is D. Congenital impatency of the lacrimal duct should not be expected to be resolved physiologically until 9 months of age. Bacterial conjunctivitis is treated with antibiotic drops, but this diagnosis is much less likely in the described situation. Viral conjunctivitis is more likely to be bilateral and is usually associated with other symptoms of a viral syndrome such as coryza and other symptoms of upper respiratory infection. Congenital impatency is a diagnosis of inference, and although it is usually treated with topical antibiotics, they would not be effective in this case. Iritis does not manifest equal pupillary size. Foreign body would manifest lid spasm, which is not found here. If present, it is diagnosed first by an inspection that usually requires double-lid eversion to be carried out effectively.

10. The answer is D. Angle closure glaucoma is characterized by rapid onset of pain that is in the eye and that exhibits a fixed mid-positioned pupil. Intraocular pressure, normally ≤ 25 mm Hg, is elevated to anywhere from 40 to

80 mm Hg. Failure to rapidly lower intraocular pressure will result in chronic uncontrolled intraocular hypertension and permanent loss of vision. Immediate medical therapy includes intravenous mannitol or oral isosorbide if intravenous equipment is not immediately available, while administering pilocarpine to constrict the pupil and ease the pressure in the Schlemm canals. Ultimately, therapy is surgical, such as laser partial iridectomy.

11. The answer is E. The patient has iritis or anterior uveitis. Posterior uveitis involves the ciliary body (cyclitis), choroid, or both. Iritis is characterized by a meiotic constricted pupil and photophobia. Photophobia is a consequence of the iridospasm and the aggravation thereof by light stimulation. Vision is blurred because of the nonspecific effects of abnormal ciliary body responsiveness but especially so at distance because the spastic ciliary body may disallow relaxation of accommodation for distant vision. Most uveitis is non-granulomatous and associated with and involving autoimmune processes, which can be seen by the presence of psoriasis in this patient. Treatment of anterior uveitis usually consists of topical glucocorticoids after confirmation by an ophthalmologist. Posterior uveitis and panuveitis are often treated by systemic glucocorticoids. Rheumatological consultation would be in order in those situations as well. Infectious causes are unusual and most often associated with immune incompetence; these are treated by appropriate antibiotics.

Angle closure glaucoma is characterized by a fixed mid-positioned pupil. Foreign bodies are rarely unseen and are signaled by the history of instantaneous symptoms. With a corneal-embedded foreign body (which would be fluorescein positive), there may be iridospasm that is relieved by removal of the foreign body. Retinal detachment of the left eye would be characterized by a curtainlike loss of vision rather than blurred vision and is usually painless. Bacterial conjunctivitis manifests much purulent exudate, matting of the eyelids, and a fine "sandy" foreign body.

12. The answer is E. The vignette describes Sjögren syndrome. It is an autoimmune disease characterized by dry mouth (carious teeth as a result) and dry eyes, as well as loss of taste and smell, pancreatitis, pleuritis, and chronic obstructive lung disease in the absence of smoking. Among many associated or metachronous conditions are parotid gland enlargement and other autoimmune diseases such as Grave disease, Hashimoto thyroiditis, vitiligo, and rheumatoid arthritis. There is no increased risk of diabetes type II (although there may be an increased risk of type I, an autoimmune disease), atherosclerotic diseases, multiple endocrine neoplasia type II, or colorectal cancers (nor other cancers).

13. The answer is E. Chronic glaucoma (open angle glaucoma), caused by increased intraocular pressure that insidiously destroys vision, occurs gradually over a period of years. African-Americans are more susceptible and should be screened beginning at the age of 35, whereas those with average risk should be screened starting at the age of 40. This occurs without causing pain but eventually causing loss of vision, first in the peripheral fields and then involving central vision. A significant percentage of patients with chronic glaucoma have normal pressure open angle glaucoma. These cases are diagnosed in primary care by fundoscopy and visual field testing (see Question 14).

Being of African-American race confers nearly a fourfold risk of developing primary open angle glaucoma (4.7% prevalence vs. 1.3% for whites). In addition, African-Americans are at risk much earlier in life than people of other races, which warrants their screening at an age as young as 20 years. Otherwise, age >50 years is a risk factor (not >35 years). Neither being female nor of Mexican or Indigenous American race is listed as a risk factor for primary open angle glaucoma; nor is exposure to sunlight. However, the latter places one at risk for pterygium (a pinguecula that forms on the sclera and crosses the limbus to extend onto the cornea). Being of Eastern Asian race is a significant risk factor for closed angle or acute glaucoma. Another risk factor for chronic glaucoma is diabetes mellitus. Chronic glaucoma is best prevented by routine intraocular tension measurements, every 2 years after the age of 40 years; abnormal readings are defined as >24 mm Hg on repeated measurement. This measurement may be taken in primary care offices by use of the inexpensive Schiotz tonometer. As mentioned, these cases are diagnosed through more subtle means (see Question 14).

14. The answer is A. A significant proportion of open angle glaucoma occurs without intraocular hypertension. This is a situation analogous to normal pressure hydrocephalus. Diagnosis in most of these cases can be made early by finding a cup/disc ratio >0.3 (30%). The earliest change in vision would be a narrowing of peripheral vision rather than a decrease in central vision (visual acuity). A decrease in distant visual acuity can result from an increase in the index of refraction (refraction density) brought about by hyperglycemia as in new or uncontrolled diabetes, among other causes. Chronic glaucoma exhibits no other physical findings, and no symptoms until visual changes are apparent. Therefore, erythema is not a sign of chronic glaucoma. Papilledema does not occur with chronic glaucoma. Acute (angle closure) glaucoma, but not open angle glaucoma, results in pupil change, in the form of relative mydriasis (dilatation).

15. The answer is C. In orbital fracture, an extraocular muscle may become entrapped and limit the range of motion of the ipsilateral eye. Although diabetes is a cause of cranial nerve VI (abducens) palsy in diabetics, diabetic VI nerve palsy is not precipitated by trauma, and the gaze error is failure to follow laterally as opposed to medially. A rupture of the eye would likely result in sluggish gaze movement, but the hallmark of an eyeball contusion is hyphema. The latter may lead to secondary glaucoma. A rupture of the eyeball may cause an irregular pupil, not found here. Iritis could occur after trauma if there were a corneal injury or foreign body, but it would not be found immediately after the trauma.

16. The answer is D. 45 degrees. In this version of confrontational field checking, the acuity of the peripheral field is being testing as well as the range (i.e., discrimination adequate to count fingers). For detection of motion only, the angle from the central axis should be limited only by the anatomic barriers, which are the nose, brow, lateral orbit, and cheek below.

References

Gariano RF, Kim CH. Evaluation and management of suspected retinal detachment. *Am Fam Physician*. 2004; 69:1691–1698.

Savory LM, Krasnow MA, Terry JE. Problems of the eye. In: Rudy DR, Kurowski K, eds. *Family Medicine: House Officer Series*. Baltimore: Williams & Wilkins; 1997:57–70.

Wilson SA, Last A. Management of corneal abrasions. *Am Fam Physician*. 2004; 70:123–130.

SECTION III

Cardiovascular Diseases in Primary Care

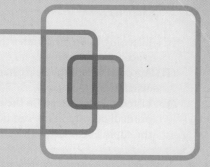

chapter 6

Cardiology

Examination questions: *Unless instructed otherwise, choose the ONE lettered answer or completion that is BEST in each case.*

1 A 45-year-old male smoker comes to his family doctor 7 days after a 4-hour bout of squeezing anterior chest pain that occurred while he was away with a group on a hunting trip, on which they traveled by canoe for 5 days away from their automobiles. He thought that he had a bout of heartburn; he has felt well since the attack and made the appointment "just in case." His electrocardiogram (ECG) shows Q waves in leads II, III, and AVF but no ST deviation nor clearly abnormal T-wave patterns. There is no prior ECG with which to compare. Which of the following available laboratory tests would be the most sensitive and specific indicator of a myocardial infarction (MI) having occurred 7 days before?

(A) Aspartate amino transferase (AST, SGOT)
(B) Myoglobin
(C) Treponin *peaks 12hrs lasts 2 wks*
(D) Creatine phosphate (CK-MB fraction)

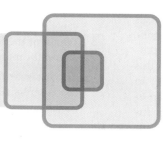

2 A 57-year-old male with symptomatic osteoarthritis of the knees and hips has had chest pains at odd times, not necessarily related to exercise, sometimes associated with emotional stress. His resting pulse rate is 52, sinus rhythm. An ECG is read as showing Wenckebach phenomenon. You decide on a cardiac stress test. Which of the following would be the most acceptable option?

(A) Phased treadmill exercise stress test
(B) Thallium sestamibi scintigraphy (scan for ischemia before and after exercise)
(C) Adenosine chemical stress test
(D) Dobutamine, radionuclide angiography
(E) Stress echo test → *ischemic areas don't dilate*

3 A 14-year-old prospective competitive athlete is scheduled for a physical examination to "go out" for junior varsity football. During the examination of the heart, a systolic murmur is heard over the left upper sternal border. Which of the following maneuvers would help the most to delineate identify the presence of infundibular hypertrophic subaortic stenosis (IHSS)?

(A) Auscultation of the heart while the candidate is performing the Valsalva maneuver phase 2 (the straining down, inspired breath holding phase)
(B) Auscultation of the heart while the patient is squatting during inspiration *↓ preload?*

(C) Listening to the heart after the candidate jogs in place for 1 minute

(D) Auscultation of the heart standing during exhalation

(E) Listening for changes in the murmur immediately upon the candidate arising from the supine position

4 A 45-year-old woman with a complaint of atypical chest pains comes to her new family physician for a checkup. Her blood pressure (BP) is 135/80; lipids results copied from the previous year are as follows: total cholesterol 150 mg/dL; high-density lipoprotein cholesterol (HDLC) 60 mg/dL: low-density lipoprotein cholesterol (LDLC) 90 mg/dL, and serum triglycerides 120 mg/dL. She has no family history of atherosclerotic vascular disease. Examination reveals a midsystolic click and a faintly perceptible systolic murmur. The doctor wants to ascertain whether prophylactic antibiotics should be prescribed for this patient before dental procedures. In an attempt to determine whether the patient has a murmur of mitral insufficiency, which of the following maneuvers would enhance that murmur for easier identification?

(A) Inspiration, squatting   *↑ venous return?*

(B) Expiration, standing

(C) Valsalva phase 3 (the release phase)

(D) Valsalva phase 4 (the rebound phase after Valsalva)

(E) Handgrip

5 A 67-year-old smoking woman with known chronic obstructive lung disease and right ventricular hypertrophy has been treated with intermittent use of a beta-adrenergic agonist drug. She now has a bout of increased coughing and shortness of breath. Which of the following blood tests might be the best indicator ruling out dyspnea caused by heart failure?

(A) Serum aldosterone level

(B) Serum cortisol level

(C) Serum pro-BNP level

(D) Serum digoxin level

(E) Serum creatinine level

6 A 63-year-old white man has had poorly controlled hypertension for at least 8 years. He has a family history of hypertension and type II diabetes. He had been on a calcium channel-blocking agent when he was last seen by you 2.5 years ago. He failed to follow up with you until he became dyspneic with exertion over the last week. BP is 160/105, apical heart rate is 110, and the rhythm is irregular. The ECG shows voltage criteria for left ventricular hypertrophy, and the chest x-ray shows a "concentric hypertrophy"

pattern in the cardiac silhouette (i.e., hypertrophy without obvious dilatation). Which of the following findings would most certainly apply to this patient?

(A) Distended neck veins

(B) Ejection fraction >50%   *Diastolic HF < asp, HTN*

(C) Pulmonary venous hypertension

(D) S_3 gallop

(E) Hepatomegaly

7 Regarding the patient in Question 6, what is the most likely type of dysrhythmia?

(A) Multiple premature ventricular contractions

(B) Primary atrial contractions

(C) Sick sinus syndrome

(D) Atrial fibrillation

(E) Second-degree heart block

8 Which of the following is the best therapeutic foundation for managing the patient in Question 6?

(A) BP control and heart-rate reduction

(B) Aggressive diuresis

(C) Angiotensin-converting enzyme inhibitors (ACEIs)

(D) Oxygen therapy

(E) Morphine sulfate injection

9 A 75-year-old man is visiting you for a routine checkup. He has seen few doctors in his lifetime and none in your city since moving there 10 years ago. You hear a diastolic murmur over the apex that radiates to the left axilla. Which of the following is the likely diagnosis?

(A) Aortic stenosis

(B) Mitral stenosis

(C) Dilated cardiomyopathy

(D) Aortic insufficiency

(E) Ventricular septal defect

10 A 17-year-old boy, upon routine preparticipation sports examination, manifests BP of 150/90 in the right arm and 110/90 in the left. Which of the following is the cause of this asymmetry of BP levels in the upper extremities?

(A) Congenital arteriovenous shunt

(B) Congenital abdominal aorta coarctation

(C) Congenital coarctation of the aortic arch

(D) Atherosclerotic blockage of the left subclavian artery

(E) Congenital stenosis of the left subclavian artery

11 In the patient in Question 10, which of the following abnormalities, if any, is most likely to be found upon examination?

(A) Systolic crescendo–decrescendo loudest over the left second interspace near the left sternal border   *aortic stenosis 2° bicuspid valve*

(B) Low-pitched holosystolic murmur at the apex radiating to the left axilla

(C) Systolic murmur at the lower left sternal border and a hepatojugular reflex

(D) Decrescendo diastolic murmur loudest at the left second interspace on the left sternal border

(E) Machinery murmur loudest along the left sternal border, both systolic and diastolic

12 A 55-year-old woman is scheduled for routine procedures by her private dentist, whose office now calls and inquires as to whether she should undergo endocarditis antibiotic prophylaxis. She has a history of mitral valve prolapse. You consult your record, which confirms mitral valve prolapse (whose evidence in her case is an audible systolic click without a murmur). Which of the following conditions is one of the indications for endocarditis antibiotic prophylaxis before dental procedures?

(A) Previous rheumatic fever without valvulitis

(B) Previous Kawasaki disease without valvular dysfunction

(C) Presence of cardiac pacemaker and implanted defibrillator

(D) Presence of mitral valve prolapse, with click and no murmur

(E) Presence of prosthetic cardiac valves, including bioprosthetic and homograft valves

13 You have followed the patient in Question 12 for another 10 years. Now she has a systolic murmur radiating to the left axilla and in fact manifests fatigue and, 3 times per week, paroxysmal nocturnal dyspnea. You decide to discuss with her the possibility of referral for mitral valve replacement. She is concerned about risks attendant to heart surgery. Which of the following cardiac procedures can you tell her is fraught with the highest perioperative mortality?

(A) Aortic valve replacement for aortic regurgitation

(B) Aortic valve replacement for aortic stenosis

(C) Mitral valve replacement

(D) Patent ductus repair

(E) Fracture of mitral valve leaflets for stenosis

14 Which of the following risk factors for coronary artery disease (CAD) is the most potent from the viewpoint of relative risk (rate of coronary disease in the person at risk compared with the rate expected in the population)?

(A) Obesity

(B) Sedentary lifestyle

(C) Hypertension

(D) Smoking

(E) HDL cholesterol <35 mg/dL

15 What time elapse is the earliest one can rule out MI by laboratory tests?

(A) 1 hour

(B) 2 hours

(C) 3 hours

(D) 4 hours

(E) 8 hours

16 Regarding a patient with a diagnosis of acute MI, in what window of time is it necessary to act to obtain the maximum value of thrombolytic therapy?

(A) 1 hour

(B) 2 hours

(C) 3 hours

(D) 4 hours

(E) 8 hours

17 A 55-year-old type II diabetic male nonsmoker is consulting you electively for the advisability of taking up a controlled exercise program. He has no history of chest pain or heart disease incidents nor symptoms of heart failure. However, a routine ECG shows a QS configuration in leads II, III, and AVF (deep Q waves; no R wave); there is no ST elevation nor depression. Each of the following statements is true about this situation except which one?

T (A) The patient has had a posterior MI of indeterminate age.

not true (B) "Silent" MIs carry a worse prognosis than symptomatic MIs.

T (C) "Silent" MI is more likely to occur in diabetics.

T (D) During the acute phase of this past MI, the patient was likely to exhibit a sinus bradycardia.

T (E) During the acute phase of this MI, the patient's symptoms were easily confused with an upper gastrointestinal syndrome.

18 A 28-year-old white male patient rushes into his doctor's office in a panic, demanding to see a doctor. He complains of heart palpitations and the doctor manages to examine his heart with a stethoscope to find a regular rate of 160. An ECG shows a supraventricular tachycardia. Which of the following methods, when effective, is the simplest way for differentiating paroxysmal atrial tachycardia (PAT) with block from atrioventricular nodal reentry tachycardia (AVNRT)?

(A) Osler maneuver

(B) Orthostatic versus sedentary BPs

(C) Digoxin level

(D) Carotid sinus massage   *No effect on PAT*

(E) Presence or absence of anginal symptoms

19 A 45-year-old man is seen in the emergency department with chest pain radiating into the left arm. He
has no atherosclerotic risk factors personally (except
his sex) and has no family history of CAD in members
before the age of 70 years; he does not smoke and has
no chronic cough or other respiratory symptoms.
Further history reveals that he complains of a sore
throat and fatigue that started 10 days ago. BP is
130/85 and the systolic pressure drops by 12 mm Hg
during inspiration. Examination finds nontender cervical adenopathy; there is no chest wall tenderness.
The heart shows systolic and diastolic murmurlike
sounds. The cardiac percussible silhouette is enlarged
to beyond the left midclavicular line. An ECG shows
ST elevation across the entire precordium. White
blood cell count is 3,500 with 60% lymphocytes and is
otherwise not remarkable. Which of the following
accounts for the described clinical picture?

(A) Acute MI
(B) Acute pericarditis
(C) Dressler syndrome
(D) Acute bronchitis
(E) Tietze syndrome

*For Questions 20 through 24, match the lettered types of
orthostatic hypotension with the numbered causes. A clinical type may apply to more than one cause.*

20 Pericarditis

21 Alcoholic polyneuropathy

22 Fever

23 Hypertensive on beta-blocker

24 Venous pooling after hot shower

(A) Neurogenic hypotension
(B) Nonneurogenic hypotension
(C) Drug-related hypotension
(D) Supine hypotension
(E) Septic hypotension

*For Questions 25 through 29, match the lettered descriptions
of heart sounds to the numbered cardiac diagnoses.*

25 Aortic stenosis

26 Mitral regurgitation

27 Hypertrophic cardiomyopathy

28 Mitral valve prolapse

29 Aortic regurgitation

(A) Holosystolic, low pitch; apex radiates to axilla
(B) Diastolic decrescendo
(C) Crescendo–decrescendo; radiates to carotids
(D) Midsystolic or late systolic click
(E) Crescendo–decrescendo; decreases with squat

*For Questions 30 through 34, match the lettered effects with
the numbered maneuver that may influence murmurs.*

30 Inspiration, squatting

31 Expiration, standing

32 Valsalva phase 3 (release)

33 Valsalva phase 4 (rebound)

34 Handgrip

(A) Decreases venous return
(B) Raises systemic vascular resistance (SVR), heart
rate, and cardiac output
(C) Increases venous return
(D) Decreases arterial BP
(E) Raises arterial BP; slows heart rate

Examination Answers

1. The answer is C. Treponin, for which lab study is most sensitive for picking up a 7-day-old MI. Treponin level peaks in 12 hours and lasts 15 days. Myoglobin peaks in 4–5 hours, lasts 7 hours; CK-MB fraction peaks in 8 hours, lasts 2–3 days; AST, known best as an indicator of hepatocellular damage, does rise in MI but is not specific enough for clinical application in cardiology.

2. The answer is D. The stress testing protocol that would be best for the described patient (atypical chest pain and resting bradycardia in a patient with symptomatic arthritis involving the knees) is D. Dobutamine, radionuclide angiography. It functions by causing vasodilatation, which is scanned by radioisotope. The injured portion of myocardium will not show the vasodilatation in response to dobutamine, and ischemic areas will fail to dilate and thus will not take up the radioactive tracer. One of dobutamine's effects is an increase in heart rate and it also increases BP. The phased treadmill exercise stress test is impractical because the arthritic patient will not likely be able to challenge cardiac output through the physical activity of the treadmill. Likewise, thallium sestamibi scintigraphy (scan for ischemia before and after programmed exercise) is not suitable for the same reasons. Adenosine chemical stress testing would be a reasonable choice if the baseline bradycardia were not present. Adenosine may reduce heart rate and especially in the face of second-degree heart block (Mobitz type 2) may cause complete arrest for varying blocks of time. Stress echo test normally involves physical exercise and thus is disqualified in patients who cannot exert normally on a treadmill.

3. The answer is B. Auscultation, while the patient is squatting during inspiration, is the maneuver that would do the most to differentiate the murmur of hypertrophic IHSS. In congenital HISS, the murmur is enhanced by any force that reduces venous return through the venae cavae, due to the hypertrophic aortic outflow tract that can progress under certain conditions to critical degrees, that is, choking off the cardiac output. Conversely, in situations that increase venous return, the outflow tract opens and turbulence is reduced. In the case presented, this results in a decreased intensity or disappearance of the murmur.

4. The answer is A. The answer to which maneuver enhances the auscultatory finding of mitral insufficiency is inspiration, squatting. This maneuver enhances venous return and thus increases mitral regurgitation when present. Expiration, standing erect, decreases venous return and effects an increase in the prominence of a mitral click. Valsalva phase 3, the release phase, produces a rapid decline in arterial BP but in a normally functioning heart has no affect on a mitral murmur. Valsalva phase 4, the rebound phase, produces a rise in arterial BP and bradycardia through its affect on the carotid sinus. Handgrip produces a rise in SVR, heart rate, and cardiac output.

5. The answer is C. The blood study that would be most helpful in delineating heart failure is serum pro-BNP level (pro-brain natriuretic peptide). BNP and ANP (atrial natriuretic peptide) are renin-angiotensin antagonists and serve as homeostatic responses to congestive heart failure (CHF). BNP has a tendency to rise with the severity of CHF. Thus, BNP is a sensitive indicator of CHF with a high negative predictive value. A recommended cutpoint for elevation is 125 pg/mL for patients under 75 years of age. On average, females' BNPs are about 15% higher than that of males (38 vs. 31 pg/mL) and people over 75 years of age roughly 10 times that of the population under 75 years (354 vs. 35 pg/mL). But even given such a wide spread, CHF results in a roughly 10-fold elevation for those under 75 years and close to 50% elevation in the over 75 population with CHF. Serum aldosterone rises in long-standing CHF, especially when there is a strong right heart failure component with great amounts of fluid retention. However, it is affected also by other fluid retention states, such as liver cirrhosis and other causes of anasarca. Serum cortisol has virtually no meaningful relationship with cardiac compensation. Digoxin, a positive inotrope, is used now most often in controlling certain supraventricular dysrhythmias. Serum creatinine level is a measure of renal function and will rise late in prerenal azotemia (long after urea nitrogen), of which CHF may be one cause.

6. The answer is B. This patient depicts diastolic heart failure (DHF). The name refers to the fact that the ventricular wall is stiff and does not fully relax during diastole. Ejection fraction is not compromised and is generally >50%, although the stroke volume is below normal. The most common causes of this type of failure are age and uncontrolled hypertension. Distended neck veins are more likely to occur with systolic heart failure, wherein the ventricles are flabby and whose contractions are weaker. Likewise, pulmonary passive congestion, although not absent in DHF, is more likely in systolic failure and its reduced ejection fraction. Both S_3 and S_4 gallops are found in a strong minority of DHF cases but are found in a majority of systolic failure cases. Hepatomegaly may be found in 15% of cases of either type of failure.

7. The answer is D. Atrial fibrillation is more likely in the presence of a stiff ventricular wall, as occurs in DHF, and is also more likely in an older patient.

8. The answer is A. Although each of the other choices except one is unassailable in the treatment of any form of heart failure, in DHF, lowering the BP to normal levels (<139/<90) and controlling the heart rate are specific and fundamental. The hypertension is the major contributing cause of the heart failure, and tachycardia (or even fast normal rates) aggravates the stiff ventricles' slowness to relax and permit adequate ventricular filling. Morphine injections are used in pulmonary edema caused by heart failure, usually of the systolic type.

9. The answer is B. Mitral stenosis produces a rumbling diastolic murmur at the apex, which in its classic presentation is associated with an "opening snap," marking the end of the murmur sound component until the next systolic cycle. The virtually sole cause of mitral stenosis is rheumatic heart disease, which is an increasing rarity. However, patients in the age range of the case presented in the vignette are still around. Many of them decompensated with pulmonary passive congestion, symptomatically very similar to that of left ventricular heart failure, and underwent mitral commissurotomy in the 1950s and 1960s. Later cases were treated by total valve replacement. The murmur of aortic regurgitation is a high-pitched diastolic murmur that starts immediately on the A_2 second sound, falling off in a decrescendo much like the sound of waves crashing on rocks. Aortic stenosis produces a systolic murmur loudest at the aortic auscultatory area. Dilated cardiomyopathy may produce mitral insufficiency and its systolic murmur, which is due to dilation of the mitral valve ring. Ventricular septal defect is a congenital lesion that causes a harsh crescendo–decrescendo left parasternal murmur.

10. The answer is C. This combination of BP levels is typical of congenital coarctation of the arch of the aorta. An arteriovenous shunt causes a widened pulse pressure (e.g., 150/60) that is distributed symmetrically throughout the vascular system. Abdominal aortic coarctation results in elevated BP levels in the upper extremities and lower BP levels in the lower extremities. Atherosclerotic blockade could occur in any part of the vascular system to produce any of the aberrations of BP discussed. However, atherosclerotic obstruction is highly unlikely in a 17-year-old patient. Although subclavian obstruction is a not rare phenomenon of atherosclerosis in likely candidates, congenital stenosis is not as likely as coarctation of the arch aorta.

11. The answer is A. This is the murmur of aortic stenosis, associated with a congenital bicuspid aortic valve (as well as with rheumatic valvulitis). This congenital lesion is present in 46% of cases of coarctation of all types. None of the other murmurs has a particular association with coarctation. The apical murmur radiating to the left axilla is that of mitral insufficiency. The murmur associate with the hepatojugular reflex is that of tricuspid insufficiency (compression of the liver produces a wave of distention of the jugular veins). The decrescendo diastolic murmur loudest at the left second interspace on the left sternal border is typical of aortic insufficiency. The systolic–diastolic murmur is, of course, the murmur of patent ductus arteriosus. Although the latter may be associated with aortic coarctation, that lesion is nearly always diagnosed and treated surgically in infancy.

12. The answer is E. The presence of prosthetic cardiac valves, including bioprosthetic and homograft valves, is an indication for antibiotic prophylaxis before dental procedures, as is the presence of mitral valve prolapse with demonstrable mitral insufficiency. Other indications include having history of bacterial endocarditis, history of rheumatic fever with valvular dysfunction, surgical systemic-pulmonary shunts, congenital and postsurgical valve deformities, and hypertrophic cardiomyopathy. All other choices are examples of cardiac-related procedures that do not involve disturbance of endocardium.

13. The answer is C. Mitral valve replacement (for mitral regurgitation) is the valve surgery fraught with the highest mortality rate. The challenge in limiting the perioperative mortality rate is met by keeping a careful eye on left ventricular size by echocardiography.

14. The answer is D. Smoking, with a prevalence of 25% in 1997, conveys a 3.5 relative risk of CAD; the next most powerful factor, family history, has a relative risk of 3.0. Having HDL <35 mg/dL is associated with a 2.0 relative risk. Obesity, with prevalence in the United States of 30% and rising, brings a relative risk of 1.4. Only central obesity constitutes a risk factor and is associated with the metabolic syndrome. These figures imply certain assumptions of degrees of intensity of the factor in question. For example, smoking as a risk factor probably finds correlation because smokers tend to be compulsive, and the great majority smoke a pack or more per day.

15. The answer is D. Creatinine phosphokinase–MB and troponin enzymes become positive within 4 to 6 hours, and troponin levels remain elevated for 4 to 5 days after the onset of MI (eliminating the need for the less-specific later- and longer-persisting enzymes such as lactate dehydrogenase). The only "false-positive" elevations of any significance occur in cases of angina, a syndrome of CAD of great seriousness in its own right.

16. The answer is C. Thrombolytic therapy, if started within 3 hours of onset of MI and when applied in cases with 0.1 mm or more ST segment elevation on ECG, reduces mortality from acute MI.

17. The answer is B. Silent MI, although more likely to occur in diabetics, does not carry a worse prognosis because of that characteristic; however, an MI suffered in a diabetic appears more likely to result in sudden death, with or without symptoms. Deep Q waves in leads II, III, and AVF are characteristic of posterior or inferior MI, and during the acute phase, an ST elevation is likely to be seen in those same leads. In the acute phase, inferior MI is more likely to present with epigastria pain and even pain that mimics "heartburn" than with the classic squeezing or pressing chest pain that radiates into the left neck or left arm.

18. The answer is D. Carotid sinus massage. This maneuver has no effect on PAT except to increase the block temporarily, which is signified by temporary prolongation of the PR interval. In the case of AVNRT, it will either have no effect or result in converting the rhythm to regular sinus. The Osler maneuver consists of testing for palpability of a pulseless radial artery with the BP cuff pressure raised above systolic BP. If present, it explains systolic pseudohypertension. Digoxin level may be helpful in differentiating the two because digoxin toxicity is a cause of PAT. However, it is a "soft" association and serves only as a basis for ruling out toxicity before evaluating the dysrhythmia further. Orthostatic BP levels have no particular value in differentiating the two rhythms but either may be associated with orthostatic symptoms, as circulation may be significantly compromised in either case as a result of the excessive rates involved.

19. The answer is B. Pericarditis is the cause of the symptoms. Chest pain may resemble that of MI, including radiation into the left arm. The ECG shows ST elevation across the precordium, more than would be seen with virtually any anterior-wall acute injury in MI. (Nevertheless, the patient would be admitted to the coronary care unit and MI would be ruled out by serial cardiac enzymes.) The drop of 12 mm Hg in systolic BP with inspiration is referred to as paradoxical pulse and is a typical finding with effusive pericarditis. It may occur also in chronic lung disease, but the patient in this vignette shows no evidence of that condition. The most common causes of acute pericarditis are viruses, including the Epstein—Barr virus (infectious mononucleosis). Nontender cervical adenopathy in the face of severe sore throat is typical, as is the leukopenia found in this case. The systolic–diastolic friction rubs may be difficult to distinguish from murmurs. The lack of chest wall tenderness rules out Tietze syndrome, a postviral costochondritis. Dressler syndrome is a postinfarction autoimmune form of pericarditis that is typically delayed by about 10 days after the MI. The enlarged cardiac percussible silhouette is caused by the fluid accumulation in the pericardial sac. Acute bronchitis neither produces ECG changes nor causes radiation of chest pain.

MATCHING THE CONDITIONS WITH THE PHYSIOLOGIC TYPES OF ORTHOSTATIC HYPOTENSION

20. Pericarditis: The answer is B, nonneurogenic hypotension. Presence of pericardial fluid or a constrictive membrane reduces the ability of cardiac stroke volume to compensate for venous pooling that occurs with orthostasis.

21. Alcoholic polyneuropathy: The answer is A, neurogenic hypotension. The neurologic pathways involved in peripheral vasomotor recovery from venous pooling fails and postural compensation is compromised.

22. Fever: The answer is B, nonneurogenic hypotension. Various possible aspects of orthostatic hypotension include dehydration and hypovolemia.

23. Hypertensive on beta-blocker: The answer is C, drug-related hypotension. Beta-blockers (and several other vasodepressive drugs) block the normal neurologic pathways for response to orthostasis.

24. Venous pooling after hot shower: The answer is B, nonneurogenic hypotension. Physiologic vasomotor response to heat involves arterial and venous dilatation that overwhelms the normal neurologic response to orthostasis.

MATCHING THE LETTERED DESCRIPTIONS OF ABNORMAL HEART SOUNDS WITH THE NUMBERED CARDIAC CONDITIONS

25. Aortic stenosis: The answer is C. This lesion causes a diamond-shaped (crescendo–decrescendo) systolic murmur at the aortic auscultatory area that radiates to the carotid arteries.

26. Mitral regurgitation: The answer is A. Mitral regurgitation (mitral insufficiency) causes a low-pitched holosystolic murmur loudest at the apex that radiates to the left axilla.

27. Hypertrophic cardiomyopathy: The answer is E. This crescendo–decrescendo decreases when the patient squats, as a result of an increase in venous return that allows greater diastolic filling in this condition in which diastolic dysfunction is a part of the pathophysiology.

28. Mitral valve prolapse: The answer is D. Midsystolic, late systolic, or pansystolic click are produced. If there is accompanying mitral insufficiency, then there is the additional murmur thereof, as described in the answer to Question 27.

29. Aortic regurgitation: The answer is B. This lesion causes a high-pitched soft diastolic decrescendo murmur that "crashes" off the second aortic sound and rapidly falls off in a decrescendo.

MATCHING THE LETTERED EFFECTS WITH THE NUMBERED MANEUVERS THAT MAY INFLUENCE MURMURS

30. Inspiration, squatting: The answer is C. This maneuver increases venous return and thus increases mitral regurgitation when present (see Question 28).

31. Expiration, standing: The answer is A. Expiration and standing erect decrease venous return and effect an increase in the prominence of a mitral click.

32. Valsalva phase 3: The answer is D. This is the release phase and produces a rapid decline in arterial BP.

33. Valsalva phase 4: The answer is E. This is the rebound phase after Valsalva and it produces a rise in arterial BP and bradycardia.

34. Handgrip: The answer is B. This produces a rise in SVR, heart rate, and cardiac output.

References

Bradley JG, David KA. Orthostatic hypotension. *Am Fam Physician.* 2003; 68:2393–2398.

Eaton CB, Cannistra AJ. Common cardiac problems in family practice. In: Rudy DR, Kurowski K, eds. *Family Medicine: House Officer Series.* Baltimore: Williams & Wilkins; 1997: 71–96.

Family Medicine Board Review 2009. May 3–9, 2009.

Gutierrez C, Blanchard D. Diastolic heart failure: Challenges of diagnosis and treatment. *Am Fam Physician.* 2004; 69:2609–2616.

Maisel AS, Zoorob R. B type natriuretic peptide in congestive heart failure. *CME Bull (Am Acad Fam Physician).* 2004; 3:1–4.

Wiviott SD, Braunwald E. Unstable angina and non-ST-segment elevation myocardial infarction: Part I. Initial evaluation and management and hospital care. *Am Fam Physician.* 2004; 70:525–532.

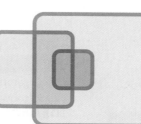

chapter 7

Peripheral Vascular Disease

Examination questions: Unless instructed otherwise, choose the ONE lettered answer or completion that is BEST in each case.

1. A 45-year-old female diabetic patient with a body mass index (BMI) of 35 has a non-healing foot ulcer, and her physician fears the development of osteomyelitis of the adjacent bony structures. Which of the following is the most sensitive test to allow realistic consideration of this diagnosis?

   (A) Computed tomography (CT) scan of the foot
   (B) Plain x-ray of the foot
   (C) White cell scan
   (D) Bone scan
   (E) MRI of the foot

   osteomyelitis ⇒ MRI

2. A 35-year-old Caucasian man comes to a family physician's office complaining of pain in the right lower leg. He has no history of similar complaints, venous thrombotic disease or pulmonary embolus. In considering non-invasive studies, which of the following is the most sensitive for phlebothrombosis?

   (A) Bone scan
   (B) Plain x-ray
   (C) Compression ultrasound study
   (D) Serum D-dimer level   *95~97% sensitive*
   (E) Examination for Homan's sign

3. Which of the following best describes the applicability of the Well's criteria in thromboembolic disease?

   (A) Differentiation of peripheral arterial occlusion versus atherosclerotic or embolic disease
   (B) Differentiation as to whether thrombotic disease is arterial versus venous disease
   (C) Assist in diagnosis of pulmonary embolism (PE)
   (D) Differentiation of hemorrhagic versus thrombotic cerebrovascular disease
   (E) Measure of right heart strain in PE

4. A 35-year-old man complains of pain and swelling of his right leg (calf, lower leg) for 3 days. History reveals that, 8 weeks ago, he was bedridden for 4 days for a severe bout of influenza. He has had no surgery requiring general anesthesia, he has never been diagnosed with cancer, and he does not have any neurologic disability. Vital signs are normal. Examination finds 1 + pitting edema and redness and diffuse swelling of the right leg. The patient has also a slight, thin, grayish discharge from the edge of his right great toenail. There are no visible superficial veins. A D-dimer test was within normal limits. Which of the following is least appropriate for the clinical disposition at this point in time?

   (A) Empirically prescribe an antibiotic effective against infection in the lower half of the body
   (B) Prescribe warm compresses and elevation of the affected extremity
   (C) Draw a white blood cell count and differential
   (D) Order a venous Doppler study of the right leg   *D-dimer ⊖*
   (E) Order culture and sensitivity test of the toe discharge

5. A 55-year-old woman who underwent cancer chemotherapy 3 months ago following surgery for breast cancer complains of left calf pain, swelling, and tenderness. The entire left leg (below the knee) is swollen with 1 to 2 + pitting edema, and there is tenderness along the distribution of the deep vein path. The D-dimer serum level is elevated. Venous Doppler study is negative for the evidence of deep vein thrombosis (DVT). Which of the following is the best approach at this time?

   ✓ (A) Venography
   (B) Serial ultrasonography
   (C) Surgical exploration
   (D) Bone scan for metastatic breast cancer disease
   (E) Prescribe cefadroxil

6. A 60-year-old male smoker complains of the acute onset of pain in the right leg. Examination shows coldness of one-third of the extremity below the knee distally. Popliteal, posterior tibial, and dorsalis pedis pulses are nonpalpable. With no additional information, which of the following is the most likely source of this arterial insufficiency?

   (A) Abdominal aortic aneurysm
   (B) Myocardial infarction

(C) Acute thrombosis of the right femoral artery
(D) Atrial fibrillation   *MCC arterial blockage*
(E) Mitral stenosis

7 Which piece of the following information would suggest thrombosis instead of embolization as the cause of a patient's acute arterial occlusion?

(A) Patient had previously been experiencing claudication in one of the calves upon walking two blocks.
(B) Patient has atrial fibrillation.
(C) Patient has mitral stenosis.
(D) Patient has no collateral circulation around the occlusion and suffers greater distal necrosis because of it.
(E) Patient has a known carotid stenosis and hypercholesterolemia and continues to smoke.

8 Regarding the patient in Questions 6 and 7, if his occlusion were chronic instead of acute, which of the following would be the *most sensitive* (i.e., earliest) indicator of chronic occlusive disease involving the patient's legs?

(A) There is an audible bruit over the femoral artery.
(B) There are symptoms of claudication after a brisk walk of half a block, which is relieved by rest.
(C) There is a decrease in the ankle-to-brachial systolic blood pressure (A/B) ratio.
(D) The patient has a 30 pack-year smoking history.
(E) There is skin atrophy and hair loss over the dorsal feet.

9 In the foregoing patient, what A/B ratio would suggest *severe* arterial occlusive disease at rest?

(A) >2.0
(B) <1.0 *nml*   *>1 nml*
(C) <0.9
(D) <0.8
(E) ≤0.4 *severe*

10 A 40-year-old man complains of 3 days of anterior and posterior chest pains. His blood pressure is 138/84, his pulse is 74 and bounding, his temperature is 98.5°F, and his respiratory rate is 16. His trachea is midline. His lungs are clear to auscultation and percussion. His cardiac examination reveals a new diastolic murmur over the right second intercostal space. A chest x-ray shows dilatation of the ascending aorta, and a CT scan of the chest confirms that there is a 4-cm aneurysm of the ascending aorta. Which of the following is the most likely cause of this patient's aneurysm?

(A) Medial cystic necrosis / *syphilis*   → *root dilation*
(B) Cigarette smoking
(C) Alcohol abuse
(D) Atherosclerosis *descending aorta*
(E) Trauma

11 On routine physical examination, a 65-year-old man reveals an expanding pulsatile mass in the midline hypogastrium. A thorough review of the patient's medical history is undertaken, and a duplex sonographic study is ordered. Which of the following is the best criterion for defining a patient with an abdominal aortic aneurysm as a potential surgical candidate?

(A) Aneurysm has 2 cm diameter.
(B) Aneurysm has 4 cm diameter.
(C) Aneurysm has 5 cm diameter.
(D) There is a coexisting coronary artery disease.
(E) There is an associated claudication of the legs.

12 The 65-year-old man in Question 11 is now 1-week status post elective surgical repair of his abdominal aortic aneurysm. In a consideration of preventive issues in this patient, which of the following is most likely to cause his death within the next 5 years?

(A) Aneurysm rupture
(B) Wound infection
(C) Stroke
(D) Postsurgical pancreatitis
(E) Coronary artery disease *CABG before AAA repair*

13 Regarding the patient in Question 11, which of the following, besides its diameter, would put him most at increased risk of rupture of this aneurysm?

(A) Obesity
(B) Age of patient >65 years
(C) Chronic obstructive pulmonary disease *COPD*
(D) Chronic hepatitis
(E) Diabetes mellitus

14 A 55-year-old man with mild to moderate hypertension who is 35 pack-year smoker is diagnosed with peripheral vascular disease (PVD) of the lower extremities after complaining of cramping deep, aching pain of the calves after walking two blocks. On examination, although the pedal and posterior tibial pulses are not palpable, the skin overlying the feet is reasonably well nourished. After various vascular studies, a vascular surgeon was consulted, and she felt that there was no solid indication for a surgical procedure. The patient and his family physician agree that the patient will make definite changes in his life style, most significantly will stop smoking, and proceeded to do so successfully. Which of the following would be the best pharmaceutical choice for medical management of the patient's claudication of the legs.

(A) Cilostazol (Pletal)   *Phosphodiesterase* (-)
(B) Nitroglycerin sublingually
(C) Pentoxifylline (Trental)
(D) Lisinopril
(E) Propranolol

15 A 65-year-old woman complains of new onset of swelling of her right lower leg and ankle. Her vital signs are normal, and she does not complain of dyspnea. There is deep calf tenderness. Which of the following would be of the most assistance in quickly determining whether there may be DVT without resorting to venogram or venous Doppler study?

(A) D-dimer serum level
(B) Complete blood count
(C) A/B measurements
(D) Serial creatine kinase levels
(E) Sedimentation rate

16 Regarding the 65-year-old woman with leg swelling, the test you ordered is reported positive for suggestion of DVT. Along with a confirmatory venous Doppler study, you wish to rule out PE. Which of the following is the most sensitive and specific method, assuming no medical contraindications?

(A) Electrocardiogram
(B) Plain chest x-ray in the interest of time
(C) Spiral CT scan of the chest
(D) Ventilation/perfusion (V/Q) scan of the chest
(E) Arterial blood gas test

17 A patient has proven DVT, and pulmonary embolus has been satisfactorily ruled out. The patient demurs regarding the option of hospitalization. You decide to commit the patient to 6 months of anticoagulation therapy. Which of the following is the most approved method?

(A) Administration of subcutaneous (SQ) heparin every 6 hours based on partial thromboplastin times (PTTs) for 5 days and immediate initiation of warfarin
(B) Initiation of warfarin and regulation of its dosage based on daily prothrombin times (PTs) over the first 5 days, followed by daily warfarin and frequency of PT determined by the results and stability of follow-up
(C) Home administration of SQ low-molecular-weight heparin (LMWH), with dosage to be regulated according to PTT follow-up

(D) Home administration of SQ LMWH for 5 days, initiating warfarin orally on day 2 of the LMWH, regulated according to serial PT   *heparin bridge to warfarin*
(E) Administration of SQ LMWH daily or twice daily for 6 months

18 Relevant to the preceding vignettes, once a patient with DVT has been diagnosed, stabilized, and anticoagulated, one should consider investigating the patient for all except which of the following issues?

(A) Occult malignancy ✓
(B) Deficiency of protein C ✓
(C) Deficiency of protein S ✓
(D) Raynaud's phenomenon
(E) Deficiency of antithrombin III ✓

19 A 58-year-old female patient was referred back to you, her family physician, by an ophthalmologist. She consulted for an episode of blindness of her left eye (only) lasting about 2 minutes that occurred 2 days ago. She denies visual disturbance since the episode and has no areas of focal weakness or numbness, nor does she have problems of mental concentration or memory. Which of the following segments of the physical examination is most likely to furnish the most helpful immediate findings?

(A) Fundoscopy   *amaurosis fugax*
(B) Cardiac segment   *→ mcc : emboli from ipsi carotid stenosis*
(C) Lung fields
(D) Neck → *carotids!*
(E) Abdominal segment

20 A 60-year-old man without specific complaints is undergoing a routine complete physical examination by you. He has not been in since his last annual examination 1 year ago. As is your custom on any patient older than 40 years, after auscultation of the heart you place the diaphragm of the stethoscope over the carotid arteries and hear a bruit over the left carotid. The pulses are palpable. No goiter is present. Further history review confirms that he has had no neurologic symptoms, including visual disturbance or motor and somatic sensory symptoms. The remainder of the history and examination are normal, and the patient is taking no ongoing medications. Which of the following is the most logical next step in disposition of the case?

(A) Refer for carotid angiogram
(B) Start aspirin 85 mg daily
(C) Order carotid Doppler studies   *Stenosis ≥ 60%*
(D) Order cardiac stress testing   *→ CEA Endarterectomy*
(E) Refer for coronary angiography

21 A 65-year-old man has recurrence of symptomatic stenosis of the <u>left iliac</u> artery after undergoing successful balloon angioplasty of the lesion 6 months earlier. Of all the following listed therapeutic interventions, which one is *not* indicated?

(A) Smoking cessation by the patient ✓
(B) Repeat balloon angioplasty ✓
(C) Mechanical atherectomy ✓
(D) Stent placement ✓
(E) Streptokinase infusion
    ↳ only in acute thrombosis

Examination Answers

1. The answer is E. MRI is the best choice among the five options given for diagnosing osteomyelitis. The CT scan is less sensitive and literally carries infinitely more radiation than the MRI (MRI has no radiation and the CT scan conveys approximately 200 times the radiation of a chest x-ray. Plain x-ray is inadequately sensitive, and the other two choices are significantly less sensitive.

2. The answer is D. D-dimer among the listed non-invasive tests would be most sensitive for venous thrombosis. D-dimer is 95% to 97% sensitive and confers a very high positive predictive value. A value greater than 500 ng/mL is the cut-point above which sensitivity is significant. Very close to this sensitivity is that found with compression venous ultrasound that is 94% sensitive and also confers a high positive predictive value. Bone scan has no applicability in vascular disease; plain x-rays, of course, have low sensitivity for soft tissue diseases. The time-honored Homan's sign, deep calf pain caused by manual squeezing of the calf, is only 50% sensitive and is associated with many false positives, for example, myositis and local infection.

3. The answer is C. The Well's criteria comprise a point system to assist in evaluating for PE. The following is a tabulation of that system:

Modified Well's criteria for PE:

Symptoms of DVT	3.0
Other Diagnosis less likely	3.0
Heart rate >100	1.5
Immobilization or surgery (<4 weeks)	1.5
Previous DVT or PE	1.5
Hemoptysis	1.0
Malignancy	1.0
A score of >6 points signifies a high probability of PE	
2–6 points signifies a moderate probability of PE	
<2 points indicates a low probability of PE	

The gold standard for diagnosis of PE is angiography. The VQ scan has high sensitivity but low specificity—that is, high negative predictive value.

4. The answer is D. Although DVT lies within the differential diagnosis of this case, the vignette places the patient in the 0% to 13% probability by the *Wells clinical decision rules* (CDRs) for assistance in diagnosing DVT. The Wells CDRs, with a maximum point of 9, show this patient to have 2 points. After 2 points are subtracted for the possibility of another diagnosis (cellulitis) that could account for the findings, the net score is 1. This confers a 0% to 13% possibility of DVT (see Table 7–1). Therefore, the patient may be followed expectantly while he is treated symptomatically or empirically. This patient may well have a case of cellulitis secondary to an infection of the great toe, for which culture, white blood cell count and differential, empiric prescription of antibiotics, and warm compresses would be appropriate. Another strong factor in a case like this, ignored in the Wells criteria, is the normal D-dimer. The latter is sensitive for the presence of intravascular thrombosis, though insignificantly specific.

5. The answer is A. According to the Wells CDR scale, this patient has a score of 4, placing her in the high-probability category for DVT (Table 7–1). Even in the face of negative ultrasonographic studies, a venogram should be ordered, although if the Wells score were in the moderate category, then serial ultrasonography would be acceptable. Prescribing cefadroxil (Duricef) would be a good choice for infection below the waist, but there is no evidence for infection in the vignette. Surgical exploration is inappropriate, and checking for metastatic disease has a secondary priority at this point.

TABLE 7–1   Wells CDR

Clinical Characteristic	Score
Active cancer (within 6 months)	1
Paralysis, paresis, or recent plaster immobilization of lower extremities	1
Recently bedridden for more than 3 days or had surgery within 12 weeks	1
Localized tenderness along the distribution of deep veins	1
Entire leg swollen	1
Calf swelling to 3 cm more expected for symptomatic side	1
Pitting edema confined to the symptomatic leg	1
Collateral superficial veins	1
Previously documented DVT	1
Alternative diagnosis at least as likely as DVT	−2

Source: Modified from Smucny J, Cohania R. *American Family Physician* (2004;70:565).

Notes: To determine the probability of DVT, calculate the score and place the patient in one of the following categories: 0 = low probability (0% to 13%); 1 to 2 = moderate probability (13% to 30%); ≥3 = high probability (49% to 81%).

6. The answer is D. Atrial fibrillation is the most common cause of acute peripheral arterial blockage. Acute obstruction is virtually always embolic in origin. Thus, acute thrombosis as a cause of acute arterial obstruction is unusual, and when it occurs it implies pre-existing atherosclerotic disease with superimposition of a thrombotic process. All other choices are valid causes of peripheral arterial embolism but not in the incidence of embolism that is due to atrial fibrillation. Myocardial infarction is the second-ranking cause of acute occlusion. When the latter occurs, it can be inferred that there is a significant portion of ventricular wall that is relatively flaccid, adjacent to which there is relative stagnation of blood flow.

7. The answer is A. The patient had previously been experiencing claudication in one of his calves when he walked two blocks. Patients with acute arterial thrombosis typically have some risk factors (including male gender) for the development of atherosclerosis and signs or symptoms of *chronic* arterial occlusive disease such as claudication.

8. The answer is C. A decrease in the A/B systolic blood pressure ratio is the earliest and most sensitive indicator for peripheral arterial occlusion. To obtain the A/B ratio, one obtains a systolic blood pressure reading on the posterior tibial artery and divides this by the systolic blood pressure reading in the brachial artery. Cigarette smoking is the strongest risk factor for peripheral arterial occlusive disease development but is not an indicator for it. Symptoms, bruits, and skin changes and loss of distal pulses occur later as the occlusive disease progresses.

9. The answer is E, <0.4. A ratio of >1 is normal, as systolic blood pressure is normally slightly higher in the legs than in the arms. A ratio <0.9 is consistent with some degree of arterial occlusive disease and <0.4 would indicate severe disease.

10. The answer is A. Descending aortic aneurysms are usually caused by atherosclerosis, although some are caused by trauma. Ascending aneurysms that are presented here are usually secondary to cystic medial necrosis or syphilis.

11. The answer is C. As the diameter of an abdominal aortic aneurysm exceeds 5 cm, the chances of rupture rise from 3% to 12% at 4 to 5 cm to 25% to 41% for over 5 cm. Coexisting coronary artery disease is a common coexisting pathology, as is claudication of the legs. However, these factors have no direct bearing on the chances of rupture. Note that the abdominal aorta, being "downstream" in the blood distribution from the thoracic aorta, is normally of a smaller diameter and thus is a smaller diameter tolerated in abdominal aneurysmal dilatation, as compared to thoracic aortic aneurysm.

12. The answer is E. Coronary artery disease is the most likely cause of death within 5 years of a patient who has undergone aortic aneurysm surgery. This is the reason aggressive search for underlying coronary artery disease is indicated before elective abdominal aortic aneurysm repair. If coronary artery bypass is indicated, it should be done before repair of the aneurysm.

13. The answer is C, chronic obstructive pulmonary disease. Rupture of an abdominal aortic aneurysm is associated with larger-diameter aneurysms, hypertension, and chronic obstructive pulmonary disease. Advanced age and possibly diabetes mellitus correlate with an increase in the incidence of abdominal aortic aneurysm but are not identified risk factors for rupture.

14. The answer is A. The best choice among those listed for medical management of claudication is Cilostazol (Pletal). Cilostazol's (Pletal) most prominently mentioned effect is its inhibition of cAMP phosphodiesterase Type III, but its clinical effects are not well understood. The drug improves walking distance statistically, in controlled studies, from 28% to 100%. Although nitroglycerin is clinically applicable in coronary artery disease, it has not been applied in PVD; pentoxifylline has been in vogue in the treatment of claudication in the distant past (i.e., 30 to 40 years ago and again 5 to 10 years ago after a rebirth), but it has not proven out well in controlled studies. Lisinopril, perhaps the most popular angiotensin-converting enzyme inhibitor, is useful in achieving relaxation of muscular arterioles; thus, effecting after load reduction and protection of kidney function in diabetes, it has not been applied in atherosclerotic PVD. Propranolol, a nonselective beta-adrenergic blocking agent, is relatively contraindicated in PVD.

15. The answer is A. D-dimer is quite sensitive for significant thrombus formation. However, it is not greatly specific because it may be elevated in the presence of soft tissue injury. Complete blood count and sedimentation rate give no specific information regarding an inflammatory process. A/B blood pressure readings are helpful in determining the presence and severity of arterial insufficiency (see Question 6). Creatine kinase enzyme levels are elevated in myocardial infarction.

16. The answer is C. For accuracy and speed, the spiral CT has become the community standard in most areas. A plain film has nothing to offer in the acute phase, although it may show a recognizable infiltrate after a few days—too late in many cases to prevent further embolism. An electrocardiogram shows nonspecific changes in 70% of cases (e.g., sinus tachycardia and nonspecific T-wave changes). Only 5% may show more specific right-sided changes such as the new appearance of right axis deviation, right ventricular hypertrophy, or P pulmonale. Thus, these are found only in cases of large emboli. A V/Q scan depends on lack of uptake of macro-aggregates of radioactive albumin in embolized areas of the lung, while the ventilation is unaffected. In lung disease, wherein ventilation is obstructed to affected segments of the lung, parenchyma perfusion may or may not be affected. This test was the standard diagnostic approach until the past 5 years. It is not specific enough, though quite sensitive in high-risk cases. Arterial blood gases may show hypoxia and respiratory alkalosis that is due to hyperventilation, when present in severe cases. The gold standard is pulmonary arteriography. It is 97% sensitive. Routine use of this study is somewhat controversial but is indicated in the following situations: intermediate or high pre-test probability when other studies leave doubt of the diagnosis; non-diagnostic V/Q scans; and when diagnosis must be established with certainty, when there are relative contraindications to anticoagulation. V/Q scan is not lost to the diagnostic armamentarium for PE as it is quite applicable when elevation of serum creatinine constitutes a contraindication for the use of contrast medium.

17. The answer is D. Anticoagulation of the patient with DVT and without pulmonary embolus for 6 months reduces the risk of recurrence of DVT and PE by 80% to 90%. The points of this question to be appreciated are the following. First, LMWH (e.g., Lovenox, enoxaparin) is as effective as intravenous therapy for this type of case and has a therapeutic onset of action comparable thereto and requires no monitoring of PTT. Second, warfarin therapy needs several days to be brought into therapeutic levels as regulated according to PT values, and it must be started virtually concurrently with the LMWH; some believe that warfarin should be started 1 day later because of the possibility of initial increase in coagulability caused by warfarin before its anticoagulation effect takes hold.

18. The answer is D. The Raynaud's phenomenon does not involve thrombosis principally; it is an arteriolar process involving vasospasm in the manual digits that results in color changes to white, bluish purple, and red, usually cycling over a relatively short period in minutes. If it is an isolated phenomenon, it is called Raynaud's disease. Otherwise it is associated with vasospastic phenomena attendant to autoimmune diseases. DVT may be associated with occult (or overt) malignancy (20% of cases, of which 25% are lung cancer) and deficiency of proteins C or S and of antithrombin III. In addition, it may be associated with factor V Leiden mutation, homocystinuria, and paroxysmal nocturnal hemoglobinuria. Mutation in factor V causes a poor anticoagulant response to activated protein C. This defect will not be detected in standard activated PTT, PT, or protein C assays. Proven superficial thrombo-

sis, after DVT and PE have been ruled out, may be treated by surgical ligation or chemical ablation.

19. The answer is D. The patient in this vignette has had a classic bout of amaurosis fugax (transient blindness), always in one eye. The vast majority of cases are due to small emboli from ipsilateral carotid artery stenosis, exceptions being in (usually) young people without vascular disease. In those cases amaurosis may be caused by choroidal or retinal artery vasospasm. The amaurosis associated with carotid artery disease may be partial (e.g., in the form of a quadrantanopsia), though often in medical school the syndrome is described as a complete loss of vision in one eye. Examination of the carotid arteries nearly always reveals auscultatory bruits. With or without a bruit the carotids must be subjected to Doppler studies or carotid artery angiography. Such examination should be done on an urgent basis concurrently with vascular surgery consultation. This syndrome is classified under transient ischemic attack. Timely carotid endarterectomy (CEA) markedly reduces the chances of stroke. Funduscopy would be abnormal only in cases of retinal vasospasm. The remainder of the physical examination, albeit always a worthy endeavor, is not particularly relevant to the complaint.

20. The answer is C. A carotid Doppler study should be done. If the stenosis is ≥60%, then a firm indication for CEA exists. This case is different from that of Question 19 in two main regards: Whereas the patient in Question 18 was symptomatic, this patient is asymptomatic. The symptomatic patient with a transient ischemic attack secondary to carotid disease, male or female, merits urgent CEA. However, as an asymptomatic man, this patient deserves a more aggressive therapeutic approach than would an asymptomatic woman. The Asymptomatic Carotid Atherosclerosis Study (ACAS) and other subsequent research showed that for ≥60% stenosis, interdictive CEA reduces the odds of stroke from roughly 11% over 10 years (≥2% per year) by roughly up to 53% (≈1% per year) for the population at large. It has been estimated that about 50% of strokes are due to extracranial pathology, accessible to the surgical knife. If men are considered separately, stroke reduction by pre-emptive CEA is an impressive 66%. However, if asymptomatic women are considered separately, the results are inconclusive. Carotid angiography is reserved for cases in which surgical indication is less than clear. Daily aspirin is a normal part of secondary prevention (and primary prevention for disease-free adults over the age of 50 or so), for the inhibition of platelet aggregation. Before any vascular surgery is to be performed, studies of the coronary circulation are a part of preoperative evaluation but not a part of the specific diagnosis of bruits or amaurosis.

21. The answer is E. A streptokinase infusion has no place in the treatment of an established plaque, whereas it may be employed in treatment of an acute thrombosis.

References

Chestnut M, Prendergast TJ. Lung disorders of the pulmonary circulation. In: Tierney LM, McPhee SJ, Papadakis MA, eds. *Current Medical Diagnosis and Treatment*, 43rd ed. New York: McGraw-Hill/Appleton & Lange; 2004:212–305.

Ebell MH. Evidence-based initiation of warfarin (Coumadin). *Am Fam Physician*. 2005; 71:763–770.

Executive Committee for Asymptomatic Carotid Atherosclerosis Study. Endarterectomy for asymptomatic carotid artery stenosis. *JAMA*. 1995; 273:1421–1428.

Family Medicine Board Review 2009. May 3–9, 2009.

Formon JJ, Kurzweg FT, Broadway RK. Aneurysms of the aorta: A review. *Ann Surg*. 1967; 165:557–563.

Kurowski K. Peripheral vascular disease. In: Rudy DR, Kurowski K, eds. *Family Medicine: House Officer Series*. Baltimore, MD: Williams & Wilkins; 1997:97–122.

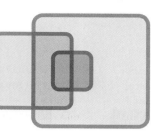

chapter 8

Cerebrovascular Disease

Examination questions: Unless instructed otherwise, choose the ONE lettered answer or completion that is BEST in each case.

1 A 65-year-old man with a history of poorly controlled hypertension and a 45 pack-year smoking history falls down returning to the bedroom from the bathroom. His wife finds him to be unable to move his right arm, and his face is drooping on the right. His speech is garbled. She calls 911, and the man is taken to an emergency department where he arrives 45 minutes after the onset of his symptoms. A decision was made to consider thrombolysis. Which of the following is not a satisfied criterion for going forward with the process of thrombolysis to interrupt a thrombotic stroke?

(A) Treatment with thrombolysis within 3 hours
(B) Computed tomography (CT) scan of the head negative for signs of hemorrhage
(C) Neurologic defect neither too small nor too large
(D) Blood pressure (BP) of 185/105   *185/110*
(E) Patient underwent herniorraphy 10 days ago *14/3*

2 A 67-year-old female reports a bout of apparent paralysis of the right upper extremity, a feeling of "totally dead" right arm, unable to be moved, that lasted for about 2 minutes. Which of the following is true regarding this attack?

(A) The majority of people who suffer such an attack will manifest infarction on MRI.
(B) If such an attack resolves within 1 hour, the risk of stroke is minimal in the foreseeable future.
(C) Anticoagulation therapy should begin forthwith.
(D) The involvement of the upper extremity indicates anterior cerebral artery pathology.
(E) A carotid duplex scan is indicated.   *TIA (< 1 hr)*

3 Regarding hypercoagulable states in cerebrovascular disease, which of the following is true?

(A) Testing for protein C should be carried out as soon as possible.
(B) Testing for protein S should be accomplished but not until 2 months after the stroke onset.

(C) Testing for antithrombin III is not relevant in the clinical setting of acute stroke.
(D) Warfarin therapy should always begin immediately after hemorrhage has been ruled out.
(E) Prothrombin gene mutation is an indication for immediate anticoagulation therapy, once hemorrhage has been ruled out.

4 A 65-year-old man successfully underwent carotid endarterectomy after discovery of a carotid bruit and a duplex ultrasound. His family physician decides to prescribe clopidogrel (Plavix). Which of the following drugs would decrease the platelet deaggravation effectiveness of clopidogrel?

(A) Motrin (Ibuprofen) *multiply the effects*
(B) Protonix (pantoprozole) *just this PPI, not others*
(C) Naprosyn (naproxen)
(D) Prilosic (omeprozole)
(E) Coumadin (warfarin)

5 A 45-year-old white man comes to you for the first time for a "complete physical." He is concerned that both his father and paternal grandfather died in their fifties of stroke; further, a paternal uncle recently had a stroke leaving him left hemiparetic but functional. After a complete review of systems and examination of all sectors, he returns to review the results, including those of comprehensive laboratory testing. You have found that he has a BP of 155/98 averaged over three determinations. His total cholesterol (TC) is 240 mg/dL, his high-density lipoprotein cholesterol (HDL-C) is 35 mg/dL, and his low-density lipoprotein cholesterol (LDL-C) is 140 mg/dL. He has smoked a pack of cigarettes per day for the past 25 years. He is employed in a high-tension occupation, that of stock trader, in which his income depends on his success on behalf of his clients. Which of the following risk factors are most prevalent in cerebrovascular (stroke) disease?

(A) Elevated LDL-C
(B) Reduced HDL-C
(C) Elevated TC
(D) Cigarette smoking
(E) Hypertension

55

6 For the person rendered hemiparetic by a stroke, secondary prevention is a critical aspect of his overall management. Which of the following risk factors, if present and corrected by the specific treatment plans listed, would be the most potent in secondary prevention of stroke?

(A) Antihypertensive drug therapy for hypertension
(B) Statin therapy for TC
(C) Smoking cessation in a one pack per day smoker
(D) Daily dosage of aspirin
(E) Warfarin (Coumadin) anticoagulation therapy

33%↓

7 Risk of stroke with *untreated* nonrheumatic (nonvalvular) atrial fibrillation varies greatly according to age, presence of risk factors, and history of prior stroke. With all categories thrown together, what is the average annual risk of stroke in the presence of nonvalvular atrial fibrillation?

(A) 1%
(B) 2.5%
(C) 5%
(D) 10%
(E) 17%

5 troke

8 In an emergency department, each of the following may be included in the differential diagnosis of acute onset monoplegia, in addition to stroke, if considered within the first few minutes of neurologic symptoms except for which one?

(A) Migraine syndrome
(B) Hypoglycemia
(C) Metastatic cancer
(D) Seizure
(E) Amyotrophic lateral sclerosis (ALS) → *gradual, not acute*

9 Knowing that control of hypertension is the most productive of therapeutic measures available for secondary prevention of stroke, within 48 hours after a patient has an acute cerebrovascular event, you would be least aggressive in control of elevated BP in which of the following clinical situations?

(A) BP of ≥200/≥120 mm Hg
(B) Concurrent acute myocardial infarction with left ventricular failure
(C) Concurrent renal failure
(D) Acute hemiplegia with a BP of 180/95 *only lower*
(E) Hypertensive encephalopathy *c̄ BP ≥ 200/120*

10 A 65-year-old white woman has seen you for her yearly gynecologic examination. You have seized the opportunity to pursue other preventive health measures and draw lipids. On the return visit, you note her lipids are at reasonably good levels. Earlier she smoked, but you talked her into successful

cessation 5 years ago. Her past medical history is significant for stenosis of her left femoral artery secondary to atherosclerosis. She has no history of hypertension or diabetes mellitus. On cardiac auscultation, you detect sinus arrhythmia but no murmurs. You do not appreciate any carotid bruit. An electrocardiogram reveals sinus arrhythmia with a rate of about 74 and a left anterior hemiblock. Which of the following features from her history or examination is a risk factor for stroke?

(A) Caucasian race
(B) Femoral artery stenosis secondary to atherosclerosis
(C) Sinus arrhythmia
(D) Female sex
(E) Left anterior hemiblock

11 With regard to stroke prevention, which of the following is the most accurate statement about ticlopidine?

(A) Ticlopidine is the best drug available for inhibition of platelet aggregation.
(B) Ticlopidine functions through a thrombolytic mechanism.
(C) The best application of ticlopidine is for platelet deaggregation in patients who are allergic to aspirin or in whom aspirin is contraindicated.
(D) Ticlopidine therapy must be monitored through serial prothrombin time.
(E) Ticlopidine therapy must be monitored through serial partial thromboplastin time.

12 Which of the following patients listed would most warrant an evaluation for vasculitis and the antiphospholipid antibody syndrome as cause(s) of stroke as opposed to the more common atherosclerotic or embolic cause?

(A) A 40-year-old woman with an ischemic stroke
(B) A 54-year-old man with known atherosclerosis of his iliac arteries and who has had two myocardial infarctions
(C) A 20-year-old patient who has had an intracerebral hemorrhage secondary to the rupture of an arteriovenous malformation
(D) A 60-year-old diabetic patient with hypertension
(E) A 70-year-old patient with chronic atrial fibrillation

13 A 65-year-old white man complains of the worst headache he has ever experienced. The headache had its onset at 3:15 PM today, and his wife has brought him to you. The patient can speak and walk and is stable as to cardiorespiratory status. Which of the following tests would you order first?

(A) A noncontrast CT scan of the head - SAH ?
(B) A CT scan of the head with contrast
(C) A magnetic resonance imaging (MRI) study of the brain
(D) Skull x-rays
(E) Lumbar puncture to look for red blood cells in the cerebrospinal fluid

14 A 65-year-old hypertensive white man who smokes has developed right hemiplegia and expressive aphasia over a period of 15 minutes while on a hunting trip. The attack occurred 30 hours ago, and his condition has not changed in the interim. He had complained of headache at the time of onset. At this time he is unable to communicate his symptoms and seems confused aside from his aphasia. Which of the following features is the most probable cause of this clinical condition?

(A) Thrombotic stroke ⊘HA
(B) Metastatic carcinoma from the lung
(C) Hemorrhagic stroke → rapid onset neuro Sx + HA
(D) Neurologic migraine
(E) Transient ischemic attack (TIA)

15 Which of the following orders would be most appropriate for a 67-year-old male patient with a BP of 160/95 who suffered an ischemic thrombotic stroke 2 hours earlier and who has a pronounced left hemiparesis and a noncontrast CT scan of the head that reveals no intracerebral hemorrhage?

(A) Coumadin
(B) A low-salt, low-cholesterol diet
(C) Rapid reduction of his BP with labetalol until it is about 120/80
(D) Ticlopidine
(E) Intravenous tissue plasminogen activator   tPA   give w/in first 3 hrs

Examination Answers

1. The answer is E. The one choice among the five given as an exclusion criterion for cerebral thrombolysis is a major surgical operation within 14 days of the onset of the stroke. The list of exclusion criteria includes no previous stroke within 3 months, small stroke in terms of neurological signs, recent major surgery (2 weeks), SBP >185/110, blood sugar <50 mg/dL. Given the stringent criteria, only 4% to 5% will qualify. The procedure results in a 30% decrease in disability at the 3 months point and no change in mortality at 1 year. Negative sequelae of thrombolysis to reverse stroke include a 10% increase in symptomatic intracerebral hemorrhage as complication.

2. The answer is E. Regarding the TIA described in this vignette, a carotid duplex scan is indicated. The chances of a stroke in a TIA by the newest definition (neurological symptoms that last less than 1 hour) is 15% within 3 months, the greatest risk being within 48 hours. By the older definition, if neurological symptoms resolve in less than *24 hours*, 50% will manifest infarction on MRI, and if symptoms persist for more than 1 hour, only 14% will recover completely. Thus, this distinction is significant; the older definition appears to overlook a strong possibility of completed stroke, albeit with minimal or no clinical evidence. Anticoagulation therapy, begun in timely fashion and after appropriate study, reduces the chances of stroke after TIA by the new definition (15% as stated) will be reduced by 80%. However, anticoagulation should not proceed until after a CT or MRI scan has ruAled out hemorrhagic stroke or certain other conditions been ruled out. Involvement of the upper extremity indicates *middle* cerebral artery pathology, as does involvement of the face. Anterior cerebral artery occlusion or TIA tends to result in neurological symptoms in the legs.

3. The answer is B. Testing for protein S should be accomplished but not until two months after the stroke onset. In fact, due to the suppression of clotting factors that occurs during the acute phase after stroke, proteins C and S as well as antithrombin III and the presence of prothrombin gene mutation, all of which are relevant for study in the presence of cerebrovascular disease, should await testing until 2 months have passed after the incidence of stroke.

4. The answer is B. Protonix (pantoprozole), proton pump inhibitor, reduces the effectiveness of clopidogrel. Apparently this is not true of other PPIs. NSAIDs such as ibuprofen and naproxen multiply the antiplatelet effects and can lead to bleeding problems when taken at the same time as clopidogrel and other antiplatelet preparations.

Warfarin anticoagulation therapy is a contraindication to antiplatelet drugs because of enhancing the danger of hemorrhage.

5. The answer is E. Hypertension is the most prevalent of modifiable risk factors for stroke, as it is present in 25% to 40% of patients who have suffered stroke and confers a relative risk (RR) of three to five times the risk of stroke in the population at large. The second most prevalent risk factor in stroke patients is hypercholesterolemia, which occurs in 6% to 40% and confers a RR of 1.8 to 2.6.

6. The answer is C. Smoking cessation is the most powerful tool in secondary stroke reduction (33% RR reduction). Aspirin antiplatelet aggregation therapy is more effective than the more expensive thienopyridine class of drugs, which are designed also as antiplatelet therapy (28% reduction in RR vs. 13%). Antihypertensive therapy is the most powerful modality in risk reduction for primary prevention of stroke (42%). However, it reduces RR by 28% in secondary prevention, similar to aspirin therapy. Statin therapy for hypercholesterolemia (and necessarily for the subgroups of dyslipidemia, i.e., elevated LDL-C and inadequate levels of HDL-C) reduces RR on an average of 25%. Warfarin therapy, although the strongest tool in secondary prevention of thromboembolic stroke caused by atrial fibrillation (66% secondary stroke RR reduction), is less effective than aspirin for thrombotic–ischemic stroke. Another special circumstance is that of secondary prevention of cerebrovascular disease after a TIA in a patient with moderate or severe carotid artery stenosis. Preemptive carotid endarterectomy reduces RR for recurrent stroke by 44% to 50% according to the American Carotid Artery study. Although it is useful to know the rank order of risk factors and of treatment thereof, it goes without saying that all known risk factors should be aggressively addressed in secondary prevention of stroke.

7. The answer is C. When all risk and demographic categories are thrown together, the overall risk of stroke in untreated nonvalvular atrial fibrillation is 5% per year. When the categories are broken down, patients younger than 65 years without risk factors ("low risk") have a 1% chance of stroke per year; those 65 to 75 years ("low moderate risk"), 1.5% per year; those 65 to 75 years who have diabetes or diagnosed coronary artery disease ("high moderate risk"), 2.5% per year; those of any age younger than 75 years with hypertension or left ventricular dysfunction but no other risk factors ("high risk"), 6% per year; and, finally, those >75 years with hypertension, left ventricular dysfunction, history of previous stroke, TIA, or systemic embolism ("very high risk") have a risk of stroke of 10% per year. Atrial fibrillation associated with rheumatic or other mitral valve disease carries a 17-fold increase in the risk of stroke over age- and sex-matched control subjects.

These ostensibly dry statistics should be appreciated in their rank order (but not memorized specifically) because of the implications for management. Persons of low and low moderate risk status should be treated with aspirin; those of low moderate risk should be treated with either aspirin or warfarin anticoagulation therapy, with a target international normalized ratio of 2 to 3; high moderate, high, and very high risk patients should be treated with aspirin, warfarin anticoagulation therapy, or both, with a target international normalized ratio of 2 to 3.

8. The answer is E. ALS would have a gradual not an acute onset. There would be motor symptoms only, and, although bulbar paralysis is one of the types of ALS, problems speaking involve dysarthria rather than expressive aphasia. Migraine aura may take the form of focal neurologic symptoms, from homonymous scotomata to hemiparesis and nearly any temporary focal neurologic lesion in between. Being a transient syndrome, migraine aura may be difficult to differentiate from TIA. The former is more likely to occur in a younger person than is the latter. Hypoglycemia may present with diplopia along with disturbed consciousness and may be briefly confused with TIA or stroke. Metastatic cancer to the brain, with hemorrhage, may present as indistinguishable from a completed stroke until an MRI or CT scan with contrast is done. However, metastatic cancer would be expected to present with a more gradual onset of more subtle neurologic symptoms before the acute event associated with the hemorrhage. Seizures may present with focal symptoms, usually with shaking movements.

9. The answer is D. In an acute stroke or TIA in the presence of significant hypertension but with BP <220/120, BP should not be lowered too aggressively. Generally, BP level immediately after a completed stroke is lower than the previous baseline, sometimes even in the normotensive range, often not recovering the previous level for up to 2 weeks. For this reason and because cerebral and coronary arterial circulation may depend on elevated pressures, generally BP should be treated rather gingerly immediately after stroke or TIA, allowing for "resetting" of autoregulatory mechanisms in the cerebral circulation. A TIA may even be precipitated by an orthostatic drop in BP. Thus, only when BP ≥220/120 (or if there is concomitant renal failure, acute myocardial infarction with left ventricular failure, or hypertensive encephalopathy), should it be aggressively lowered within the first few days after stroke or TIA.

10. The answer is B. Femoral artery stenosis secondary to atherosclerosis is a risk factor for stroke, as would be known coronary or carotid artery disease. African-American race is a risk factor, but neither Caucasian nor Asian race is a risk factor. As to sex, maleness is a risk factor. Other risk factors for stroke have been discussed in previous questions and their answer sections.

11. The answer is C. While ticlopidine functions as an inhibitor of platelet aggregation to prevent intravascular thrombus formation, it is not superior to aspirin and, by some reports, is inferior in that regard. No monitoring of clotting functions is required. Its best indication is for substitution for aspirin in patients who cannot take aspirin.

12. The answer is A. In a 40-year-old normotensive woman (especially one with no strong family history of atherosclerotic disease), an ischemic stroke is a definite "outlier." In other words, this is a person one would normally place in a low-risk status for stroke. A workup for vasculitis or antiphospholipid antibodies is normally reserved for patients who have other features of these disorders (e.g., evidence of systemic lupus), or those who are on medications that are associated with these disorders (such as procainamide), or those who have suffered ischemic strokes at a young age (age <45 years) with no risk factors for atherosclerosis and no other explanation (such as an atrioventricular malformation) for this stroke.

13. The answer is A. A noncontrast CT scan of the head. This patient has a classic presentation for subarachnoid hemorrhage (SAH). Ninety percent of SAH cases will show intraventricular blood on a noncontrast CT. Contrast adds nothing to the sensitivity of this study for SAH and takes more time and is more expensive. Contrast also requires assurance that the patient's renal function shows no elevation of serum creatinine; the latter may not be assumed in people with atherosclerotic vascular disease, which is the most common cause of SAH in the group of individuals who are 50 years or older. Cerebrospinal fluid is obtained only if the CT scan is negative in the face of suspected SAH and shows no lesions that could cause herniation when the cerebrospinal fluid is withdrawn. Skull x-rays are of no value. A CT scan is more sensitive and faster than an MRI.

14. The answer is C. Headache in the presence of rapid onset of neurologic symptoms is a prominent feature of hemorrhagic stroke and may be severe. The mechanism for this is the edema and swelling that develops in response to the hemorrhage and the resultant increase in intracranial pressure. Vomiting and a clouded sensorium are also typical features. Ischemic strokes do not produce this marked edema and produce either no headache or a very minimal headache. In the latter case, the onset is usually not so rapid unless the cause is an embolic thrombus. Brain metastases are always a possibility in a long-time smoker. However, the onset of symptoms is not likely to be rapid. A TIA by the newest definition lasts less than 1 hour (it is less than 1 hour and even by the old rule, less than 24 hours). Although migraine may be heralded by a neurologic aura (neurologic migraine), the aura is short lived, a matter of minutes to an hour, followed by neurologic recovery and, only then, the headache.

15. The answer is E, intravenous tissue plasminogen activator. Acute use of warfarin or ticlopidine, although used in tertiary prevention of stroke, is not effective in acute stroke as clotting factors tend to be suppressed for two months after the acute phase of a stroke. Tissue plasminogen activator will decrease the neurologic defect if given within the first 3 hours after ischemic stroke, but it increases the risk of hemorrhagic stroke development. Patients should initially be allowed nothing by mouth because of the frequency of associated swallowing difficulties and risk for aspiration. Rapid reduction of BP is contraindicated because this may drastically compromise cerebral blood flow. BP is lowered gradually so that homeostatic mechanisms may readjust to the new systolic pressures. Low salt and low cholesterol are primary and secondary prevention strategies but have no place in acute care of stroke.

References

Aminoff J. Nervous system. In: Tierney LM, McPhee SJ, Papadakis MA, eds. *Current Medical Diagnosis and Treatment*, 43rd ed. New York: McGraw-Hill/Appleton & Lange; 2004: 941–1000.

Coletta EM. Cerebrovascular disease and brain injury. In: Rudy DR, Kurowski K, eds. *Family Medicine: House Officer Series*. Baltimore: Williams & Wilkins; 1997:123–132.

Family Medicine Board Review 2009. May 3–9, 2009.

Solenski NJ. Transient ischemic attacks: Part I. Diagnosis and evaluation. *Am Fam Physician*. 2004; 69:1665–1674.

Solenski NJ. Transient ischemic attacks: Part II. Treatment. *Am Fam Physician*. 2004; 69:1681–1688.

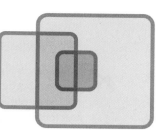

chapter 9

Pediatric Cardiology

Examination questions: *Unless instructed otherwise, choose the ONE lettered answer or completion that is BEST in each case.*

1 A 4-year-old male patient is brought to the family doctor by his mother after 5 days of fever (101°F), because of cracking and fissuring lips and bilateral painless conjunctivitis. On examination he manifests a "strawberry tongue," unilateral cervical adenopathy, and redness and swelling of the palms of the hands. A rapid strep flocculation test and, 2 days later, a throat culture were "negative" (latter meaning no beta-hemolytic streptococcus growth). The fever remains over the next 2 days. Each of the following complications may occur during the next few days except for which one?

(A) Coronary aneurysm — *not acute* [Kawasakis]
(B) Myocarditis
(C) Pericarditis
(D) Valvular heart disease
(E) Coronary arteritis

2 A 10-year-old boy is brought to the family physician by his parents because of the onset of involuntary and random jerking movements of the extremities, incoordination of purposeful movements and slurred speech, Sydenham chorea. Further history reveals the boy to be atopic with asthma that he "outgrew," pneumonia on one occasion treated outside the hospital, and an episode characterized by upper respiratory symptoms during a family vacation 4 years ago that was never treated but was followed by several weeks of mild to moderate changing joint pains and transient "bumps" under skin. The boy has been asymptomatic since and has participated heartily in outdoor play and athletics. Which of the following is the most likely diagnosis?

(A) Huntington chorea
(B) Sydenham chorea → *rheumatic fever*
(C) Parkinson disease
(D) Cerebral embolism from the heart
(E) Seizure disorder

3 Each of the following statements is true regarding normal electrocardiogram tracings in infancy and childhood except for which one?

(A) Heart rate decreases with age during the first year.
(B) The PR interval increases during the first year.
(C) Left ventricular dominance prevails at birth. *RV b/c PDA*
(D) Leads I and AVF show QRS that is net positive in the 1-year-old.
(E) The P wave deflection is positive in II, III, and AVF.

4 On a routine well child examination of a 9-year-old boy, you hear a grade III/VI systolic murmur along the left sternal border. You believe it is a functional murmur. Which of the following would assist you in making that determination by decreasing the intensity of a functional murmur?

(A) Temperature of 102°F
(B) Hemoglobin level of 8
(C) Anxiety
(D) Performing a Valsalva maneuver *↓ CO*
(E) Cutaneous vasodilatation

5 A 4-year-old boy is brought to you for routine well child examination after his family moved into the area, seeking a new physician for their care. The boy has manifested normal growth and development. He has normal energy output, playing outdoors with his age peers without difficulty. He manifests no cyanosis. On examination you notice a grade IV/VI smooth-sounding (i.e., not harsh) systolic murmur, which is loudest at the pulmonic auscultatory area. The second sound has a fixed split, not varying with inspiration. Which of the following is the most likely diagnosis of this murmur?

(A) Pulmonic stenosis (PS)
(B) Ventricular septal defect (VSD)
(C) Functional murmur
(D) Atrial septal defect (ASD) *systolic at pulm area c̄ split S2*
(E) Patent ductus arteriosus (PDA)

6 Regarding the patient in Question 5, which of the following is the most significant complication, besides congestive heart failure (CHF), that may result from late diagnosis?

(A) Frequent and severe upper respiratory infections
(B) Right ventricular CHF

(C) Shunt reversal → *will produce cyanosis*
(D) Clubbing of the fingernails
(E) Left ventricular CHF

7 A 15-year-old girl complains of chest pains and palpitations. Her mother is concerned that the girl may have mitral valve prolapse (MVP). In what position(s) is a click that is attendant to MVP most likely to be heard upon auscultation? *thin girls*

(A) Supine
(B) Sedentary
(C) Standing
(D) Prone
(E) Reverse Trendelenburg position

8 You are examining a 4-year-old boy for routine well child care. You hear a soft grade I/II murmur loudest in the left second intercostal space. Which of the following would most reassure you and the parents that this is a venous hum and *not* the murmur of pulmonic valvular stenosis?

(A) A venous hum has only a diastolic component.
(B) A venous hum has a coarse, harsh sound.
(C) The murmur stops with compression of soft tissue. *can compress veins*
(D) With PS, cyanosis is present.
(E) In venous hum, S$_2$ is normal.

9 While examining a 3-week-old male infant for his first well child visit, you notice that he has a harsh, pansystolic loud murmur at the lower left sternal border. There is also a heave over the left precordium. The child has been eating normally and the family has not observed any episodes of cyanosis or dyspnea. You find no cyanosis. You had examined this child at birth and before his discharge from the newborn nursery and did not discern any murmurs during these examinations. S$_2$ is normally split (increases with inspiration). Which of the following lesions is the most likely to account for the murmur?

(A) Tetralogy of Fallot
(B) ASD
(C) PDA
(D) VSD *Most common type*
(E) Venous hum

10 Regarding the child in Question 9, for which of the following complications is the child at risk?

(A) Heart failure
(B) Eisenmenger syndrome   ↑ *pulm flow*
(C) Bacterial endocarditis
(D) Failure of the defect to spontaneously close
(E) All of the above   *ALL*

11 You detect a grade III/VI harsh murmur over the left sternal border and second right intercostal space in a 13-year-old adolescent boy. He has no dyspnea, orthopnea, syncope, or chest pains. You suspect he has congenital aortic stenosis. Each of the following findings on physical examination correlates with that diagnosis, except which one?

(A) There is radiation of the murmur to the neck.
(B) There is presence of an ejection click.
(C) The murmur is loud and harsh both at the base and left sternal border.
mitral insuff (D) There is radiation of murmur to the left axilla.
(E) There is presence of a palpable thrill in the suprasternal notch.

12 On a routine examination of a new patient, diminished blood pressure readings are found in an adolescent's legs, relative to that found in the upper extremities. You suspect coarctation of the aorta. Each of the following may be associated with coarctation except for which factor?

✓(A) This may be an XO female patient. *Turners*
✓(B) There may be notching of the ribs seen on x-ray.
✓ (C) A delay in the femoral pulse may be found.
(D) Cyanosis of the lips and clubbing of the fingernails may be observed.
✓ (E) The patient is more likely to be male than female.

13 A 16-year-old boy is brought to you for the first time by his parents, complaining of increasing fatigability. Auscultation of the heart reveals a grade III/VI systolic ejection murmur and thrills at the right second intercostal space and in the suprasternal notch. S$_2$ is not split, either in inspiration or in expiration. The murmur is heard neither over the carotid arteries nor in the left axilla. Which of the following lesions explains these findings?

(A) PS
(B) Aortic stenosis (AS)
(C) ASD
(D) VSD
(E) Mitral valve prolapse (MVP)

14 A baby is born prematurely, at a weight of 3.64 lb (1.65 kg). What is the treatment of choice for a hemodynamically significant PDA in this infant that persists for longer than 48 hours?

(A) Observation for clinical deterioration
(B) Thrombosing the patent ductus through cardiac catheterization
(C) Surgical ligation
(D) Vasodilators
(E) Indomethacin

15 You hear a carotid bruit in a 3-year-old girl who has otherwise been healthy and has been growing and developing appropriately for her age. She is on no medications. Which of the following would you recommend?

(A) Aspirin 325 mg by mouth daily
(B) Persantine by mouth three times daily
(C) A carotid Doppler study
(D) A cerebral angiogram
(E) Observation only *common physiologic murmur in children*

16 You see a newborn boy after a few hours of birth. His weight is 8.5 lb (3.85 kg). You hear a loud murmur along the lower left sternal border. You delay his discharge home with the mother, pending evaluation of the cardiac status. On day 3 the nursery reports that the baby manifests cyanosis. Which of the following most likely accounts for this picture?

(A) PDA
(B) Transposition of the great vessels → *delayed onset cyanosis*
(C) Coarctation of the aorta
(D) ASD

Examination Answers

1. The answer is A. Coronary aneurysms are not likely to be present during the acute phase of this illness, which is classically presented as Kawasaki disease. The illness occurs in children under the age of 5 years, diagnosed (albeit arbitrarily as so many rheumatologic diseases are) by the following criteria: fever for more than 5 days and at least four of the following: bilateral painless nonexudative conjunctivitis; lip or oral cavity changes, for example, lip cracking and fissuring and strawberry tongue; unilateral cervical adenopathy; polymorphous exanthems; extremity changes such as swollen and red palms. Each of the cardiac complications mentioned may occur *acutely* except for aneurysms. However, aneurysm may indeed occur (15% to 25%) but no sooner than 10 days after the onset. Although there is neither a clear-cut group of diagnostic criteria nor a single specific or sensitive test to make the diagnosis, the disease must be diagnosed early to minimize chances of carditis through the institution of intravenous immune globulin and *high-dose aspirin therapy.* Aneurysms generally disappear within 5 years, but the resolution phase is when they may obstruct and cause acute myocardial infarction. Although the question may appear to be an example of pedantic trickery, the foregoing information in the aggregate may facilitate making the diagnosis in this rather ill-defined disease.

2. The answer is B. Sydenham chorea, well known to students as a sequela of rheumatic fever. What is less well known is that this syndrome may occur years after the acute phase of rheumatic fever. Huntington chorea, though inherited, rarely occurs during childhood and the choreiform movements are more sinuous. Parkinson disease virtually never occurs in childhood, and the tremor is the well-known slow pill rolling motion. Cerebral embolism from the heart would produce a neurologic syndrome that would suggest a mass lesion, and seizures have a beginning and an ending. Sydenham chorea follows a benign and self-limited course.

3. The answer is C. The incorrect statement is that "left ventricular dominance prevails at birth." In fact, at birth, as the ductus arteriosis (PDA) in the fetus has been shunting right to left. Thus, the right ventricle carried much of the load for the left-sided circulation. Thereafter, of course, the shunt shifts from left to right. Heart rate decreases with age during the first year; the PR interval increases during the first year; leads I and AVF show QRS that is net positive in the 1-year-old, commensurate with the left ventricle, assuming the major cardiac output load after the PDA has closed; the P wave deflection is positive in II, III, and AVF.

4. The answer is D. Performing a Valsalva maneuver will reduce the intensity of functional murmurs. Functional murmurs increase in intensity in situations that increase cardiac output, such as with fever, anemia, anxiety, or cutaneous vasodilatation. The Valsalva maneuver diminishes end-diastolic left ventricular volumes and diminishes cardiac output, and it either diminishes the murmur or produces no change in the murmur.

5. The answer is D. ASD is a not uncommon congenital anomaly. It is characterized by a systolic murmur located at the pulmonic auscultatory area and fixed split second heart sound. The murmur is caused not by flow through the ASD but by increased flow through the pulmonary artery outflow tract; thus, the murmur sounds very much like that of PS. VSD is the most common congenital heart defect. Like ASD, PDA, and PS, it is a noncyanotic condition because the shunt is from left to right in ASD, VSD, and PDA, and PS is not characterized by a shunt of any kind (though in advanced cases there may be cyanosis). ASD usually causes no symptoms until the second decade, except in the complete form. In the latter there is not only an ostium primum defect but also a VSD and mitral insufficiency as well. Such cases are usually symptomatic in childhood. In any event, the diagnosis needs to be made to effect repair before CHF compounds the issue.

6. The answer is C, shunt reversal (from left to right toward right to left) that produces cyanosis. Right ventricular CHF and ultimately cyanosis and nail clubbing are direct results of shunt reversal. Left ventricular CHF usually does not occur in this disease. Frequent upper respiratory tract infection and even pneumonia are early complications of ASD and other left-to-right shunts, but they are not the most dire consequences.

7. The answer is C. Standing position is the most likely among the choices to allow auscultation of the MVP click. MVP in adolescents is most likely to occur in thin girls. Chest pains and palpitations are reported with MVP, but it has not been proven that these symptoms are more common in MVP patients than in the population at large. In the Trendelenburg position, the patient is supine with head tilted upward; the reverse Trendelenburg position has the patient prone with the head end tilted down. The latter is a quick treatment for neurogenic hypotension to increase cerebral circulation.

8. The answer is C. A venous hum is blocked by the compression of the soft tissue just cephalad to the maximum point of audibility of the murmur. One accomplishes this by placing one or two fingers in a transverse position in the aforementioned position. The murmur is also said to dissipate when the child lies supine, but this is not reliable. Furthermore, the venous hum often dissipates with the turning of the child's head. The quality of the murmur is soft, not harsh. The murmur tends to be both systolic and diastolic in timing; that is, it is machinery like. Neither PS nor venous hum may manifest cyanosis with the exception that, in the case of PS, cyanosis may occur in advanced and symptomatic cases (this patient manifested no other signs or symptoms). S_2 is normal not only in venous hum, of course, but also in mild-to-moderate cases of PS. Jugular venous hum occurs after the age of 2 years, often in preschoolers, but never as late as adolescence.

9. The answer is D. VSDs account for 30% of congenital heart defects and are the most common type. Tetralogy of Fallot manifests cyanosis early on, as there is a right to left shunt from the beginning. ASDs cause a murmur that is located more cephalad, at about the second left intercostal space near the left sternal border, and is characterized by a fixed split second sound. Patent ductus is characterized by a continuous murmur that is loudest in systole (the machinery murmur). Venous hum has been described. It does not make an appearance until about 2 years of age.

10. The answer is E, all of the above. Patients with VSD may develop several complications, most of which relate to the increased pulmonary blood flow. This can lead to pulmonary hypertension, the more likely the larger the defect. The latter, of course, leads to a reversal of the shunt, then becoming right to left (the Eisenmenger syndrome). Smaller VSDs often spontaneously close in the first few years of life, but this is less likely with larger defects and in older children. Patients with VSD are prone to bacterial endocarditis, and prophylaxis is recommended.

11. The answer is D. Radiation of a systolic murmur to the left axilla is virtually pathognomonic of mitral insufficiency. The murmur of aortic stenosis is loud and harsh, both at the base and at the left sternal border, and radiates to the carotids. There may be palpable thrills in the suprasternal notch, the right base (point of S_2), and over the carotid arteries. The intensity of the suprasternal notch thrill best correlates with the size of the gradient across the area of stenosis. An ejection click is common (thus, not all clicks are caused by MVP). Of all cases, 75% are of the valvular stenosis type, 23% are subvalvular, and 1% to 2% are supravalvular.

12. The answer is D. Cyanosis of the lips and clubbing of the fingernails will not be observed in coarctation. Male individuals are significantly more often affected than female individuals. However, if a phenotypic female is affected, she is quite likely to be an XO genotype. The

femoral pulse delay and collateral formation are usually not evident in children. Although delayed femoral pulses are not usually found in children, by the age of adolescence this finding is common. Also, by adulthood, rib notching is commonly found in coarctation. The most common locus of coarctation is the thoracic aorta just distal to the origin of the left subclavian artery.

13. The answer is A. PS occurs most often as valvular stenosis, comprising 10% of congenital heart disease lesions. In mild to moderate cases, an opening click may be heard more prominent during expiration than inspiration. In severe cases, S_2 is not heard at all, and hence, no split is discernible. In the most severe cases, there is early cyanosis, often caused by right to left shunting through a patent foramen ovale. Other cases do not become symptomatic until later in life, constituting an indication for balloon valvuloplasty and occasionally valve replacement, which is best accomplished before the individual reaches the age of 20 years. Aortic stenosis, 75% of which cases are of the valvular type, do not become symptomatic until the fourth or fifth decades, if ever. The murmur radiates to the carotids. ASD manifests a fixed split S_2. VSD exhibits a systolic ejection murmur, loudest along the lower left sternal border. MVP murmur radiates to the left axilla.

14. The answer is E, indomethacin. Most hemodynamically significant PDAs in premature infants will close with the use of intravenous indomethacin if they do not spontaneously close within the first 2 days with supportive care. Indomethacin is dosed orally at 0.1 to 0.3 mg/kg every 8 hours or intravenously at 0.1 to 0.3 mg/kg every 12 hours. Indomethacin does not usually effect closure of PDA in full-term infants. If indomethacin is not successful, then surgery is advised.

15. The answer is E, observation only. Carotid bruits are a common physiologic murmur in children and can be heard in conjunction with a still murmur. There are also murmurs that occur within the first 2 days of life, *transitional murmurs*, a nonspecific term for benign and transient functional murmurs often present in newborns within minutes to hours (but not at the moment) of birth, one of which may be the PDA.

16. The answer is B. Transposition of the great vessels accounts for delayed onset of cyanosis in a newborn. Transposition of the great vessels presents with cyanosis early in life. A patent ductus is necessary along with the transposition to allow any oxygenated blood to reach the systemic circulation. Without either a patent ductus or other pathway for shunting of oxygenated blood into the left side of the heart, the condition is incompatible with life. The ductus arteriosus serves the purpose but closes within a few days. Those cases that are associated with

VSD (thus the loud murmur typical of that lesion) begin shunting unoxygenated blood into the right ventricle, and mixed systemic oxygenated and unoxygenated blood goes into the systemic circulation. When transposition is associated with ASD, there is only a soft murmur, but cyanosis occurs at about the same time. Although an isolated ASD could be associated with cyanosis, the cyanosis would not occur in infancy. Rarely in adulthood, pulmonary hypertension can develop, which then can change the shunt from a right to left and produce cyanosis, but this is much less likely to be seen in ASD as it is in VSD or if a patent ductus persists. Whether associated with ASD or VSD, cyanosis is worse when there is also PS. Hypoplastic left heart is not characterized by a shunt and therefore is not associated with cyanosis. Transposition of the great vessels occurs in male to female infants 3:1 and tends to occur in larger than average-sized babies. Repair through reversal of the great vessels surgically must occur within the first 7 days.

References

Bricker JT, Anderson JC. Cardiovascular problems in children. In: Rudy DR, Kurowski K, eds. *Family Medicine: House Officer Series*. Baltimore, MD: Williams & Wilkins; 1997:133–144.

Bashore TM, Granger CB, Hranitzky P, Patel MR. Heart disease. In: *Current Diagnosis and Treatment*. McGraw Hill-Lange; 2010:294–387.

Thilo EH, Rosenberg AA. The newborn infant. In: May WW, Levin MJ, Sondheimer JM, Deterding RR, eds. *Current Pediatric Diagnosis and Treatment*, 19th ed. McGraw Hill; 2010:1–60.

Sondheimer HM, Darst JR, Shaffer EM, Miyomoto SD. Cardiovascular diseases. In: May WW, Levin MJ, Sondheimer JM, Deterding RR, eds. *Current Pediatric Diagnosis and Treatment*, 19th ed. McGraw Hill; 2009.

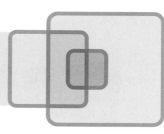

chapter 10

Hypertension

Examination questions: *Unless instructed otherwise, choose the ONE lettered answer or completion that is BEST in each case.*

1 Each of the following is one of the actions of hydrochlorthiazide except for one. Which among those listed does not apply to hydrochlorthiazide (hctz)?

(A) Distal loop diuresis
(B) Reduction of insulin resistance (↑resistance)
(C) Kaliuresis (excretion of potassium)
(D) Natriuresis (excretion of potassium) sodium
(E) Preservation of bone calcium

2 A 55-year-old Caucasian man has a history of poorly controlled hypertension with blood pressure (BP) running 165±/105±. He is presently on lisinopril 20 mg bid. A routine chemical battery of blood tests shows a blood urea nitrogen (BUN) test result of 40 mg/dL, serum creatinine 2.1 mg/dL, and serum potassium 5.1 mEq/L. Which of the following might be the most effective as an antihypertensive adjunctive to the current regimen?

(A) Hydrochlorthiazide
(B) Capoten
(C) Furosemide → renal Fxn compromised, so good choice
(D) Triampterene
(E) Amiloride

3 The antihypertensive category of "alpha$_2$ receptor stimulants" includes *clonidine*, methyldopa, and many others. Each of the following is true about this classification except for which one?

(A) Antihypertensive effects of alpha$_2$ stimulants are wrought through reduction of central sympathetic outflow ✓
(B) At high dosages, alpha$_2$ stimulants elevate BP ✓
(C) Alpha$_2$ stimulants are characterized by predisposition to a hypertensive discontinuance syndrome ✓
(D) Beta-adrenergic blockade works well in conjunction with alpha$_2$ stimulants ✗
(E) Alpha$_2$ stimulants work well in conjunction with antihypertensive diuretics ✓

4 You have been following a 35-year-old Caucasian man for 5 years as his primary care physician. During those years, the patient has "spiked" his BP several times to levels such as 150/100 when he first arrived at the office, most often when he was on a tight schedule. Usually the BP has subsided to 110 to 120/70 to 80. However, over the past year, more and more time elapses after the patient's arrival at the office before the BP subsides to normal range, and over the past 2 months, the lowest systolic BP level you have found has been 145 and the lowest diastolic BP level has been 98. This has occurred despite the patient's compliance with your prescribed no-salt-added diet. The patient denies headaches, focal weakness, numbness, and bouts of confusion. The man weighs 165 lb (74.74 kg) at a height of 5 ft 10 in (1.77 m). Which of the following medication classes would be the least likely to be effective as single-drug therapy?

(A) Thiazide diuretic ↑ peripheral resistance (↓Nat no help)
(B) Angiotensin-converting enzyme inhibitor (ACEI)
(C) Beta-blocking agent
(D) Angiotensin-converting enzyme (ACE) receptor blocking agent
(E) Verapamil (calcium channel blocker [CCB])

5 A 48-year-old African-American man has manifested BP levels of 150/100, 145/95, and 170/105 on consecutive separate days over a 3-week period. He has a family history of deaths by stroke and renal failure. Which of the following may be the single most propitious choice as the first drug to be prescribed?

(A) Hydrochlorthiazide HCTZ
(B) Lisinopril (an ACEI)
(C) Propranolol (beta-adrenergic blocker)
(D) ACE receptor blocking agent
(E) Hydralazine (vasodilator)

6 Normal BP is presently defined as <140/<90. However, therapeutic targets vary with special circumstances. Regarding the black male patient with hypertension, what should be the targeted therapeutic level of BP?

(A) ≤100/50
(B) ≤139/89
(C) ≤130/80
(D) ≤125/75   AA MAP < 100
(E) ≤100/60

7 Regarding a patient to be placed on a diuretic to control BP, which of the following has the most special significance in ancillary studies to obtain *before* starting the patient on the chosen drug therapy?

(A) Electrocardiogram (EKG)
(B) BUN, creatinine
(C) Electrolytes   ✓ aldosteronism
(D) Complete blood count
(E) Liver function battery

8 Hypertension is the most potent risk factor for which one of the following conditions?

(A) Myocardial infarction
(B) Peripheral vascular disease
(C) Stroke
(D) Lung cancer
(E) Renal failure

9 A 75-year-old woman is seeing you for the first time; it is the first time she has seen any doctor for the past 30 years. She had three random, consecutive BP determinations over a 1-week period, which were measured at 180/80, 170/75, and 183/85. You decide that her isolated systolic hypertension should be treated with a pharmaceutical agent. Which of the following would be the best first-line drug?

(A) Hydrochlorthiazide
(B) Lisinopril (an ACEI)
(C) Propranolol (beta-adrenergic blocker)
(D) ACE receptor blocking agent
(E) Verapamil (CCB)

10 A 52-year-old obese man has a BP of 160/100; he has been under treatment for the past 25 years, presently consisting of an ACEI and a CCB, and he has a creatinine level of 2 mg/dL and a BUN level of 38 mg/dL. Although he has a brother with diabetes mellitus type II, his 2-hour postprandial blood sugar is 90 mg/dL. You ordered a C-peptide test and find that the level is elevated. In discussion of his renal function, you must teach the patient what he must do to retard the accelerated reduction of renal function. You begin by telling him that which of the following diseases is the leading cause of end-stage renal disease (ESRD)?

(A) Diabetes   #1 in ESRD
(B) Pyelonephritis
(C) Hypertension
(D) Chronic glomerulonephritis
(E) Polycystic kidney disease

11 A 45-year-old white man with a multiple family history of hypertension weighs 180 lb (81.54 kg) at a height of 5 ft 10 in. (1.77 m) and presents with a BP of 145/95. You place the patient on a no-salt-added diet with a resultant fall in BP to 130/85, that is, consistent for the next 6 months. The BP then rises again as the patient gains weight to 195 lb (88.33 kg) and lapses on the low-salt diet. This time the BP responds dramatically to hydrochlorthiazide 25 mg/triamterene 37.5 mg once daily. As first-line drugs for therapy in essential hypertension, thiazide diuretics are effective in approximately what percentage of cases of hypertension in white individuals?

(A) 10% to 20%
(B) 20% to 30%
(C) 30% to 40%   30–40
(D) 40% to 50%
(E) 60% to 70%

12 A 35-year-old woman presents to you with BP readings of 150/100, 145/98, and 160/95 on three successive days. A routine metabolic profile shows normal BUN, creatinine, blood sugar, sodium, chloride, and bicarbonate, but a potassium level of 2.8 mEq/L. She denies diarrhea, vomiting, past or present fistulae or enterostomy, or taking any prescription medications. Which of the following types of hypertension is most likely present?

(A) Essential hypertension of the vasoconstrictive type
(B) Essential hypertension of the salt-retentive type
(C) Pheochromocytoma
(D) Primary aldosteronism   ↓ K+
(E) Renovascular hypertension

13 Which of the following may be an important part of making the diagnosis in the case of Question 12?

(A) 24-hour urine catecholamine levels
(B) 24-hour urine vanillylmandelic acid (VMA) levels
(C) 8 AM supine overnight and 12 PM upright serum aldosterone levels
(D) BP levels sitting followed by BP levels standing every 15 seconds for 2 minutes
(E) Urinary metanephrine levels   Pheo

14 Each of the following statements regarding pheochromocytoma is true except which one?

(A) Patients with paroxysms of anxiety are often tested for pheochromocytoma
(B) Ten percent of cases are bilateral (found in both adrenals)
(C) Familial cases tend to be bilateral
(D) Sensitivity and specificity for 24-hour urine metanephrine, free catecholamine, and VMA levels are sufficient to diagnose pheochromocytoma alone
(E) Virtually all cases are curable through surgery

75–80%, NOT ALL

⭐ **15** In hypertensive patients with no other risk factors (e.g., diabetes) and who are not ethnically African-Americans, which of the following is the therapeutic target for BP levels?

(A) ≤120/80
(B) ≤130/85
(C) 130 to 140/≤89
(D) 140 to 159/90 to 99
(E) ≤210/≤120

16 A 29-year-old woman has become hypertensive and BP levels are difficult to control. You have her on 10 mg lisinopril twice daily, hydrochlorthiazide/

triamterene once daily, and 80 mg verapamil 3 times daily. BP levels run 160/105 despite the foregoing. Serum potassium was normal before therapy was started. The 24-hour urine studies for VMA, metanephrine, and free catecholamines were within normal limits. Which of the following may be helpful in further elucidating the diagnosis?

(A) EKG
(B) Liver function profile
(C) Lipid screen
(D) Abdominal examination ✓ for bruit (renal a. stenosis)
(E) Complete blood count

Examination Answers

1. The answer is B. Hydrochlorthiazide does not reduce insulin resistance. In susceptible individuals, hctz can precipitate type II diabetes mellitus, albeit reversible upon discontinuance. Hctz is a distal loop diuretic, which is a quite serviceable antihypertensive, tending to function thereby in people who have a tendency to retain salt and whose hypertension may respond to dietary salt restriction. Hctz does cause excretion of sodium and potassium, the latter to pathological proportions on occasion. Hctz causes a slight elevation of serum calcium and in that respect tends to preserve bone calcium, for example, in those that might be susceptible to osteoporosis.

2. The answer is C. Furosemide, as a proximal loop diuretic, does not normally have an antihypertensive pharmacologic effect. However, as renal function is compromised from whatever cause, it becomes an antihypertensive diuretic. Capoten, as an ACE inhibitor, would be redundant along with lisinopril; triampterene, a weak diuretic, has virtually no effect on BP but works well with other diuretics due to its potassium-saving effect. Hydrochlorthiazide has been discussed. Amiloride is a potassium-saving weakly antihypertensive diuretic.

3. The answer is D. Beta-adrenergic blockade *does not work well* in conjunction with alpha$_2$ stimulants; thus, that is the incorrect statement. In fact, particularly because clonidine remains a popular antihypertensive drug, it is important for the clinician to know that both beta-blockers and alpha$_1$-blocking agents do not work well with alpha$_2$ blockers. Alpha$_2$ stimulants may be misnamed because their therapeutic application is the sympatholytic/antihypertensive effect. At high dosages, alpha$_2$ stimulants do stimulate peripheral alpha$_2$ receptors and raise BP, as do reflexly both alpha$_1$ and beta-blockers. Alpha$_2$ stimulants are characterized by predisposition to a hypertensive discontinuance syndrome that features also tachycardia, anxiety, and tremulousness. Alpha$_2$ stimulants as antihypertensive agents work well in conjunction with antihypertensive diuretics.

4. The answer is A. A thiazide diuretic is the least likely of the choices given, to be effective in the case presented. This patient manifests the characteristics of hypertension based on the elevated peripheral resistance as a preponderant mechanism. The patient's vignette suggests that the person is sensitive to or responsive to sympathomimetic mechanisms (i.e., the "hot reactor"). As such, the patient's BP is more likely to respond to ACEIs, ACE receptor blockers, beta-blockers, or CCBs rather than to diuretics. Failure of the patient to respond to salt restriction supports the theme, as diuretic responsive hypertension is based on salt and water retention that increases volume. Thirty-five percent of whites and Asians, if hypertensive, respond to diuretics, particularly thiazides. All others respond to the other drugs to varying degrees, often in combination with the other classes mentioned. Ultimately, many cases manifest mixed pathophysiology, because homeostatic mechanisms tend to protect BP on the low side with the passing of time.

5. The answer is A. African-Americans with hypertension have an approximately 65% chance of sodium/water retention and therefore would have about that likelihood of responding to a simple diuretic, such as hydrochlorthiazide, generally compounded with triampterene or spironolactone to titrate the potassium loss due to untrammeled hydrochlorthiazide.

6. The answer is D. All hypertensive patients must have their BP levels controlled to normal levels not only to reduce stroke and other atherosclerotic disease risk status but also for protection of renal function over time. African-Americans, along with diabetics, among others, have renal function that is more vulnerable to deterioration with elevated BP levels, even at high normal levels; 125/75 is calculated to a mean arterial pressure (MAP) of 100. Nephrologists actually recommend that African-Americans' BP levels (MAP) be controlled to an MAP of 98 mm Hg.

7. The answer is C. Electrolytes should be checked before starting a hypertensive patient on any drugs, but particularly a diuretic. The reason for this is that one of the causes of secondary hypertension is primary aldosteronism. It causes not only hypertension of a salt-retentive type but also hypokalemia. Once the diuretic is started, the serum potassium is unreliable for several days. The other studies mentioned, except for the liver function battery, are all part of a proper database for initiation of therapy in hypertension but may be obtained after the drug therapy has begun.

8. The answer is C. Hypertension is the most powerful risk factor for stroke, including both hemorrhagic and thrombotic types. Of course, hypertension is a contributing risk factor for all the atherosclerotic diseases as well but is not a risk for lung cancer. Of course, hypertension is a contributing risk factor for all the atherosclerotic diseases.

9. The answer is A. hydrochlorthiazide is the best single first drug therapy for aged individuals with isolated systolic hypertension, as it is in a majority of African-Americans at any age. Elderly people with hypertension, too, have a tendency for salt-retentive, volume-dependent hypertension. Moreover, hctz and other thiazides, in the elderly, have a vasodilation effect.

10. The answer is A. Diabetes is the chief cause of ESRD, accounting for up to 50% of cases, whereas hypertension is the cause in 27% of cases of ESRD. The pathophysiological mechanisms of diabetes type II are under way for years before the onset of hyperglycemia occurs. This is a result of insulin resistance and resultant hyperinsulinemia. C-peptide levels are directly related to endogenous insulin levels. Therefore, this patient, being a prediabetic (elevated C-peptide) with imperfectly treated hypertension, has a double dose of risk factors and must get immediately to work towards preservation of renal function (see chapter 17).

11. The answer is C. As mentioned in a variety of ways in this publication, about 35% of whites, Asians, and most other ethnic groups in the United States (but 65% of African-Americans) with hypertension have a primarily salt- and water-retention mechanism and thus respond to both salt restriction and diuretic therapy.

12. The answer is D. Hypertension in the face of hypokalemia and in the absence of diuretic medication or gastrointestinal or other pathologic loss of potassium is primary aldosteronism until proven otherwise.

13. The answer is C. In primary aldosteronism, the serum baseline aldosterone level is >20 μg/dL. The level does not rise after 4 hours of erect posture. A 24-hour urine study for aldosterone is also measured and indicates hyperaldosteronism when the excretion is >20 μg/24 hours. VMA, catecholamines, and metanephrine are measured to diagnose pheochromocytoma. Sitting and standing BP levels are done to diagnose orthostatic hypotension.

14. The answer is E. Only about 75% to 80% of cases are cured. Not only are 10% of cases bilateral but another 10% have metastases at the time of diagnosis. The majority of patients presenting to the primary care physician with paroxysms of anxiety have a phobic reaction or anxiety neurosis by other names; however, many of these indi-

viduals have elevated BP levels during attacks of anxiety and are logically evaluated for pheochromocytoma. Sensitivity and specificity for 24-hour urine metanephrine levels alone are not sufficient to diagnose pheochromocytoma. However, if the specimen is tested also for free catecholamines and VMA, then they are sufficient, provided the symptoms occur on the day of the collection or the tumor excretes norepinephrine, which appears on a constant basis. Familial cases tend to occur in association with multiple endocrine neoplasia, types II A and II B, and the familial cases tend to be bilateral.

15. The answer is B. The BP target for therapy and follow-up of essential hypertension is ≤130/85. This is true only for nondiabetic individuals and persons who are not African-American. The upper limit of normal systolic BP is 139; the pressure definition of stage 4 hypertension is ≥210/≥120 mm Hg, according to the Joint National Committee on Detection, Evaluation and Treatment of High Blood Pressure.

16. The answer is D. The patient should be examined for an abdominal bruit, specifically a bruit deep in one flank that could be generated by renal artery stenosis. Essential hypertension, be it volume dependent or based more on peripheral vascular resistance, usually has its clinical onset in a person's late 30s or 40s. Hypertension significantly earlier or that which comes on after a person reaches the age of 60 must be evaluated for other causes, of which renovascular type is one. When a person is at a younger age, the cause is most likely due to a congenital fibrous band, which has a 2:1 female-to-male occurrence ratio. After a person reaches the age of 60, the cause is more likely an atherosclerotic one, which has a 2:1 male-to-female occurrence ratio. None of the other choices has any specific relevance to the diagnosis of the pathophysiology of hypertension.

References

Family Medicine Review. Kansas City, Missouri; May 3–9; 2009.

Joint National Committee on Detection. *Evaluation and treatment of high blood pressure (JNC-V). Arch Intern Med* 1993;153:161.

Rudy DR. Hypertension. In: Rudy DR, Kurowski K, eds. *Family Medicine: House Officer Series.* Baltimore: Williams & Wilkins; 1997:145–168.

Neurology in Primary Care

chapter **11**

Neurology

Examination questions: Unless instructed otherwise, choose the ONE lettered answer or completion that is BEST in each case.

1 A 46-year-old Caucasian woman complains of increasingly severe fatigue that she believe emanates from poor sleep quality. Her husband notes that she moves frequently during her sleep, and the patient notes that recently as she begins to ready herself for sleep she has discomfort in her legs that is momentarily relieved by moving them. Each of the following may be helpful in the treatment of this condition except?   *Restless Leg Syndrome*

(A) Two month trial of ferrous sulfate ✓
(B) Stretching exercises before bedtime ✓
(C) A glass of red wine before bedtime
(D) Gabapentin ✓
(E) Oxycodone 5–10 before bedtime ✓

2 A 12-year-old boy has been brought to the family physician with the history that his parents discovered a tick on his body after his return from a Boy Scout camp in rural Wisconsin. Which of the following statements about the possibilities of Lyme disease is true?

(A) Erythema migrans (EM) always begins at the tick bite site.
(B) Serological tests of Lyme disease will be positive by the time of the onset of EM.
(C) Neurologic features occur in a minority of cases.   *10%*
(D) The occurrence of carditis is most often in late Lyme disease.
(E) Any of the macrolide antibiotics are as good as other antibiotics in effectiveness.

3 In the treatment of epilepsy, defined as two documented seizures of any type (e.g., partial, absence, generalized) without known cause, which of the following antiepileptic drugs is the most broadly applicable?

(A) Valproate (Depakene)   *Mixed type / Uncertain sz*
(B) Phenytoin (Dilantin)
(C) Gabapentin (Neurontin)
(D) Oxycarbazepine (Trileptal)
(E) Pregabalin (Lyrica)

4 A 65-year-old white man complains that he has a tremor in the right hand. It is best displayed when he reaches for a pen and is manifested easily in the finger-to-nose test. In which of the following locations is the lesion?

(A) Right brachial plexus
(B) Right cerebellum   *Intention tremors - cerebellum*
(C) Left motor cortex
(D) Left cerebellum
(E) Left basal ganglia

5 A 16-year-old boy has developed a movement disorder. When he abducts his arms, they begin to flap like beating wings. Which of the following disease processes is likely to be the cause?

(A) Hemochromatosis
(B) Drug-induced tremor
(C) Amyotrophic lateral sclerosis (ALS)
(D) Wilson disease   *Wilsons gives you WINGS*
(E) Essential tremor

6 A 67-year-old man has had a gradual onset of a rest tremor over the past 2 years. On examination you note a 4- to 6-Hz flexion–extension tremor at the elbow and pronation–supination movement of the forearm. This patient may manifest each of the following additional findings except for which one?

(A) Tremor worsens with stress. ✓
(B) Tremor diminishes with volition of the movement. ✓
(C) Tremor improves with alcohol ingestion.   *Parkinsons*
(D) Patient exhibits bradykinesia (slow, shuffling gait and decreased arm swinging). ✓
(E) Patient exhibits cogwheel rigidity. ✓

7 A 68-year-old white woman has been a patient of yours for 2 years and is a lively conversationalist. She has had unexpected falls recently and complains of "weakness" of her legs. As she enters the office for the first time in 3 months, she manifests a wide-based gait that you have not noted in the past. She complains also of urinary urgency incontinence. She answers questions correctly but often takes long to speak and is not as spontaneous in her responses as she had been in the past. She can carry out sequential tasks upon request. Which of the following conditions explains these findings?

(A) Subdural hematoma
(B) Multiple-infarct dementia
(C) Multiple sclerosis (MS)
(D) Normal pressure hydrocephalus (NPH)   *wet, wobbly*
(E) Alzheimer disease (AD)

8 Regarding the patient in Question 7, which of the following is the mainstay of therapy?

(A) Ventriculoperitoneal shunt ✓
(B) Glucocorticoid therapy
(C) Nonsteroidal anti-inflammatory drug therapy
(D) Physical therapy
(E) Aspirin 85 mg daily

9 A 25-year-old white female patient of German and Danish descent had an episode 3 months ago consisting of several days of urinary hesitancy, blurred vision in the left eye, and some difficulty in sureness of gait. She was visiting away and waited for her family's return so as to be able to consult you, her primary physician. However, by the time she had returned from vacation, the symptoms had disappeared. Now, these symptoms are recurring in a slightly different form. She now complains of diplopia, hypesthesias, paresthesias, and an electrical sensation down the spine when she flexes her neck. Her gait is again disturbed, and she manifests hyperreflexia on the left lower extremity along with a Babinski sign. Which of the following is the most sensitive test for diagnosing her condition?

(A) Computed tomography scan of the head
(B) Lumbar puncture
(C) Serologic test for Lyme disease
(D) Test for vitamin B_{12} blood level
(E) Magnetic resonance image (MRI) of the brain
    MS

10 Regarding the patient in Question 9, each of the following is an approved disease-modifying drug for the condition *except* for which one?

(A) Interferon 1a
(B) Interferon 1b
(C) Glatiramer
(D) Infliximab   *TNFα   for RA*
(E) Mitoxantrone

11 A 78-year-old woman is brought by her family for gradual loss of the ability to care for herself. Although she is fully ambulatory and her level of consciousness is full, she has left her kitchen stove on without knowing it and has lost total control of her checkbook, whereas in the past she had been assiduous in the management of her financial affairs. The family physician diagnoses dementia. Which of the following lists of ancillary studies would be the most propitious for diagnosing reversible causes of her dementia?

(A) Complete blood count, thyroid-stimulating hormone, noncontrast computed tomography scan of the head, mental status examination
(B) Serum electrolytes, liver function battery
(C) Chest x-ray, upper endoscopy
(D) Liver biopsy and serum iron, total iron-binding capacity, and ferritin levels
(E) Carotid angiogram

12 A 67-year-old man is brought to you by his family because of rigid gait and lack of facial expression coming on over a period of several months. You suspect Parkinson's disease (PD). Many aspects of PD can mimic other neurological syndromes. Which *one* of the following features is seen in patients with PD?

(A) Choreiform movements ✗
(B) A resting tremor that is unilateral at its onset
(C) A loud, widely variable tone speech ✗
(D) Spastic gait ✗
(E) A bilateral resting tremor ✗

13 You are examining a 65-year-old patient with PD, complaining mainly of a very annoying tremor of the dominant right hand. She is on no medication. Although she has some symptoms of bradykinesia and demonstrates some cogwheeling on physical examination, she states that her tremor is the only feature that disturbs her functioning. Which of the medications listed here would be most likely to improve her tremor?

(A) Bromocriptine
(B) Carbidopa/levodopa
(C) Orphenadrine *anticholinergic for rigidity/tremor*
(D) Selegiline
(E) Amitriptyline

14 A 48-year-old man had suffered from a gastroenteritis-like syndrome 3 weeks before experiencing a rapid onset of paralysis that began with his lower extremities and progressed to involve the upper extremities as well. He complains also of fingertip numbness and hypesthesias. As you hospitalize him for close monitoring, you obtain no history of recent industrial toxin exposure, recent ingestion of any canned foods or shellfish, or recent tick bite. The patient's vaccine immune status is totally up to date. This syndrome is an example of which of the following pathologic processes?

(A) Chronic inflammatory neuropathy
(B) Combined upper and lower motor neuron disease
(C) Neuropathy associated with malignant disease
(D) Autoimmune polyneuropathy *Guillain-Barré*
(E) Mononeuropathy

C. jejuni

15 A 72-year-old man who remains athletic, boats in the summer, and skis in the winter comes to you 2 weeks after his latest winter vacation. He complains of increasing fatigue and drowsiness. His daughter urged him to come in when she found him increasingly difficult to arouse. Although he admits to taking several falls, he is unaware of any head injury. Furthermore, his neurological examination discloses no lateralizing or focal findings. Head and scalp examinations are negative for focal tenderness and deformity. Plain x-ray of the skull is negative. Complete blood count and comprehensive chemical profile as well as thyroid-stimulating hormone levels are within normal limits. Which of the following is the likely diagnosis?

(A) Postconcussion syndrome
(B) Chronic subdural hematoma *accel/decel*
(C) Medical condition *forces in elderly*
(D) Subarachnoid hemorrhage
(E) Stroke

Examination Answers

1. The answer is C. A glass of red wine before bedtime does not relieve symptoms of *restless leg* syndrome, obviously described in the vignette. Restless leg syndrome (RLS) is classified as a sleep disorder. Alcohol and tobacco should be avoided. All the other choices are valid in empiric trial for symptom relief, as may be dopamine agonists such as ropinirole (Requip) and pramipexole (Mirapex); opiates (e.g., oxycodone, benzodiazepines, and gabapentin [Neurontin]). RLS is statistically associated with iron deficiency anemia and when diagnosed by low serum ferritin, iron supplementation is appropriate and may be helpful. The syndrome is also statistically associated with B_{12} deficiency, depression, uremia, rheumatoid arthritis, and polyneuropathy. PT modalities such as stretching before bedtime have been helpful to some patients as has been Sinemet CR 50/200.

2. The answer is C. Neurologic features occur in a minority of cases of Lyme disease, that is, about 10%. While EM usually begins at the tick bite site (70% to 80%), it may occur well away from the entry site. Serological tests of Lyme disease will not necessarily be positive by the time of the onset of EM. The most sensitive test early is the ELISA, which is good for screening but is not adequately specific. The IgM antibodies rise 2–4 weeks after the onset of EM; IgG antibodies occur late and can signify past or active chronic disease. Carditis occurs most often in early Lyme disease rather than in late disease. The same applies to neurologic disease, a common form of which is facial nerve palsy. Macrolide antibiotics, which are effective to a degree, cannot match the success of doxycycline or amoxicillin in effectiveness.

3. The answer is A. Valproate (Depakene) has broad application. Others that are so classified include the newer drugs felbamate (Felbatol), lamotrigine (Lamictal), levetiracetam (Keppra), topiramate (Topomax), and zonisamide (Zonagran). The implication of the classification is that they are most likely to be appropriate for seizures of apparently mixed types or those not diagnosed with certainty. Phenytoin was for years a mainstay for generalized seizures but now is categorized as applying to partial seizures, as is the newer preparation gabapentin, also in increasing use for radicular and peripheral neuralgic pain, for example, tic douloureux. Oycarbazepine like its cousin carbamezepine is listed as being indicated in partial seizures. Pregabalin (Lyrica) is also listed for use in partial seizures.

4. The answer is B. Right cerebellum. Intention tremors, examples of kinetic tremor, originate in the cerebellum, ipsilateral to the symptomatic extremity, unlike what occurs in upper motor neuron lesions in the cortex. Of course, upper motor lesions do not produce tremors but do produce spasticity as well as hyperreflexia on the contralateral side, the latter resulting on occasion in clonus. Right brachial plexus lesions, being peripheral neuropathic, would produce flaccid paralysis. Basal ganglia lesions are the site of Parkinsonian tremor.

5. The answer is D. Wilson disease is caused by abnormally elevated gastrointestinal absorption and decreased hepatic excretion of copper, resulting in liver buildup as well as depositions in the brain, cornea, and kidney. The wing beating tremor is a classic sign. Hemochromatosis causes liver damage but not tremor. Drug-induced tremors vary with the type of drug involved and may be fine tremors of sympathomimetic enhancement, resembling a benign essential tremor; mimic in some ways athetoid tremors, as in tardive dyskinesia; may be rest tremors, associated with neuroleptics, metoclopramide, or phenothiazines; or the intention tremors of alcoholism. ALS does not cause tremor per se (see discussion of Question 3).

6. The answer is C. The tremor described, that of PD, does not improve with alcohol ingestion. Benign essential tremor improves with alcohol ingestion. The patient has PD and manifests the tremor typical of that condition (although 10% to 20% of cases show no tremor while manifesting all the other findings mentioned in the vignette). Classically, PD exhibits the rest tremor described (decreasing with consciously intended movements of the involved extremity), the cogwheel rigidity, and bradykinesia.

7. The answer is D. NPH is within the differential diagnosis of dementia. Classically and fairly reliably, the triad of gait instability, urinary incontinence, and dementia distinguish this condition as opposed to AD (positive predictive value, 65%). The dementia is usually not the presenting complaint and is characterized by lack of spontaneity, inattention, and latency in response. Correctness of statements and fact recall are not usually positive findings in NPH but problems that are encountered in AD. Gait abnormality is a later finding in AD, as is urinary incontinence, and AD more often involves agnosia, aphasia, and apraxia, abnormalities that are not encountered in NPH. Apraxia refers to discoordination of learned movements such as strike, step, and arm swing in gait. In addition, AD features difficulty with word formation and failure to interpret stimuli within an appropriate context. Chronic subdural hematoma may manifest symptoms of dementia, headache, and drowsiness but not usually urinary incontinence. Multiple-infarct dementia mimics AD.

8. The answer is A. The only therapy that may change the course of the disease is ventriculoperitoneal shunt to decompress the cerebrospinal fluid (CSF; however, part of the definition of NPH is a "normal" pressure of CSF). Success is best achieved when the symptoms have been of relatively short duration such as in the presented case. Even then, estimates of success vary widely, from 33% to 90%.

9. The answer is E. This clinical picture in a young woman of Northern European descent, that of scattered neurologic findings that exacerbated and remitted and recurred 3 months later, fits the classic picture of multiple sclerosis. Females are affected twice as frequently as males. The MRI of the brain is nearly completely sensitive, though not perfectly specific. The MRI performed with a high-field magnet (≥ 1.5 T) should show areas of high signal in the white matter of the brain and spinal cord on T2-weighted images, characteristic of demyelinating lesions in MS. Therefore, the demyelinating process affects both sensory and motor fibers. Lumbar puncture is also very helpful in disclosing CSF immunoglobulin-G concentration increased relative to other CSF proteins, such as albumin with oligoclonal bands (90% sensitive and less specific than MRI). Lyme disease and subacute combined degeneration (as in pernicious anemia) should be entertained and ruled out, the latter by the B_{12} level, but they have no value in the diagnosis of MS per se. Other tests that address diseases in the differential diagnosis include thyroid-stimulating hormone, sedimentation rate, antinuclear antibodies, and a serologic test for syphilis. A more refined list would address more rare conditions, not likely to be relevant in the early stages of this syndrome encountered in primary care.

10. The answer is D. Infliximab is a tumor necrosis factor inhibitor used in rheumatoid arthritis and other autoimmune diseases. Of interest is the fact that, as understanding of MS has developed, it has emerged as an autoimmune disease. The other drugs mentioned are all capable of a roughly one-third reduction in the rate of exacerbation of the disease and appear to address the autoimmune aspects of MS. A new drug, now approved for Phase II testing, is natalixumab (Antegren, Tsar), whose early studies indicate a 90% reduction in acute activity and 50% reduction in number of relapses.

11. The answer is A. Reversible causes of dementia include pernicious anemia, hypothyroidism (especially in the elderly population), and depression. Serum electrolytes would diagnose hyponatremia, a cause of stupor, not dementia; liver function blood tests or biopsy would diagnose hepatic coma; carotid angiogram would elucidate cerebral arterial blood flow, which is important in focal neurological symptoms as in transient ischemic attack or stroke. The other modalities and tests offer no significant

information for diagnosing dementia or disturbance of consciousness.

12. The answer is B. The tremor in PD is initially unilateral, only later involving both sides. Choreiform movements are rapid, purposeless movements that occur in Huntington chorea (wormlike movements) and Sydenham chorea (jerky movements of the extremities, particularly hands and feet), but not in PD. About 20% of PD patients eventually develop a dementia, and autonomic features including orthostatic hypotension are common. Constipation and impotence can also be seen. The gait is shuffling with little arm swing. The speech is very soft and monotonal but delirium is not a part of the picture.

13. The answer is C. Orphenadrine (Disapal, Norflex) is an anticholinergic medication. This class of drugs is most helpful when the main goal of therapy is to control rigidity and tremor. Other examples of this class used in PD include benztropine mesylate (Cogentin), biperidin (Akineton), procyclidine (Kemedrin), and trihexylphenidyl (Artane). Although other medications are superior in improving rigidity and bradykinesia such as bromocriptine, a dopaminergic drug, the anticholinergics are more effective in diminishing the tremor. Dopaminergic drugs are effective in relieving rigidity and bradykinesia. Levodopa alleviates all aspects of PD but does not alter the progression of the disease. Sinemet is a fixed combination of carbidopa and levodopa. Selegiline is a monoamine oxidase inhibitor that is sometimes used as an adjunct to levodopa to control the fluctuations in its effect. Amitriptyline is an antidepressant with strong anticholinergic side effects but is not used in the treatment of PD.

14. The answer is D. This patient has Guillain–Barré syndrome, which is thought to be based on an autoimmune process. The condition is also called demyelinating polyradiculoneuropathy. Twenty percent of cases appear to have links with *Campylobacter jejuni* infection. Most other cases have followed apparent viral gastroenteritis, viral upper respiratory tract infection, or influenza by about 1 to 3 weeks. The disease, though potentially life threatening (3% to 5% case mortality) because of the involvement of respiratory and deglutition functions, is usually self-limited and reverses within a few weeks. The differential diagnosis includes botulism, intermittent porphyria, diphtheria, Lyme disease, poliomyelitis, heavy metal poisoning, and tetrodotoxin poisoning from contaminated shellfish. Chronic inflammatory demyelinating neuropathy is similar in symptomatology and signs except that it is chronic, remitting, and exacerbating. Combined upper and lower motor neuron disease is a description of ALS. Both sensorimotor and pure sensory polyneuropathies can occur as nonmetastatic complications of malignancies. On some occasions, this syndrome may precede the diagnosis of cancer. Therefore, occult malignancy must be considered initially in the differential diagnosis of Guillain–Barré syndrome as well. Mononeuropathies involve just one peripheral nerve, for example, cranial nerve VI palsy occurring in diabetes, usually type I.

15. The answer is B. This history fits that of chronic subdural hematoma from acceleration–deceleration forces that cause tearing of bridging veins in a closed head injury. Such injuries are more likely to occur in older people and often without a definite history of head injury. Whether they should be evacuated surgically depends on the clinical situation and the thickness of the hematoma. Postconcussion syndrome presents similarly clinically but would hardly be expected to be devoid of a clear history of head trauma, complete with a healing scalp contusion. Subarachnoid hemorrhage is arterial and as such is sudden and dramatic (see chapter 7). Strokes virtually always result in focal and lateralizing neurological findings; also, their onsets are rapid, not subtle.

References

Aminoff MJ. Nervous system. In: Tierney LM, McPhee SJ, Papadakis MA, eds. *Current Medial Diagnosis and Treatment*, 43rd ed. New York: McGraw-Hill/Appleton & Lange; 2004:941–1000.

Calabresi PA. Diagnosis and management of multiple sclerosis. *Am Fam Physician.* 2004; 70:1935–1944.

Family Medicine Board Review 2009. Kansas City, May 3–9.

Rowland LP, ed. *Textbook of Neurology.* Baltimore, MD: Williams & Wilkins; 1995.

Smaga S. Tremor. *Am Fam Physician.* 2003; 68:1545–1552.

Verrees M, Selman WR. Management of normal pressure hydrocephalus. *Am Fam Physician.* 2004; 70:1071–1078, 1085–1086.

Respiratory Diseases in Primary Care

chapter **12**

Pneumonia and Bronchitides

Examination questions: *Unless instructed otherwise, choose the ONE lettered answer or completion that is BEST in each case.*

1 To assist in the decision whether to hospitalize a patient with community acquired pneumonia (CAP), each of the following may be a factor in favor of hospitalization except for which one?

(A) The patient is confused ✓

CURB-65

(B) Serum creatinine >2.0 mg/dL

(C) Respiratory rate >30 ✓

(D) Blood pressure <90 mm Hg ✓

(E) Age >64 years ✓

2 A 35-year-old African-American woman complains of red and irritated eyes with photophobia for about 2 months. Visual acuity is 20/25 for each eye separately, and she says this is her "normal." On questioning she admits to shortness of breath with exertion, which she attributes to neglecting physical training and advancing age. A chest x-ray shows perihilar adenopathy. A lung biopsy finds noncaseous granuloma. Angiotensin-converting enzyme is elevated. On spirometry, FEV_1 is 80% of predicted normal for her (percent of vital capacity expired in 1 second). Which of the following would be the best therapeutic approach.

(A) Non-steroidal anti-inflammatory drugs (NSAIDs)

(B) Bronchodilators

(C) Inhaled glucosteroids

(D) Observation for 4–6 months while treating the eyes symptomatically   *Sarcoid*

(E) Systemic glucosteroids

3 A 47-year-old atopic individual (constitutionally subject to eczema, allergic rhinitis, or allergic asthma) makes an appointment with the family doctor complaining of onset within the past 36 hours consisting loose cough, sharp chest pains with deep breath in the upper anterior chest. These symptoms occurred in the absence of preceding sore throat or coryza. He has never been in the hospital nor has he had a course of antibiotics within 5 years. Vital signs reveal respiratory rate to be 16/minute, BP 128/78 and regular pulse at 90, temperature 99°F. Physical examination discloses percussive dullness corresponding to the right upper lobe. Within that area auscultation reveals fine moist rales while the remainder of the lung fields show only normal breath sounds. The doctor diagnoses pneumonia. The list of possible bacterial organisms as causative (the most likely 95% of cases) includes all the following except for which one?

79

(A) *Moraxella catarrhalis* → otitis media
✓ (B) *Legionela pneumophila*
✓ (C) *Streptococcus pneumoniae*
✓ (D) *Mycoplasma pneumoniae*
✓ (E) *Hemophilus influenzae*

4 A 32-year-old previously healthy and athletic male, resident of Portsmouth, Ohio, is diagnosed as having CAP based on setting, fever to 101°F (38.3°C), cough, physical findings, and clinical stability. He is treated with clarithromycin by prescription for a ten day course. On the 5th day, he still has a fever of 100.8°F (38.2°C), unchanged cough and continued malaise. After a chest x-ray reveals miliary distribution of bilateral pulmonary infiltrates a tuberculosis skin test is read as negative. Further history reveals that he had been spelunking 2 weeks before the onset of the symptoms. Histoplasmosis is now a consideration. Which of the following would be the best test at this point to confirm that diagnosis?

(A) Histoplasmosis skin test
(B) Lung biopsy for histopathological study
(C) Urine test for Histoplasma polysaccharide antigen
(D) Biopsy to obtain silver methenamine stain for *Histoplasma capulatum*
(E) Blood fungus culture

5 A 19-year-old man has asthma. He is a nonsmoker, and there are no smokers in his home. He has attacks 3 to 4 times per week and takes the short-acting beta$_2$ agonist albuterol, inhaled two sprays every 6 hours (q 6 h) for symptoms when they occur. What is the best next regimen to institute for this patient?

(A) High-dose inhaled corticosteroids
(B) Increase the frequency of the short-acting inhaled beta$_2$ agonist
(C) Systemic corticosteroids
(D) Low-dose inhaled corticosteroids
(E) Long-acting beta$_2$ agonist

6 A 45-year-old male, 30-pack-year smoker complains of exertional dyspnea and dry cough increasing over the past year. He denies orthopnea. He has been a schoolteacher all his adult life, was athletic in his 20s and 30s, and has lived in homes built after 1975. You ordered spirometry testing. The results are as follows: forced vital capacity (FVC), 40% of expected FVC for age and weight (normal 80% to 120%); forced expiratory volume in 1 second (FEV$_1$), 90% of FVC; FEV$_1$/FVC, 95%. Which of the following conditions accounts for these findings?

(A) Acute asthma
(B) Chronic obstructive pulmonary disease (COPD)
(C) Restrictive lung disease

↓ FVC   FEV$_1$/FVC : nml

(D) Pneumonia
(E) Mesothelioma

7 A 58-year-old man who has smoked all his adult life at the rate of one pack per day (38 pack-years) complains of acute dyspnea. He has had a cough, producing half a cup (118.26 mL) of sputum each morning. After the onset of a bout of coryza, on the third day, he became short of breath. Physical examination reveals no definite wheezes, but rather just a reduced percussible diaphragmatic excursion; the patient purses his lips during expiration. His spirometry results are as follows: FVC, 90% of expected FVC for age and weight (normal 80% to 120%); FEV$_1$, 50% of expected; FEV$_1$/FVC, 50% of the predicted ratio. Which of the following conditions best explains these spirometry findings?

(A) Acute asthma
(B) COPD →   ↓ FEV$_1$ / FVC
(C) Restrictive lung disease
(D) Pneumonia
(E) Mesothelioma

8 A 55-year-old man and his wife complain that for a year he has been constantly clearing his throat and frequently coughs just as he is falling off to sleep or on occasion while asleep. He has never smoked and is on no prescription medications, and he has not seen other doctors for the cough. Which of the following is the least likely cause of this problem?

✓ (A) Postnasal drainage drip (PND)
✓ (B) Incipient asthma
✓ (C) Gastroesophageal reflux disease (GERD)
(D) Eosinophilic bronchitis
✓ (E) Bronchiectasis

Match the findings in the numbered items with the lettered causes of acute or severe dyspnea (adapted from Karnani).

9 Intermittent breathlessness; triggering factors exist; allergic rhinitis; prolonged expiratory phase

10 Smoker; barrel chest; prolonged expiratory phase

11 History of hypertension, coronary artery disease, diabetes; orthopnea, paroxysmal nocturnal dyspnea; pedal edema, jugular venous distention

12 History of generalized anxiety, panic disorder, sighing breathing

13 Postprandial dyspnea

(A) Gastroesophageal reflux, aspiration, or food allergy
(B) Anxiety disorder, hyperventilation

(C) Congestive heart failure (CHF)
(D) COPD
(E) Asthma

Unless instructed otherwise, choose the ONE lettered answer or completion that is BEST in each case.

⍟ 14 A 25-year-old man who was previously healthy has a rapid onset (over 10 hours, starting during mid-morning) of severe sharp, stabbing, chest pain and a temperature of 102°F when he consults you at 6 PM. He has otherwise been in good health, does not smoke, and denies any high-risk activities for HIV acquisition. He has no allergies. Physical examination reveals a temperature of 102°F, a pulse of 110, and a blood pressure of 124/82. He appears to be in great distress, being both toxic and in much pain with each inspiration. Chest examination reveals bronchophony, egophony, and dullness to percussion in the right posterior chest. There are some "sticky" rales in this area also. There is no accessory muscle use, clubbing, or cyanosis, but there is definite splinting of the right lung field with inspiration. A sputum Gram stain reveals gram-positive diplococci. Chest x-ray reveals a right lower lobe infiltrate. Which of the following therapeutic intervention is likely to benefit this patient the most?

(A) Penicillin → lobar PNA (S. pneumonia)
(B) Trimethoprim/sulfamethoxazole
(C) Postural drainage
(D) Tetracycline
(E) Cefadroxil

15 A 19-year-old male college student has experienced a gradual onset of a dry cough over a period of 1 week. He complains of headache. The white blood cell count is 11,500 with normal differential except for three band forms. Chest examination is negative for rales ("crackles") and percussible dullness. The chest x-ray shows patchy bronchopneumonic infiltrates. Which of the following is the most likely cause of this condition?

(A) *S. pneumoniae*
(B) *Klebsiella pneumoniae*
(C) *M. pneumoniae*   atypical PNA
(D) *Gram-negative sepsis*
(E) *Staphylococcus aureus*

⍟ 16 A 65-year-old man has developed a cough with low-grade fever and comes to see you on the fourth day. He complains of headache and difficulty focusing mentally. His vital signs reveal an apparent sinus bradycardia at 56. A complete blood count shows a low-grade leukocytosis with an unremarkable differential; electrolytes manifest a hyponatremia at 128 mEq/L.

Chest x-ray shows diffuse patchy infiltrates weighted toward the bases. Which of the following is the most likely diagnosis?

(A) *Pneumococcal pneumonia*
(B) *K. pneumonia*
(C) *M. pneumonia*
(D) *Legionella pneumonia*
(E) *Viral pneumonia*

⍟ 17 Which of the following scenarios would suggest alertness to the possibility of an anaerobic organism as a cause of pneumonitis?

(A) Pneumonia in a long-time smoker with COPD
(B) A stroke patient in the acute phase with bulbar symptoms and dysphagia   Aspiration PNA
(C) A 45-year-old woman who had an influenza infection 1 week earlier
(D) A 30-year-old nonsmoker with a cough who recently travelled to Arizona   coccidio
(E) A 34-year-old nonsmoker with AIDs

18 In which of the following clinical situations would a determination of alpha₁ protease inhibitor (formerly called alpha₁ antitrypsin) level be most appropriate?

(A) There is a 75-year-old patient with severe emphysema and cor pulmonale. The person is now home bound and on continuous O_2 with an FEV_1 of 0.9 L; the patient has marked hypoxemia, mild CO_2 retention, and a 35-pack-year smoking history.
(B) There is a 70-year-old male patient with increasing shortness of breath for 10 years and a 30-pack-year smoking history.
(C) There is a 32-year-old patient with mild shortness of breath with heavy exertion for 1 year and with a distant past history of 1-pack-year smoking history.   COPD in absence of smoking
(D) There is a 48-year-old male patient with mild shortness of breath with exertion for 1 year and a 40-pack-year smoking history.
(E) There is a 55-year-old patient with shortness of breath for 5 years who has a 20-pack-year. History of smoking, but who quit 5 years ago. Her husband smokes two packs of cigarettes per day in the house.

19 Assuming no contraindications, which of the following medications is the first-line pharmacologic agent of choice in treating mild to moderate COPD?

(A) Inhaled corticosteroids
(B) Oral corticosteroids
(C) Inhaled beta-agonist
(D) Oral theophylline
(E) Inhaled tiotropium bromide   Spiriva
    ↳ anticholinergic

Examination Answers

1. The answer is B. Serum creatinine >2.0 mg/dL is *not* a criterion for hospitalization of a patient with CAP. This question addresses well laid out guidelines for hospitalization. They are: patient confused; *BUN* >20 mg/dL (addressing hypovolemia and circulation rather than renal function); respiratory rate >30, blood pressure <90 mm Hg, and age >64 years. The acronym for memory aid is CURB-65.

2. The answer is D. Observation for 4–6 months while treating the eyes symptomatically if warranted. The patient has classic sarcoidosis, which is known to remit and exacerbate. Sarcoidosis is diagnosed on the basis of preponderance of evidence rather than by specific and sensitive testing. Lifetime incidence is said to be 0.85% for the white population and 2.4% for African Americans. Both figures are certainly far too high for reality and doubtlessly reflect tertiary care center experience. About 30%t to 60% remain symptomatic. While pulmonary involvement can be life threatening, this case did not seem to definitely symptomatic on that regard. The uveitis was treatable symptomatically. NSAIDs are appropriate when arthritis symptoms exist that respond to them. The lung disease can be symptomatic, restrictive disease with symptoms or obstructive. Either inhaled glucosteroids or bronchodilators may be needed, but the spirometry findings and mild symptoms did not justify that approach; systemic glucosteroids would be reserved for life-saving urgency and for as short a period as possible.

3. The answer is A. *M. catarrhalis*, while common in community acquired otitis media, as a cause of CAP, it is highly unusual. *S. pneumoniae* accounts for 20% to 70% of CAP; *M. pneumoniae* causes 1–40% of cases, depending on the time and place; *H. influenzae* and *L. pneumophila* each between 2% and 10% of cases in an outpatient community setting. Needless to say, if the case of CAP does not meet the CURB-65 criteria and need not be hospitalized, the foregoing dictates the empiric choice of antibiotics.

4. The answer is C. Urine test for Histoplasma polysaccharide antigen is positive in up to 92% of cases of disseminated histoplasmosis, a likely diagnosis even in this healthy young man, given his possible heavy exposure to the fungus in his cave exploration within the 3–21 days incubation period for acute pulmonary infection. The test is noninvasive and more sensitive than the blood test for the same antigen, not to mention the biopsy and tissue collection and culture routes and much faster to obtain a result. The other methods mentioned are valid methods and quite well indicated, if the clinical setting calls for such invasion as entailed in tissue collection.

5. The answer is D. The category of low-dose inhaled corticosteroids would be appropriate for this patient who has asthma in the mild persistent stage. Other choices could include cromolyn or nedocromil, basophil stabilizing agents (see Table 12–1). While *mild* intermittent asthma requires no maintenance medication, the other three levels of severity are indications for long-term pharmacologic agents, that is, maintenance medications. Mild persistent cases may be maintained on low-dose corticosteroids (glucocorticoids) or basophil stabilizers. Medium- and high-dose inhaled glucocorticoids are reserved for moderate persistent and severe persistent severity, respectively. Quick relief agents such as rapid acting beta$_2$ agonists are to be used only as rescue medications, not for long-term therapy. Moderate persistent and severe persistent cases are indications for the alternate agents, long-acting bronchodilators as well. Systemic glucocorticoids are to be used only in severe persistent cases.

TABLE 12–1 Classification of Severity of Asthma

	Mild I	Mild P	Mod P	Severe P
Symptoms	≤2×/wk ≤2 nights/mo	>2×/wk >2 nights/mo	<1×/d >1 night/wk	Constant Night (often)
Pulmonary tests	FEV$_1$, PEF ≥80% predicted	FEV$_1$, PEF ≥80%	FEV$_1$ or PEF >60%, <80%	FEV$_1$ or PEF ≤60
Medicines	None daily	Low-dose Inh corticost Or cromolyn Or nedocromil	Medium-dose Inh corticost LA Br LA beta$_2$ agonist	High- dose Inh corticost LA Br LA beta$_2$ agonist Systemic corticosteroid

Notes: Mild I, mild intermittent; Mild P, mild persistent; Mod P, moderate persistent; Severe P, severe persistent; Inh corticost, inhaled corticosteroid; LA, long-acting; Br, bronchodilator.

6. The answer is C. Restrictive lung disease. The reduced FVC, the amount one can exhale in one breath after full inspiration, defines restrictive lung disease. FEV_1 is the proportion of the FVC (as a percentage) that can be exhaled in 1 second and can be normal in restrictive lung disease. FEV_1/FVC is normal if 95% of the predicted ratio is achieved (i.e., 75% of the FVC exhaled within 1 second). Poor effort is not a likely explanation in this case, as the patient has a history of athleticism and determination. The chronicity rules out pneumonia. Both acute asthma and COPD manifest prolonged FEV_1 on spirometry, not reduced FVC. Mesothelioma occurs virtually solely in people who have worked around and have inhaled dust from asbestos. Pulmonary fibrosis has several causes, among which is respiratory bronchiolitis-associated interstitial lung disease. It occurs in this age group in heavy smokers. It remits in 20% of cases and may respond to glucocorticoids. The median life expectancy with the diagnosis is more than 10 years. Smoking cessation is necessary. The other major cause is idiopathic pulmonary fibrosis, a disease that comes on in a person's late 50s, has no known treatment, and whose prognosis is approximately 3 years after diagnosis.

7. The answer is B. The reduced FEV_1 and FEV_1/FVC ratio are indicative of COPD. Actually, the spirometry findings are also compatible with acute asthma, as both conditions are characterized by reduced capacity to exhale air. The clinical information given in the vignette rules against asthma in the chronicity, the absence of wheezing, and the pursed lips during expiration, a nearly pathognomonic finding for COPD. (Although advanced and critically severe asthma may not exhibit wheezing, that combination occurs in association with far advanced and acute illness compared with the case presented.)

8. The answer is D. Eosinophilic bronchitis, though not a rare disease in pulmonary clinics, is uncommon in primary care practice. PND, asthma, and GERD, the "pathogenic triad of chronic cough," account for a significant majority of chronic cough in nonsmoking, immunocompetent cases. There may be two causes in 18% to 62% of cases. Chronic cough is defined as persistent for more than 8 weeks. Bronchiectasis is a strong fourth cause. In smokers, of course, chronic bronchitis and COPD come to the fore. Angiotensin-converting enzyme inhibitors cause cough in 5% to 20% of cases. PND appears to have an atopic basis and may respond to an H1 antihistamine. PND may be associated with sinusitis; sinus x-rays may be negative in some 20% to 40% of cases. It should be appreciated that asthma may manifest cough without wheezing in up to 57% of cases. A methacholine challenge test is recommended in possible asthma cases as being virtually 100% sensitive so that a negative test effectively rules out asthma. Although a 24-hour esophageal pH monitor is the gold standard for diagnosis of GERD, empiric treatment with H+ pump blocking agents such as omeprazole is a more practical approach. Chest x-ray is abnormal in 87% of cases of bronchiectasis, although a computed tomography scan of the chest is superior.

9. The answer is E, asthma. Intermittent breathlessness and the existence of triggering factors, allergic rhinitis, and a prolonged expiratory phase describe asthma. Unlike with COPD, the prolonged expiratory phase is caused by a dynamic spasm of the bronchiolar musculature and is reversible by medication.

10. The answer is D, being a smoker and having a barrel chest and prolonged expiratory phase. COPD is evidenced by these findings and is statistically likely, given the history of smoking. Both asthma and COPD exhibit a prolonged expiratory phase of respiration. However, that abnormality in COPD is virtually fixed while in asthma it occurs in bouts.

11. The answer is C, congestive heart failure. In this situation (history of hypertension, coronary artery disease, diabetes; orthopnea, paroxysmal nocturnal dyspnea; and pedal edema, jugular venous distention), CHF is a statistical likelihood; however, the cause of dyspnea is not diagnosed by the symptomatology given.

12. The answer is B, hyperventilation syndrome. For history of generalized anxiety, panic disorder, and sighing breathing, the cause is anxiety disorder, hyperventilation. The attendant respiratory alkalosis aggravates the symptoms of anxiety. However, care must be taken not to assume that all anxious hyperventilation is functional, as pulmonary embolus and acute CHF certainly can be associated with apprehension and anxiety.

13. The answer is A, GERD. For postprandial dyspnea, the cause is gastroesophageal reflux, aspiration, or food allergy. Always there would be an accompanying cough.

14. The answer is A. Penicillin remains the drug of choice in this typical community-acquired case in a previously healthy person with lobar pneumonia. The etiologic agent maybe assumed to be caused by *S. pneumoniae*. Because of the acuteness of the case, this patient will need to be hospitalized for a day or two but should respond dramatically. Trimethoprim/sulfamethoxazole (Bactrim, Septra), although theoretically effective against the gram-positive side of the spectrum, is bacteriostatic, not bacteriocidal. If the patient is allergic to penicillin, then most clinicians would employ a macrolide antibiotic, such as clarithromycin. In the acutely ill patient who is to be in treatment for acute pneumonitis, tetracycline is not powerful enough for this clinical situation. However, of subacute progression of a lower respiratory infection, where mycoplasma may be considered, both the tetracyclines and the macrolides may be better choices than penicillin. Cefadroxil is classified as a first-generation cephalosporin but is generally more effective against the gram-negative spectrum and usually considered in "below the waist" infections.

15. The answer is C. *M. pneumonia* has been named one of the atypical pneumonias, based on x-ray findings out of proportion to clinical findings. Headache is a hallmark of mycoplasmal respiratory infection. The course is slow and symptoms fairly mild, although mycoplasmal infections may be associated with a multitude of extrapulmonary involvements, such as the Raynaud phenomenon, related to cold agglutinins present during the acute infection and cardiac involvement in dysrhythmias, CHF, and EKG abnormalities. Streptococcal (pneumococcal) pneumonia is classically the opposite of the picture presented here (i.e., rapidly developing course, discrete or lobar x-ray findings, significant leukocytosis and fever). Pneumonia from *K. pneumoniae* is uncommon, being a gram-negative infection that produces lobar pneumonia in its classic form, and found as an opportunist in people who are immunologically defenseless such as diabetics, alcoholics, and COPD patients. *S. aureus* is also found as a pathogen in the lungs only as an opportunist. Gram-negative sepsis is, of course, a systemic critical condition in which pneumonia is not particularly a prominent finding.

16. The answer is D, Legionella. The case illustrates several points: Bradycardia is common and headache and stupor not uncommon in Legionella disease; early laboratory findings are nonspecific. However, diagnosis is ultimately made by the 3- to 5-day growing culture in buffered charcoal yeast extract agar or less often by acute and convalescent antibody titers in a fourfold rise to 1:128, requiring 4 to 12 weeks for the change, earlier for immune globulin M (IgM) and later for immune globulin G (IgG) types; hyponatremia reflects a phase of syndrome of inappropriate anti-diuretic hormone (SIADH), associated often with lung disease but is often out of proportion to the clinical severity of the disease, and *V. pneumonia* is characterized by one of the most severe nonproductive coughs encountered in primary care medicine. The other choices have been discussed elsewhere.

17. The answer is B. The stroke patient with bulbar signs and symptoms is at risk of aspiration pneumonia. Aspiration pneumonia is usually produced by aspirated oral anaerobes. Neurologic deficits that are associated with dysphagia, level of consciousness, seizures, drug overdose, alcoholism, and recent dental procedures may all cause aspiration. Influenza pneumonic complications are most likely to be pneumococcal or staphylococcus. The Southwest U.S. traveler must be considered to have coccidioidomycosis. AIDs patients may have any of the pneumonitides discussed, depending on their clinical status, but their specific susceptibility is to *Pneumocystis carinii*.

18. The answer is C, a 32-year-old with mild shortness of breath with heavy exertion for 1 year and with a distant smoking history of 1 pack-year. The question emphasizes that not all COPD is caused by smoking. When COPD presents in the absence of a severe smoking history or significant other environmental air pollution history, alpha$_1$ protease inhibitor deficiency must be considered as an etiology. If present, the enzyme can be given exogenously.

19. The answer is E. Inhaled tiotropium (Spiriva) an anticholinergic agent, is the first-line drug therapy for COPD. Tiotropium has some incremental advantages over ipratropium, such as once-daily dosing and a marginal therapeutic edge as measured by the amount of supplemental beta$_2$ agonists and Transitional Dyspnea Index scores. Otherwise ipratropium is equally effective. All the listed agents are sometimes used in COPD patients (although inhaled corticosteroids have been shown to have little effect), but inhaled anticholinergics such as discussed should be the starting agent because of its better therapeutic profile.

References

Holmes RL, Fadden CT. Evaluation of the patient with chronic cough. *Am Fam Physician.* 2004; 69:2159–2166, 2169.

Karnani NG, Reisfield GM, Wilson GR. Evaluation of chronic dyspnea. *Am Fam Physician.* 2005; 71:1529–1537, 1538.

Lipsky MS, Sternbach M. Pneumonias, bronchitides and chronic lung disease. In: Rudy DR, Kurowski K, eds. *Family Medicine: House Officer Series.* Baltimore, MD: Williams & Wilkins; 1997:185–200.

Mintz M. Asthma update: Part I. Diagnosis, monitoring and prevention of disease progression. *Am Fam Physician.* 2004; 70:893–898.

National Asthma Education and Prevention Program. *Expert Panel Number 2.* Washington, DC: National Institutes of Health/National Heart, Lung, and Blood Institute; 1997 (NIH publication 97–4951).

Rakel RE, Bope EP, eds. *Conn's Current Therapy.* Philadelphia, PA: Saunders; 2009.

chapter 13

Respiratory Diseases in Children

Examination questions: *Unless instructed otherwise, choose the ONE lettered answer or completion that is BEST in each case.*

1 A 4-year-old boy is brought to the family doctor for inspiratory stridor that began last evening, 3 days after the onset of coryza and evolving tracheobronchial cough. His temperature was 99.8°F orally (37.7°C). He demonstrates inspiratory stridor at rest after a temporary response to nebulized racemic epinephrine (2.25%). Lateral neck x-rays were read as normal. Which of the following would be the best next step, assuming hospitalization would not be necessary?

(A) Send the child back to the urgent care center
(B) Arrange for home-delivered oxygen
(C) Inject 50 mg of ceftriaxone IM
(D) Dexamethasone 0.6 mg/kg IM   *persistent*
(E) Advise cool mist therapy at home   *Croup*

2 A 10-year-girl, assumed to have viral croup, failed to respond to racemic epinephrine and other standard treatments; she developed fever to 104°F (40°C) the evening of the visit with the family physician. A lateral x-ray of the neck shows no enlarged epiglottis but a stenotic subglottic lumen. Which of the following is the most critical likely diagnosis?

(A) Bacterial tracheitis
× (B) Severe viral
⌄ (C) Epiglottitis
⌄ (D) Status asthmaticus
⌄ (E) Bronchiolitis

3 A 6-year-old boy is brought to the family doctor for a recurrence of attacks of productive coughing. The boy has a history of "asthma" and chronic diarrhea and is small for his age. Further history reveals that as a newborn baby the boy had a serious bout of "bowel obstruction." On examination the patient has rhonchi and wheezes and hepatomegaly. Which of the following may be most likely to be diagnostic of this child's condition?

(A) Complete blood count (CBC)
(B) Serum proteins
(C) Sputum culture
(D) Blood immunoreactive trypsin level
(E) Sweat chloride   *Cystic Fibrosis*
               >60

4 A 2-week-old full-term baby boy has developed cough and exhibits fever, cyanosis, and tachypnea. Which of the following organisms should be considered in the choice of antibiotic therapy of this community-acquired pneumonia (CAP)?

(A) *Streptococcus pneumoniae* and beta-hemolytic streptococci
(B) *Staphylococcus aureus* and Hemophilus organisms
(C) Chlamydia organisms and *Staphylococcus albus*
(D) Group B streptococci and coliform bacteria *GBS*
(E) *Chlamydia trachomatis* and *Mycoplasma pneumoniae* *in first 3 wks*

5 A 2-month-old baby girl who lived at home since her normal birth and delivery has respiratory distress, although she manifests no fever. You suspect pneumonitis. Which of the following is the likely best choice of antibiotics, assuming the girl has a CAP and is to be treated as an outpatient?

(A) Penicillin
(B) Azithromycin
(C) Amoxicillin
(D) Ceftriaxone
(E) Ampicillin

6 A previously healthy 1-year-old child has a rapid onset of a rattling cough without preceding coryza. Temperature is 101°F. He has a dull facial expression. Which of the following is the best first choice of antibiotic for this CAP in an outpatient setting?

(A) Penicillin V potassium
(B) Amoxicillin
(C) Erythromycin or other macrolide antibiotic
(D) Gentamycin
(E) Methicillin

7 A 7-year-old boy is diagnosed with pneumonia. Which of the following is the least likely among expected bacterial causes to be considered?

(A) *Chlamydia pneumoniae* ✓
(B) *M. pneumoniae*
(C) *S. pneumoniae*
(D) *Hemophilus influenzae type B*
(E) *C. trachomatis*

8 There are occasions when it appears to be worthwhile to obtain a sputum sample for culture or smear. Which of the following criteria would allow confidence that the sputum sample was valid for study?

(A) Cough is clearly productive.
(B) Patient has a temperature >101°F.
(C) The specimen is obtained from the nasopharynx.
(D) The ratio of WBCs to epithelial cells in the specimen is greater than 1:1.
(E) The patient has not suffered from recent vomiting.

9 Which of the following agents is the cause of the vast majority of cases of bronchiolitis?

(A) Influenza A
(B) Influenza B
(C) Adenoviruses
(D) Respiratory syncytial virus (RSV)
(E) *S. pneumoniae*

10 Which of the following is the peak season of RSV infection?

(A) May through June
(B) July through August
(C) November through March   WINTER
(D) March through May
(E) April through June

11 Which of the following is an accepted method of prophylaxis against RSV in the present state of technology?

(A) Vaccination with live attenuated RSV
(B) Vaccination with killed RSV preparation after exposure
(C) Pooled gamma globulin
(D) Monoclonal antibody given monthly   Palivizumab
(E) Amoxicillin through the peak season

12 Which of the following is established as effective in hospitalized RSV infection?

(A) Nebulized furosemide
(B) RSV immune globulin (RSV-IG)
(C) Aerosolized ribovirin
(D) Supportive care and supplemental oxygen
(E) Antibiotics

13 Which of the following organisms accounts for the vast majority of cases of croup (laryngotracheobronchitis [LTB], laryngotracheitis, or laryngotracheobronchopneumonitis)?

(A) RSV
(B) Parainfluenza viruses   75%
(C) Mycoplasma organisms
(D) Chlamydia organisms
(E) Ureaplasma organisms

14 Which of the following best differentiates, by history, LTB (croup) from epiglottitis?

(A) Temperature
(B) Presence of inspiratory stridor
(C) Length of time from onset to defining symptom   12~24
(D) Lung field auscultation   coryza-
(E) Presence or absence of dyspnea   str

15 What is the most likely age range of an infant or child with croup?

(A) Birth to 3 months
(B) 3 months to 6 months
(C) 6 months to 12 months
(D) 12 months to 6 years
(E) 6 months to 12 years

16 The parents of a 6-year-old boy report that he has developed rapidly a temperature of 103°F at the same time as he complains of dyspnea, drooling, inability to swallow well, and soft inspiratory stridor. On examination he manifests intercostal retractions. The child is taken to the emergency department and met by an otolaryngologist to examine the patient in the operating room, where a tracheotomy could be performed as the epiglottis and larynx were to be examined. After the emergency has been dealt with, which of the following antibiotics is appropriate?

(A) Penicillin
(B) Amoxicillin
(C) Clarithromycin
(D) Ceftriaxone   Epiglottitis → Rocephin
(E) Dihydrostreptomycin

Examination Answers

1. The answer is D. Dexamethasone 0.6 mg/kg IM in a single dose to treat persistent croup (LTB), rebounding after epinephrine. Once controversial, systemic glucosteroids are now known to be effective in croup to reduce the time in the hospital and earlier discharge from emergency departments (or orally 0.15 mg/kg). Oxygen therapy is the standard of care if admission becomes necessary, signaled by inspiratory stridor, air hunger, or cyanosis. Antibiotics are not directly indicated as croup is viral, assuming the stridor is not caused by epiglottitis or bacterial tracheitis, addressed in later items in this chapter. Cool mist therapy at home is officially now said to be unsupported by objective data. This does fly in the face of experienced physicians' impressions over years.

2. The answer is A, bacterial LTB, an unusual disease that may be life threatening. Management is similar to that for epiglottitis. Diagnosis is confirmed by bronchoscopy showing a normal epiglottis, irregular membrane formation, and purulent tracheal secretions. Both asthma and bronchiolitis involve bronchospasm (expiratory wheezing or expiratory crackles) – not tracheal inspiratory stridor. Intubation is often required and intravenous antibiotics to cover *S. aureus* and *H. influenzae*.

3. The answer is E. Sweat chloride, elevated above 60 mmol is diagnostic of cystic fibrosis (CF). The complete blood count is not sensitive or specific in any way to help in diagnosis. Serum protein would likely show hypoalbuminemia, commonly found in cystic fibrosis but not diagnostic of anything except for malnutrition. Sputum culture would likely yield upper respiratory flora. Blood immunoreactive trypsin level is a first step screening examination in the newborn period, but then diagnosis would have been confirmed by the sweat chloride.

4. The answer is D. Group B streptococci and coliform bacteria are the flora to be expected in pneumonia of the newborn within the first 3 weeks. The antibiotic of choice is amoxicillin, and the patient should be admitted to a hospital.

5. The answer is B. Azithromycin is the antibiotic of choice for respiratory disease of the infant between the ages of 3 weeks and 3 months. This is based on the fact that the most likely organisms to be encountered in a CAP in this age group are *C. trachomatis* and *S. pneumoniae*. *C. trachomatis* is significant in its involvement of the eyes. Thus, empiric coverage must be designed to cover that organism as well as *S. pneumoniae*.

6. The answer is B. Amoxicillin is recommended as the empiric choice in this age group, even though chlamydial pneumoniae is one of the two most commonly found etiologic agents, along with *S. pneumoniae* (amoxicillin is not effective with chlamydia). Chlamydial pneumonia is more slowly developing, and the second tier of likely agents to be found in this age group includes *H. influenzae* B and Moraxillae. Thus, especially in acutely developing illness, amoxicillin is a wiser first choice here than a macrolide.

7. The answer is E. *C. trachomatis* has virtually disappeared from the pathogenic flora by the time a child reaches the age of 4 years, whether as a cause of pneumonia or of other infections. From the age of 5 years into adolescence, the most common organisms to be found in pneumonia in the outpatient setting are *C. pneumoniae*, *M. pneumoniae*, and *S. pneumoniae*. *H. influenzae* B is a less common cause and much more so as increasing numbers of children are immunized against this organism in the first year of life.

8. The answer is D. If white blood cells in the sputum specimen are greater than 25/low-power field for example and epithelial cells less than 25/low-power field, one can have confidence in the validity of a sputum specimen. A productive cough is a more propitious sample but that does not guarantee a valid sample. Fever has no predictive value in obtaining a specimen. A nasopharyngeal source is less secure for validity than is an oral source because the bacteria that colonize the nasopharynx are no more likely than oral sources to reflect the pulmonary contents.

9. The answer is D. RSV is the predominant cause of bronchiolitis, though other organisms that may be implicated are mycoplasma, chlamydia, ureaplasma, and pneumocystis. Bronchiolitis may be responsible for chronic lung disease in children and life-threatening disease in children under 3 months of age, especially those who were born at gestational ages of ≤ 28 months. Although case fatality is less than 1%, the mean length of illness is 12 days, and in 10% of cases the illness lasts longer than 4 weeks. RSV results in later wheezing in 34% to 40% of cases. Bronchiolitis occurs in children throughout the first year and even up to age of 2 years.

10. The answer is C. November through March, the typical winter season, is the annual span of disease from RSV.

11. The answer is D. The monoclonal antibody given monthly throughout the season of RSV is palivizumab.

This is recommended in monthly intramuscular injections in the winter months for high-risk patients. Another method of prophylaxis is intravenous RSV-IG, such as RespiGam.

12. The answer is D. Supportive care and supplemental oxygen are effective according to research evidence. None of the others are proven to be effective in hospitalized children with RSV disease. Of interest is that RSV-IG, although recommended for prophylaxis, is not felt to be effective in acute disease. Said to be "possibly effective" are nebulized ipratropium with or without a beta-2 agonist (e.g., albuterol); oral, inhaled, or parenteral glucosteroids; and nebulized epinephrine. Confounding the question of efficacy of glucosteroids and epinephrine is that many patients who respond may have atopic disease with an asthmatic component.

13. The answer is B. Parainfluenza viruses (human parainfluenza viruses 1, 2, and 3 account for 75% of all cases). Of interest is the fact that parainfluenza viruses have exhibited a pattern of biennial epidemics during the autumn months of odd-numbered years since 1973.

14. The answer is C. Croup, a viral illness with subglottic involvement, typically exhibits the symptoms of inspiratory stridor only after 12 to 24 hours of coryza, typical of a viral "cold." Epiglottitis, a much more serious condition, begins suddenly. Epiglottitis is caused by bacterial infection with supraglottic involvement, classically by *H. influenzae* but also by *S. aureus* and *Corynebacterium diphtheriae*. Although epiglottitis is characterized more by high fever than is croup, this appears to be a weak factor on which to base a preliminary diagnosis. Whereas croup virtually always includes a cough, epiglottitis rarely does so. Epiglottitis typically includes dysphagia while croup does not. The child with croup is comfortable in all positions, whereas the patient with epiglottitis will be sitting forward with the mouth open. Both conditions are characterized by inspiratory dyspnea. Croup is benign and epiglottitis is potentially critical.

15. The answer is E. Six months to twelve years is the wide range of age within which a child can be afflicted with croup. In contrast, epiglottitis can affect infants, older children, or adults. In adults, epiglottitis is not the potentially life-threatening disease as it is in younger people.

16. The answer is D. The vignette describes typical epiglottitis, a respiratory emergency. Of note is the fact that the stridor of epiglottitis is not as dramatic as that of croup. Examination to confirm the diagnosis must be made by an expert who will recognize the cherry red epiglottis and erytenoids. The antibiotic must be chosen to be effective against *H. influenzae* B as well as the less frequently involved organisms *Neisseria meningitidis* and Streptococcus species. Ceftriaxone is the antibiotic of choice.

References

Kerby GS, Deterding NR, Balasubramaniam V, et al. *Respiratory tract and mediastinum.* In: Hay WH, Levin MJ, Sondheimer JM, Deterding RB, eds. *Current Diagnosis and Treatment Pediatrics.* 19th ed. New York: McGraw-Hill Lange; 2007.

King MS. Respiratory diseases in infants and children. In: Rudy DR, Kurowski K, eds. *Family Medicine: House Officer Series.* Baltimore, MD: Williams & Wilkins; 1997:201–216.

Ostapchuk M, Roberts DM, Haddy R. Community acquired pneumonia. *Am Fam Physician.* 2004; 70:899–908.

Steiner RWP. Treating acute bronchiolitis with RSV. *Am Fam Physician.* 2004; 69:325–330.

SECTION VI

The Gastrointestinal Tract in Primary Care

chapter 14

Medical Problems of the Gastrointestinal Tract

Examination questions: Unless instructed otherwise, choose the ONE lettered answer or completion that is BEST in each case.

1. A 35-year-old woman has returned from a prolonged stay due to business in the Caribbean islands with a complaint of severe and unrelenting diarrhea. She had not been taking antibiotics and had no history of diarrhea in the past. She has lost weight and complains of fatigue. Her blood count shows hemoglobin level of 10 g/dL with a mean cell volume measured at 101 μm^3 (normal 80 to 96). The stools are bulky, particularly foul smelling and they float. Which of the following is most likely the best treatment, assuming confirmation of the diagnosis?

   (A) Loperamide orally 4 times per day as needed
   (B) Clear liquids only for 3 days followed by low-residue diet for 1 week
   (C) Tetracycline course orally for 3 weeks   *tropical sprue*
   (D) Vancomycin 500 mg 4 times per day for 10 to 14 days
   (E) Azithromycin 500 mg daily for 3 days

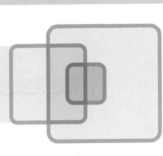

2. A 45-year-old female enters an urgent care center with a complaint of acute abdominal pain. She relates two attacks of less severe abdominal pain within the past 3 months that radiated around the right flank to the mid-thoracic dorsal area. On examination, she exhibits spider angiomata and dilated flank veins. The pain has rapidly built over a period of about 36 hours. The pain radiates through to the back opposite the epigastric area and seems to be relieved by leaning forward. Each of the following is true regarding this case except for which statement?

   ✓ (A) The most sensitive diagnostic test is the serum amylase.
   ✓ (B) Lipase elevation begins within 4 to 8 hours and remains elevated 8 to 14 days.
   ✓ (C) The vast majority of attacks are mild and not fatal.
   ✗ (D) The severity of disease is directly proportionate to the size of the amylase elevation.
   ✓ (E) This patient must be treated to prevent delirium tremens while managing the underlying condition.

3 Which of the following colorectal cancer screening recommendations would be acceptable for a 35-year-old woman whose father had colon cancer at the age of 55 years and an older brother who had 6 adenomatous polyps discovered on routine dual contrast barium enema (DCBE) at the age of 48 years?

✗ (A) Colonoscopy beginning now and every 10 years

(B) Colonoscopy starting at age 40 and every 5 years thereafter

✗ (C) Flexible sigmoidoscopy every 5 years; consider colonoscopy if positive

✗ (D) Fecal occult blood test annually, followed by colonoscopy or DCBE if positive

✓ (E) DCBE now and every 5 years; consider colonoscopy if positive

4 A 38-year-old woman has complained of abdominal pain and variably changing bowel habits consisting of cramps, bloating, and diarrhea alternating on occasion with constipation (lack of bowel movements for a day or so) for about 5 years. There are no specific foods that seem to be associated with either diarrhea or constipation. Between bouts, stool are well formed and of normal size. She has not lost weight and her height and weight are as expected, given her parents' anthropometrics. She has no family history of colorectal cancer; flexible sigmoidoscopy and later colonoscopy, indicated on the basis of her lower bowel symptoms, have been negative on two occasions. Which of the following regimens is the most likely to provide relief from the diarrhea, constipation, and abdominal pain?

(A) Hyoscyamine (Levsin)

(B) Tricyclic antidepressants, for example, amitriptyline

(C) Alosetron (Lotronex)   IBS → 5HT₃ agonist

(D) Loperamide (Imodium)

(E) Serum serotonin reuptake inhibitor (fluoxetine, Prozac; paroxetine, Paxil)

5 Which of the following parasite is capable of causing intestinal malabsorption?

(A) *Enterobius vermicularis*

(B) *Giardia lamblia*   Steatorrhea !

(C) *Ancylostoma duodenale*

(D) *Necator americanus*

(E) *Entamoeba histolytica*

6 A 75-year-old white woman with presumptive recurrent pneumonia was readmitted to the hospital where she had been kept for 2 weeks as a result of her prolonged course. She had been discharged on levofloxacin. After a period of recovery, she began to have fever again plus weakness, dyspnea, and watery diarrhea with mucus. Upon readmission, she was placed on moxifloxin and doxycycline, based on x-ray findings of pneumonia. A complete blood count showed a leukocytosis level greater than that which had been found on the previous admission, $30,000/mm^3$ with a neutrophilia and a left shift toward young cells (band nuclei). Which of the following is the likely cause of her illness?

(A) Recurrent pneumonia

(B) Irritable bowel syndrome (IBS)

(C) Pseudomembranous colitis

(D) Carcinoma of the descending colon

(E) Ulcerative colitis

7 Which of the following is the best choice of therapeutic agents among those presented for the treatment of pseudomembranous colitis?

(A) Clindamycin

(B) Third-generation cephalosporin

(C) Amoxicillin-clavulanate

(D) Metronidazole   Vanc #2

(E) Doxycycline

For Questions 8 through 12, match the numbered causes of occult gastrointestinal (GI) bleeding with the lettered settings in which the cause is most likely to be found.

8 Carcinoma of the colon
≥ 50

9 Vascular ectasia (angiodysplasia)
Chronic renal failure

10 Blue rubber bleb nevus syndrome
Cutaneous Hemangiomas

11 Celiac sprue
Chronic diarrhea/abd pain

12 Kaposi sarcoma, cytomegalovirus colitis   AIDS

(A) Chronic renal failure

(B) Cutaneous hemangiomas

(C) Chronic diarrhea, abdominal pain

(D) Age ≥50 years

(E) Acquired immunodeficiency disease

For Questions 13 through 17, match the numbered conditions commonly associated with nausea and the lettered recommended pharmacologic agents or combinations for treatment thereof.

13 Migraine headache   DA's 5A's

14 Vestibular nausea   H1 block, anticholinergics

15 Pregnancy-induced nausea   Ginger, B6, promethazine

16 Gastroenteritis   DAs, SAs

17 Postoperative nausea, vomiting

DAs, SAs
Dexamethasoa

(A) Dopamine antagonists (DAs), serotonin antagonists (SAs)
(B) DAs, SAs, dexamethasone
(C) Metoclopramide, prochlorperazine
(D) Histamine 1 blocker, anticholinergics
(E) Ginger, vitamin B$_6$, promethazine

Resume choosing the one lettered answer or completion. A nausea treatment choice may be used for more than one cause of nausea.

18 A 74-year-old man being treated for chronic renal failure has the rapid onset of hematochezia consisting of frequent maroon-colored stools. Upper endoscopy was negative to the ligament of Treitz, as was colonoscopy except for bleeding brisk enough to obscure visibility. Radioisotope-tagged red cell scan (Technetium 99) revealed a small bowel source. Which of the following is the most likely cause of brisk GI bleeding, given the foregoing scenario?

(A) Meckel diverticulum
(B) Lymphoma
(C) Crohn disease
(D) Angiodysplasia
(E) Jejunoileal diverticulum

19 The patient in Question 17 has not stopped bleeding and you consider angiography as a therapeutic approach. Which of the following is the most significant disadvantage with that plan?

(A) It is specific only for a bleeding Meckel diverticulum.
(B) There is a risk of intestinal infarction with embolization.
(C) There is no intervention capability.
(D) It misses mucosal lesions.
(E) Physician interpretation is time consuming.

20 A 35-year-old male graduate student complains of intermittent difficulty swallowing for the last 3 months. He notes that this happened 6 years ago and lasted for about 7 months. Which of the following symptoms would most enable you to reassure the patient that he does *not* have an organic basis for the dysphagia?

(A) Rapidly progressing dysphagia with weight loss
(B) Slowly progressing dysphagia, over months or years
(C) Intermittent acute symptoms or even acute obstruction
(D) Dysphagia for both solids and liquids
(E) Odynophagia

21 Ulcerative colitis is a systemic disease and involves many extraintestinal processes. They include all of the following except which one?

(A) Uveitis
(B) Sclerosing cholangitis
(C) Arthropathies
(D) Pyoderma gangrenosum
(E) Erythema nodosum

Examination Answers

1. The answer is C. A tetracycline course orally for 3 weeks will treat successfully *tropical sprue.* The symptoms are not only those of diarrhea but of malabsorption, based on weight loss and bulky floating stools. It occurs in people who have resided long periods in a tropical region. It is felt to be caused by changes in the bowel flora and responds to tetracycline or sulfonamides after a few weeks. Loperamide is a popular over counter medication used for symptomatic relief for self-limited causes of community-based diarrheas. The same applies to the clear liquids and "BRAT diet." Vancomycin is used for *Clostridium difficile*-caused pseudomembranous colitis, a disease that complicated antibiotic therapy; azithromycin is prescribed for diarrhea caused by *Campylobacter jejuni.*

2. The answer is D. The severity of disease is *not* directly proportionate to the size of the amylase elevation, so the statement that it *is* directly related thereto is the incorrect one. The Ranson criteria consist of five statistical indicators of severity upon admission. They are age >55 years, white blood count (WBC) >16,000 cells/mm^3, serum glucose >200 mg/dL, serum lactic dehydrogenase (LDH) >350 IU/L, and aspartate transaminase (AST) >250 U/dL. Acute biliary pancreatitis, which this patient could have, with her past symptoms suggestive of gallbladder disease, usually features much higher amylase levels, although the attack clinically may be relatively mild. (Her alcoholism is a more likely cause of the disease in the illustrated case.) The most *sensitive* diagnostic test is the serum amylase, which rises virtually with the onset of illness and remains elevated for about 4 days. However, amylase is not the most specific, given the fact that other conditions, such as perforated peptic ulcer, are characterized by elevated serum amylase. Lipase elevation begins within 4 to 8 hours of the onset in acute pancreatitis and remains elevated 8 to 14 days. Seventy to eighty percent of attacks are fairly mild and lead benign courses. This patient must be treated to prevent delirium tremens while managing the underlying condition, given her clear stigmata of alcoholism and cirrhosis.

3. The answer is B. Colonoscopy starting at age 40 and every 5 years thereafter. This fits the criterion based on the index patient having two first-degree relatives with either colon cancer or adenomatous polyps before the age of 60 years. Colonoscopy every 10 years is appropriate for a person of average risk beginning at the age of 50 years. Flexible sigmoidoscopy every 5 years also is approved for people of average risk, again beginning at the age of 50 as is fecal occult blood test annually (certainly the least advised routine method due to the numerous false-positive and false-negative examinations but often the most palatable for apprehensive patients). DCBE is appropriate, as is colonoscopy, for

the high-risk patient featured but not necessary until she attains the age of 40 years, and every 5 years thenceforth.

4. The answer is C. Alosetron (Lotronex), most likely among the choices to give global relief from the woman's symptoms. This vignette describes perfectly IBS. Alosetron, a 5-HT$_3$ antagonist, is a member of the family of serum norepinephrine reuptake inhibitors (SNRIs), subtypes of which being studied are 5-HT$_3$, 5-HT$_{1A}$, 5-HT$_4$, and 5-HT$_{2B}$ antagonists. IBS is defined as a chronic noninflammatory condition characterized by abdominal pain, altered bowel habits (diarrhea or constipation), or bloating without known organic basis. The condition should not be diagnosed in the face of alarm symptoms (e.g., hematochezia, persistent pencil stools, and unexplained anemia), and IBS patients over 50 years of age with average risk based on family history should undergo standard screening for colorectal cancer according to American College of Gastroenterology guidelines. Alosetron presently is approved in the United States only for "women with severe diarrhea-predominant IBS," because of serious adverse effects in some cases. However, in contrast to traditional treatment modalities for IBS, alosetron has an A rating for evidence-based recommendations. Hyocyamine, an anticholinergic, showed benefit in relieving global IBS symptoms in only one of three studies; tricyclic antidepressants have shown benefit in relieving abdominal pain but are not superior to placebo in mitigating global symptoms of IBS; loperamide has been shown to reduce the number of stools in diarrhea but is of no benefit in relieving global; IBS symptoms; serum serotonin reuptake in inhibitors' effectiveness has not been documented. A medication not among the choices, the 5HT4 antagonist tegaserod is known to be effective against constipation-predominant IBS in women, not diarrhea-related IBS.

5. The answer is B. Giardia is a protozoan that causes numerous GI symptoms, including nausea, vomiting, diarrhea, and steatorrhea. Giardiasis is the most common (i.e., prevalent) parasite worldwide and second in the United States after *E. vermicularis* (pinworm). The protozoan is passed by the fecal–oral route and therefore occurs where water processing is less than optimal (being relatively resistant to chlorination), such as in developing countries and outdoor camping situations. In the latter scenario, it is enhanced in its communicability by its survivability in cold water. The pinworm, whose only host is humans, lives in the large intestine and lays eggs on the perineum. It rarely results in more than perineal pruritus, but occasionally can cause weight loss, urinary tract infection, and appendicitis. *A. duodenale* and *N. americanus* are the "Old World" and "New World" hookworms, respectively. Hookworm causes pruritus on occasion and, after attainment of a large worm load in the intestines, may cause microcytic, hypochromic anemia through consumption of host blood. *E. histolytica* is the etiology of amebiasis and acutely causes diarrhea, dysentery, and severe abdominal pain and may ultimately result in chronic systemic disease. Each of the parasites discussed here that are passed through the fecal–oral route are more incident and prevalent in groups that practice oral–anal sex.

6. The answer is C. Pseudomembranous colitis is the most likely diagnosis in view of the woman's recent and continuing treatment with antibiotics and the watery diarrhea. The leading bacterial causation is *C. difficile.* A hospital stay of 4 weeks or longer results in a 50% rate of *C. difficile* acquisition, compared with a 3% prevalence of GI colonization in the general population; a 2-week stay appears to present a risk of 13% for acquisition. Although pneumonia may be recurrent or persistent and antibiotics continue to be indicated, the diarrhea and marked leukocytosis require a working diagnosis of pseudomembranous colitis. Neither IBS nor carcinoma of the colon causes watery diarrhea or leukocytosis. Ulcerative colitis is unlikely in view of the clinical setting.

7. The answer is D. Metronidazole is effective against *C. difficile* and is inexpensive; the most important side effects are neurologic. The second choice of antibiotics is vancomycin, the chief caveat being nephrotoxicity. Each of the other antibiotics mentioned is a risk factor for the disease, being broad spectrum and not specifically effective against *C. difficile.* Among the antibiotics, clindamycin is fraught with the greatest risk of *C. difficile* disease. Only 20% of antibiotic-related diarrhea is caused by *C. difficile,* but virtually all cases of pseudomembranous colitis result from *C. difficile.* Pseudomembranous colitis carries a 1% to 2.5% case mortality.

MATCHING QUESTIONS 8 THROUGH 12

8. The answer for carcinoma of the colon is **D,** age ≥ 50 years.

9. The answer for vascular ectasia (angiodysplasia) is **A,** chronic renal failure.

10. The answer for blue rubber bleb nevus syndrome is **B,** cutaneous hemangiomas.

11. The answer for celiac sprue is **C,** chronic diarrhea, abdominal pain.

12. The answer for Kaposi sarcoma, cytomegalovirus colitis is **E,** acquired immunodeficiency disease.

MATCHING QUESTIONS 13 THROUGH 17

13. The answer for migraine headache is A, DAs, SAs.

14. The answer for vestibular nausea is D, histamine 1 blocker, anticholinergics.

15. The answer for pregnancy-induced nausea is E, ginger, vitamin B_6, promethazine.

16. The answer for gastroenteritis is A, DAs, SAs.

17. The answer for postoperative nausea, vomiting is B, DAs, SAs, dexamethasone.

DISCUSSION OF QUESTIONS 13 THROUGH 17

These recommendations are based on the theories of the mechanisms involved in production of nausea associated with the five conditions. The nausea of migraine is associated with the neurotransmitter dopamine, antagonists of which are used for headache with nausea, such as metoclopramide (Reglan) or prochlorperazine (Compazine). For nausea alone in migraine are recommended the foregoing classes of drugs as well as serotonin antagonists, such as ondansetron (Zofran). Vestibular nausea is mediated by histamine and by acetylcholine, and hence, it is treated by histamine 1 blocking agents ("antihistamines") and by anticholinergic agents. The mechanism of nausea associated with pregnancy is poorly understood, but the recommendations made, that is, ginger and vitamin B_6, are based on empiric response and safety for use during the first trimester of pregnancy. Hyperemesis gravidarum is treated by either promethazine (Phenergan) or an SA and, as a second-line approach, glucocorticoids. Neurotransmitters associated with gastroenteritis are dopamine and serotonin; therefore, DAs are used, as just exemplified. The same applies to postoperative nausea and vomiting.

18. The answer is D. Angiodysplasia may occur throughout the GI tract but is found most frequently in older patients and those with chronic renal failure, particularly in the upper tract. This may be a result of increased platelet dysfunction associated with uremia. All other choices may be sources of small intestinal bleeding but relatively infrequently as compared with angiodysplasia.

19. The answer is B. Risk of intestinal infarction with embolization. Angiography functions as a diagnostic tool for brisk GI bleeding by the show of dye that appears in the lumen when the arterial blood supply to the bleeding segment of bowel has been cannulated. It is also a therapeutic tool that works by embolization of the vessel that supplies the bleeding area. The chief danger is that of infarction of the segment, that is, hemorrhaging. Small bowel barium follow-through is a diagnostic tool for hemorrhage but fails in cases of mucosal lesions.

20. The answer is D. Dysphagia that is due to an esophageal motor disorder is characterized by symptoms with both solids and liquids. Rapidly progressing dysphagia with weight loss is a cause for suspicion of esophageal cancer. Slowly progressing dysphagia, over months or years, is suggestive of benign stricture; intermittent acute symptoms or spasmodic acute obstruction is characteristic of symptomatic esophageal ring (the Schatzki ring, *at the lower end of the esophagus*); odynophagia, although it is due to other causes, when of recent onset, usually indicates ulcerative esophagitis caused by aphthous disease, or if longer, such ulcerative disease could be due to more serious underlying causes such as immune compromise emanating from diseases such as cancer, blood dyscrasias, cancer chemotherapy, or acquired immunodeficiency disease.

21. The answer is A. Extraintestinal processes of *ulcerative colitis* include all of those listed except uveitis. Sclerosing cholangitis, pyoderma gangrenosum, and arthropathies are well known to be associated with ulcerative colitis, although the bases for these are poorly understood. Similarly, erythema nodosum is associated but less frequently than the other entities.

References

Flake ZA, Scalley RD, Bailey AG. Practical selection of antiemetics. *Am Fam Physician.* 2004; 69:1169–1174, 1176.

Kennedy TM, Rubin G, Jones RH. Clinical evidence: Irritable bowel syndrome. *Am Fam Physician.* 2005; 71(3):525.

Kucik CJ, Martin GL, Sortor BV. Common intestinal parasites. *Am Fam Physician.* 2004; 69:1161–1168.

Manning-Dimmit LA, Dimmit SG, Wilson GR. Diagnosis of gastrointestinal bleeding in adults. *Am Fam Physician.* 2005; 71:1339–1346.

Mitchell SH, Schaeffer DC, Dubagunta S. A new view of occult and gastrointestinal bleeding. *Am Fam Physician.* 2004; 69:875–881.

Nidiry JJ. Medical problems of the gastrointestinal tract. In: Rudy DR, Kurowski K, eds. *Family Medicine: House Officer Series.* Baltimore: Williams & Wilkins; 1997:217–234.

Rakel RER, Bope EP, eds. *Conn's Current Therapy 2009.* Philadelphia, PA: Saunders-Elsevier; 2009.

Schiller L. Malabsorption. In: Rakel RE, Bope EP, eds. *Conn's Current Therapy.* Philadelphia, PA: Saunders-Elsevier; 2009.

Schroeder MS. Clostridium difficile-associated diarrhea. *Am Fam Physician.* 2005; 71:921–928.

chapter 15

Surgical Issues of the Gastrointestinal Tract

Examination questions: *Unless instructed otherwise, choose the ONE lettered answer or completion that is BEST in each case.*

1 A 25-year-old man enters the office with pain in the abdomen with the onset 36 hours ago and increasingly worse since then. Initial examination of the chest is negative and the abdomen, while in tender to deep palpation in the lower midline, manifests neither rebound tenderness nor positive Rovsig sign. However, when the doctor lays the patient on the left side and directs the patient to extend his right hip while the doctor resists the effort, the patient complains of severe pain deep in the right lumbar area. This finding may indicate each of the following diagnoses except for which one?

Psoas test

- (A) Positive in retrocaecal appendicitis
- (B) Positive in Crohn disease
- (C) Positive in perinephric abscess *pain above pelvic area*
- (D) Positive in pelvic appendicitis
- (E) May be positive, if pain is elicited by a digital rectal examination, palpating posteriorly.

2 Which of the following may exhibit purpuric discoloration in any or all of the following areas: periumbilical (Cullen sign), inguinal region (Fox sign), and the flanks (Grey sign):

- (A) Acute cholecystitis
- (B) Irritable bowel syndrome
- (C) Hemorrhagic pancreatitis
- (D) Peptic ulcer
- (E) Superior mesenteric artery insufficiency

3 A 65-year-old man, previously healthy, has noted dysphagia with both liquids and solids for about 2 months. It occurs in paroxysms that last for up to 20 to 30 minutes. The frequency of the attacks has been increasing recently. Without further history, which of the following is the most likely cause of the symptom?

- (A) Esophageal diverticulum
- (B) Adenocarcinoma of the esophagus
- (C) Stricture from peptic esophagitis

- (D) Functional motility disorder
- (E) Postradiation therapy

4 Which of the following is true about carcinomas of the upper gastrointestinal (GI) tract?

- (A) Incidence of carcinoma of the stomach is increasing in the United States. ↓
- (B) Incidence of carcinoma of esophagus and proximal stomach is increasing. *GERD*
- (C) Carcinoma of the stomach is a disease for which routine screening is appropriate. X
- (D) Vitamin C intake is a risk factor for carcinoma of the stomach.
- (E) Excess intake of fruits and vegetables is a risk factor for carcinoma of the stomach.

5 A 56-year-old man is concerned about stomach cancer because of the death of a co-worker from that disease. Each of the following is a risk factor for stomach cancer except which one?

- (A) Familial adenomatous polyposis
- (B) History of a gastric ulcer that revealed high-grade dysplasia
- (C) Atrophic gastritis
- (D) *Helicobacter pylori* infection
- (E) Hyperplastic polyps

6 Which of the following is the most important, productive, and practical reason to offer or refer for upper endoscopy in any patient over 45 years with persistent dyspepsia?

- (A) To diagnose gastric peptic ulcer
- (B) To diagnose gastroesophageal reflux
- (C) To diagnose early stomach cancer *↑risk, can screen*
- (D) To diagnose peptic duodenal ulcer disease
- (E) To diagnose atrophic gastritis

7 You suspect atypical presentation of appendicitis in a 26-year-old woman who has had abdominal pain for 2 days: There is no rebound tenderness, questionable obturator and psoas signs, and a higher white blood cell (WBC) count than is usually encountered in appendicitis. Pelvic examination reveals right adnexal area tenderness but no cervical tenderness Which of the following may be *most* helpful in determining whether the patient has appendicitis, thus making it less likely for you to commit to unnecessary surgery or missing timely intervention in the event of appendicitis?

(A) Abdominal plain films
→ (B) Helical computed tomography (CT) scan of the abdomen
(C) CT scan
(D) Ultrasonography
(E) Magnetic resonance image

8 A 40-year-old white man has been treated for peptic ulcer disease (PUD) symptoms for several weeks. The patient also has diarrhea, a problem he had not had in the past. He denies taking nonsteroidal anti-inflammatory medication either by prescription or over the counter. You treated the patient with a 3-week course of the histamine 2 receptor blocking agent (H2 receptor blocker) ranitidine, but the patient's symptoms only slightly improved and recurred fully within days after discontinuance of the drug. You then prescribed the hydrogen pump blocking agent omeprazole for 3 weeks with similar disappointing results. Esophagogastroduodenoscopy then demonstrated a large ulcer (3-cm diameter) distal to the duodenal bulb. During the procedure, studies were done for *H. pylori* that were negative. Which of the following would be the next logical action?

(A) Draw blood for a gastrin level   *refractory PUD*
(B) Refer for lower endoscopy to rule out ulcerative colitis
(C) Order barium upper GI series with small bowel follow-through to rule out Crohn disease
(D) Order stool cultures for bacterial cause of infectious diarrhea
(E) Order stool studies for ova and parasites

9 A 55-year-old man is alcoholic and has an episode of bleeding esophageal varices. The patient is impressed with your warnings regarding the dangers of alcoholism and vows to visit a local Alcoholics Anonymous chapter and to stop drinking alcohol. Which of the following is a valid medical approach to reduce the chances of repeat bleeding episodes, thus avoiding surgical emergencies caused by hemorrhage?

(A) Calcium channel blocking agent
(B) Beta-selective agonist agent
(C) H2 receptor blocker
(D) Nonselective beta-adrenergic blocking agent
(E) Proton pump blocker

10 A 70-year-old white woman is found to have a hemoglobin level of 4 g/100 mL and a macrocytosis. Serum vitamin B_{12} level is abnormally low. The patient denies history of diarrhea. Serum folic acid levels are normal. As you begin treatment of this patient, which of the following procedures comes under the heading of "best practice"?

(A) Barium enema
(B) Barium swallow with small bowel follow-through
(C) Upper GI barium series
(D) Colonoscopy
(E) Upper endoscopy *pernicious anemia r/o gastric carcinoma*

11 Which of the following sites of colon cancer, upon presentation of symptoms and signs, confers the most favorable prognosis?

X (A) Cecum
X (B) Ascending colon
X (C) Transverse colon
X (D) Iliocolic junction
(E) Sigmoid colon

12 A 35-year-old white man has had abdominal pain for the past 36 hours. Examination of the anterior aspect of the abdomen is negative for rebound tenderness, although there is some deep tenderness in the midline below the umbilicus. The WBC count is elevated to 19,000 with 80% neutrophils, of which 30% are bands. Which of the following would be helpful in establishing a diagnosis of retrocecal appendicitis?

X (A) Babinski response
(B) Obturator sign
X (C) Rovsig sign
X (D) Murphy sign
X (E) Osler sign

13 A male newborn who is 4 weeks old has begun to vomit over the past 2 days after each feeding, and the vomit is blood streaked. Last evening the vomiting became projectile. You notice a peristaltic wave in the upper abdomen moving from left to right. Deep palpation between attacks reveals an olive-sized nodule in the epigastrium. Which of the following is the likely diagnosis?

(A) Acute gastritis
(B) Iliocolic intussusception
(C) Pyloric stenosis
(D) Esophageal atresia
(E) Pneumonia

14 An 11-month-old male infant develops apparent colicky abdominal pain, as he screams and draws up his knees with each bout of pain. Within 12 hours the child exhibits vomiting and diarrhea consisting of bloody mucous stools. Deep palpation reveals a sausage-like mass in the supraumbilical area of the midline abdomen. Which of the following is the most likely cause of these findings?

(A) Meconium plug
(B) Hirschsprung disease
(C) Carcinoma of the colon
(D) Shigellosis
(E) Intussusception

15 A 45-year-old female patient has just been told that her brother, who is 3 years older than she, has been diagnosed with colorectal cancer (CRC). She has no symptoms or change in bowel habits, blood in the stool, or any abdominal discomfort. She wishes to know what measures she should take to avoid an encounter with the disease. First, you explain to her that the lifetime risk of carcinoma of the colon is about 2.5% for the average American. What would be the corresponding risk figure for her, a person who has a first-degree relative with colon cancer?

(A) 2.5% to 3%
(B) 7% to 7.5%   7~7.5%
(C) 10%
(D) 15%
(E) 20%

16 Regarding the patient in Question 15, you perform flexible sigmoidoscopy and excise a polyp that turns out histologically to be an adenomatous polyp of the tubular type. What is your next advice and disposition for her medical care?

(A) Fecal occult blood testing every year, three stools, two samples per stool, beginning at age of 50 years
(B) Dual-contrast barium enema annually starting at 50 years
(C) Flexible sigmoidoscopy every 5 years starting at 50 years
(D) Colonoscopy now and every 3 years if findings are negative
(E) No need to worry, considering the odds are overwhelmingly in her favor

Examination Answers

1. The answer is D. Pelvic appendicitis will not result in pain with the maneuver described. The doctor has performed the psoas test. It would not be positive because the psoas sign elucidates retrocaecal inflammatory processes above the pelvic area. The obturator sign, elicited by pain causation associated upon internal rotation of the right hip, should be positive in a pelvic appendicitis. The psoas sign is defined as pain elicited by the extension of the ipsilateral hip against resistance.

2. The answer is C. Hemorrhagic pancreatitis, and any other cause of hemoperitoneum, may cause any of the signs alluded to in the main stem, for example, ruptured ovarian cyst when blood escapes to sufficient extent.

3. The answer is D. Functional motility disorder is most likely the cause of dysphagia that involved both liquids and solids from the onset. Each of the other choices are causes of dysphagia, but each is an example of mechanical obstruction. Mechanical processes, except for swallowed foreign bodies, are more insidious in the development, involving solid foods early and as the dysphagia progresses to liquids become difficult to swallow as well. The course is more or less steady. Dysphagia of that type raises a red flag and must be evaluated as soon as possible to rule out carcinoma.

4. The answer is B. Although the overall incidence of carcinoma of the stomach has been decreasing in the United States for years, carcinoma of the proximal stomach, esophagogastric junction, and esophagus is increasing. Most physicians feel this is because of the increased incidence and prevalence of gastroesophageal reflux disease. The latter is related to the increasing prevalence of obesity. Vitamin C intake may be protective. Lack of fruit and vegetables may be a risk factor. Screening of asymptomatic patients of normal risk status for carcinoma of the stomach is not recommended because of the invasiveness of any effective screening method and the low incidence in low-risk populations.

5. The answer is E. Hyperplastic polyps (of the colon or elsewhere) have no malignant potential and are not associated with gastric carcinoma. However, surveillance for gastric cancer is recommended for individuals with each of the other four risk factors. Familial adenomatous polyposis, noted for CRC development in all persons by the age of 40, is also thought to be a risk factor for adenocarcinomas in other sites, as is the Lynch syndrome (family cancer syndrome II, hereditary nonpolyposis CRC).

Gastric ulcer with biopsy evidence of high-grade dysplasia (and also gastric metaplasia, but not benign gastric ulcer) is a risk factor. Pernicious anemia is a risk factor as is atrophic gastritis, without which pernicious anemia does not exist.

6. The answer is C. Perhaps of the greatest surprise, gastric cancer can be a screenable disease. Although a large proportion of patients with gastric cancer are asymptomatic, if patients are chosen for high-risk status (see the explanation given for Question 2) and upper endoscopy is utilized aggressively, the cure rate can be as high as 90%. The other choices are fruitful indications for esophagogastroduodenoscopy as well, but a degree of time urgency is conferred for early diagnosis of gastric carcinoma.

7. The answer is B. Helical CT scanning is quite accurate, with sensitivity of about 92% and specificity of 97%. This test has become nearly routine in emergency departments. A helical CT scan is especially useful in differentiating appendicitis from salpingitis in women. Although plain abdominal x-rays may identify an appendiceal fecalith (appendicolith) that occurs in only 5% of cases. Ultrasonography carries an accuracy of 71% to 97%. A magnetic resonance image is helpful in children and women.

8. The answer is A. Association of refractory PUD and diarrhea, especially when one or more ulcers include(s) a lesion larger than usual, located distal to the duodenal bulb, suggests Zollinger–Ellison syndrome. Gastrinomas occur in the pancreas, duodenal wall, or lymph nodes, or, when associated with multiple endocrine neoplasia, type 1, occur in multiples in endocrine organs such as the parathyroid glands. One-third of gastrinomas are malignant. Over 90% of patients with gastrinomas develop PUD and one-third will have watery diarrhea that can be quite severe and, of course, refractory to usual treatment. Although each of the other choices are causes of diarrhea, they would have to coexist with PUD in this case, none of which is found in that association.

9. The answer is D. Nonselective beta-blockers have been shown to reduce the chances of bleeding from esophageal varices to 15% from a 25% rate in placebo-treated control subjects. H2 receptor blockers and proton pump blockers would be good choices for reflux symptoms but are not reported to prevent hemorrhage from varices once they have developed.

10. The answer is E. The patient has pernicious anemia. Treatment consists of parenteral monthly injections of vitamin B_{12}. The reason for doing upper endoscopy at the time of diagnosis is to rule out gastric carcinoma, the risk of which is threefold that of the general population. The *prevalence* of gastric carcinoma is 1% to 3% in pernicious anemia.

11. The answer is E. A sigmoid colon (as with other descending colon) location is most likely to be discovered in Duke stage A (confinement to the mucosa) because the earliest symptom is usually hematochezia, occurring well before the primary tumor encircles or obstructs the colon. This location confers a 5-year cure rate of 90%. Blood from tumors arising from more proximal levels is digested and changed from a visible form in the early stages, thus not alerting the patient until change in bowel habits or even bowel obstruction supervenes. Fecal occult blood screening could, of course, detect early and curable tumors in the more proximal locations. Thirty-two percent of CRCs occur in the descending colon, divided into 25% in the sigmoid and 7% in the remaining descending colon. Males are more likely than females to develop cancer in the left or descending colon, whereas females are more likely to develop it in the right colon. Stage B is confined to the muscularis and if excised at that point confers a 60% to 75% 5-year survival; Stage C is defined a spread to at least one lymph node involvement and survival drops to about 25% to 50%. D is distant metastases: 5% 5-year survival.

12. The answer is B. The obturator sign is defined as pain upon internal rotation of the thigh with the right hip flexed. When it elicits pain deep in the lower lumbar area (as opposed to the hip joint proper or pain radiating down the anterior thigh), it signifies contact between the internal obturator muscle and an inflammation process, usually a retrocecal appendix. The psoas maneuver is the alternative if retrocecal appendicitis is still suspected and the obturator sign is absent (either one may be performed before the other). With the psoas sign, the ipsilateral hip is extended, and pain is elicited if there is an inflammatory process touching the psoas muscle. The Babinski sign is an abnormal plantar reflex of the foot and toes in the presence of an upper motor neuron lesion in the opposite side of the brain or any part of the corticospinal tract above the crossover level. The Rovsig sign is the presence of right lower quadrant pain upon release of deep pressure by the examining hand in the abdomen in the presence of classic appendicitis with normal positioning wherein the organ is touching the anterior parietal peritoneum. The Murphy sign is the inhibition of inspiratory effort when the examining hand is deeply placed beneath the right costal margin in the presence of an inflamed gallbladder. The Osler sign is the presence of painful petechia-sized red spots on the hands and feet pathognomonic of subacute bacterial endocarditis.

13. The answer is C. This patient has a typical presentation of pyloric stenosis. A male infant who is 2 weeks to 4 months of age most typifies pyloric stenosis. Male infants are affected four times as frequently as female infants.

14. The answer is E. Intussusception is the most common cause of bowel (as opposed to pyloric) obstruction in the first 2 years of a baby's life. Eighty percent of cases occur in the first 2 years of life, peaking in the time period from 5 to 9 months. Male infants are affected three times as frequently as female infants; presentation includes colicky abdominal pain, "current jelly stools," reflex vomiting, leukocytosis, hemoconcentration, and a palpable mass. Meconium plug is a cause of obstruction in the newborn. Hirschsprung disease is a potentially fatal condition of the newborn in which normal peristalsis is prevented by the segmental absence of ganglion cells of the mucosal and muscular layers of colon or rectosigmoid segments of bowel. Obviously, both are causes of congenital bowel obstruction. Carcinoma of the infant colon is extremely rare. Shigellosis is a form of bacterial dysentery that causes profuse bloody diarrhea.

15. The answer is B, 7% to 7.5%. The lifetime risk of carcinoma of the colon of about 2.5% is roughly tripled for a person who has a first-degree relative with either colon cancer or adenomatous polyp. This translates to a 7% to 7.5% lifetime risk. Because the incidence increases with each decade of life, all the foregoing percentages are multiplied for the upper age groups. For example, the expected incidence of colon cancer of nearly 0.4% per 1,000 per year at the age of 50 years would be more than 1.2% per 1,000 in every year for a person with such a first-degree family history.

16. The answer is D. Although A, B, and C are acceptable methods of CRC screening for patients of average risk, beginning at the age of 50 years, any patient who has a first-degree family history of CRC should begin such screening at the age of 40 years. Because this patient has now been diagnosed with a tubular adenomatous polyp, one of three precancerous types, she should undergo colonoscopy now, and this should be repeated every 3 years, assuming the study reveals no cancers (see Chapter 45). The presence of a single adenomatous polyp in any segment of the large intestine implies the strong possibility of other polyps throughout the remainder of the colon.

References

American Academy of Family Physicians. Family Medicine Board Review 2009. May 3–9, 2009. Kansas City, Missouri.

Bellows CF, Berger DH, Crass RA. Management of gallstones. *Am Fam Physician*. 2005; 72:637–642.

Brown CM. Surgical issues of the gastrointestinal tract. In: Rudy DR, Kurowski K, eds. *Family Medicine: House Officer Series*. Baltimore, MD: Williams & Wilkins; 1997:235–254.

Layke JC, Lopez PP. Gastric cancer: Diagnosis and treatment options. *Am Fam Physician*. 2004; 69:1133–1140, 1145–1146.

McQuaid KR. Alimentary tract. In: Tierney LM, McPhee SJ, Papadakis MA, eds. *Current Medical Diagnosis and Treatment*. 43rd ed. New York: McGraw-Hill/Appleton & Lange; 2004:515–622.

Old H, Dusing RW, Tap W, et al. Imaging for suspected appendicitis. *Am Fam Physician*. 2005; 71:71–78.

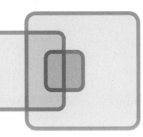

chapter **16**

Problems of the Liver

Examination questions: Unless instructed otherwise, choose the ONE lettered answer or completion that is BEST in each case.

1 A 33-year-old woman has a diagnosis of post-inflammatory cirrhosis after suffering a bout of hepatitis B. Recently, on upper endoscopy, she demonstrated presence of esophageal varices, and a decision was made to utilize nonselective beta-adrenergic blockade to prevent bleeding of the varices. Which of the following is the parameter that in follow-up indicates the therapeutic endpoint has been reached?

(A) Hemoglobin increases by 2 g/dL
(B) Pulse rate drops by about 25%
(C) Rise in blood pressure by 10%
(D) Normalization of AST and ALT
(E) Normalization of serum bilirubin

2 A man who weighs 220 pounds at a height of 5 ft 10 in. undergoes a routine physical examination. The physician finds the liver to be palpable at 6 cm (>2 in.) below the right costal margin. A chemical profile shows AST elevated threefold above normal and the ALT twice normal. A needle biopsy shows fatty infiltration (steatohepatosis). Each of the following conditions is in the top four most likely causes *except* for which one?

(A) Iatrogenic of pathophysiologic glucocorticoid effects
✓(B) Alcoholic liver disease
✓(C) Obesity
✓(D) Diabetes
✓(E) Hypertriglyceridemia

3 The list of drugs that can idiosyncratically cause severe liver toxicity, that is, not dose related and relatively unpredictable, is large. However, the commonly used antipyretic analgesic drug acetaminophen (e.g., Tylenol) causes drug-induced hepatitis in a dose-related fashion. Which of the following is the toxic single dose of acetaminophen in an average size person?

(A) 4 g
(B) 6 g
(C) 10 g
(D) 16 g
(E) 20 g

4 A 28-year-old woman who admits to a history of intravenous drug abuse is planning a serious new relationship and is concerned about the possibility of passing hepatitis to her new sex partner. A screening test for anti-hepatitis C antibody was negative. You obtain a hepatitis B panel. Which of the following sets of laboratory findings make the diagnosis of hepatitis B carrier?

✗ (A) HBsAg negative, anti-HBc negative, anti-HBs negative unexposed
✗ (B) HBsAg negative, anti-HBc positive, anti-HBs negative
✗ (C) HBsAg negative, anti-HBc negative/positive, anti-HBs positive
(D) HBsAg positive, anti-HBc positive, immunoglobulin M (IgM) anti-HBc positive, anti-HBs negative
(E) HBsAg positive, anti-HBc positive, IgM anti-HBc negative, anti-HBs negative

acutely infected
sAg +
core +
IgM −

5 Which of the following is the best indicator of a high degree of hepatitis B virus (HBV) replication, hence marker of infectivity?

(A) HBsAg
(B) HBcAg
(C) HBeAg ✓ *e = infectiviteeee*
(D) Anti-HBs
(E) Anti-HBc

6 The woman seeking testing for hepatitis B before starting a serious relationship exhibits the following results: HBeAg negative, HBc antibody positive, HBs antibody positive, ALT, and AST levels normal. What is your advice to the patient vis-a-vis her prospective fiancee'?

(A) He should take the three injection series of hepatitis vaccine.
(B) He should have hepatitis B immune globulin injection.
(C) The couple should be advised to use a barrier method of contraception for protection of the man from hepatitis B.

(D) There need be no particular protective measures for her fiancée.

(E) The fiancée should take a course of an immune modulator such as recombinant alfa-2b (Intron A).

7 A 56-year-old male patient who had transfusions 20 years ago and contracted hepatitis C comes to you as a new patient. During your examination, you notice dilated flank veins, redness of the palms, and suspicion of ascites. From a computed tomography scan, you find ascites and conclude that the patient has cirrhosis. Knowing that hepatitis C is a strong risk factor for hepatocellular carcinoma, stronger even than hepatitis B, you decide to begin with a screening baseline test for that disease. Which of the following tests serves that purpose?

(A) Carcinoembryonic antigen test
(B) Alpha-fetoprotein test   *Baseline hepatocellular CA test*
(C) Breast cancer 1, early onset (BRCA1) genetic test
(D) Human chorionic gonadotropin test
(E) Prostate-specific antigen test

8 A 45-year-old white man has undergone a routine periodic physical examination. You note that, for the past 3 years, each hepatic profile testing ordered by your office has shown ALT and AST elevations of up to two to three times normal levels. You decide to investigate in stepwise fashion. Each of the following steps would be appropriate at this time, except for which one?

(A) Inquire as to drinking habits
(B) Inquire as to intravenous street drug usage
(C) Complete review of the patient's medications
(D) Order an ultrasound study of the liver
(E) Order serologic tests for hepatitides A, B, and C and blood tests for iron studies

9 A 35-year-old woman who has had two pregnancies and is 20% overweight presents with jaundice. Serum conjugated bilirubin level is elevated to twice the upper limit of normal. Unconjugated bilirubin is normal. Which of the following, as a single procedure, is most likely to elucidate a cause of this clinical situation?

(A) Blood draw for hepatitides A, B, and C
(B) Computed tomography scan of the liver
(C) Ultrasound study of the extrahepatic biliary system   *extrahepatic obs. jaundice*
(D) Plain x-ray of the abdomen   *↓ conj bili*
(E) Blood draw for ALT and AST

10 A 46-year-old woman is evaluated for worsening fatigue and pruritus that have been present for at least 8 years. Abdominal pain has not been a major symptom. Recently, she has complained of diarrhea

with stools that float in the commode. She drinks two to three glasses of wine weekly. On examination, you find xanthomas on the extensor surfaces of the forearms. She also manifests xanthelasmas on the eyelids. There are dilated flank veins on each side of the trunkal area. There is no mass palpable. The comprehensive metabolic profile shows alkaline phosphatase elevated to twice the upper limit of normal, and direct-acting (conjugated) bilirubin is elevated to 1.5 times the upper limit of normal. The lipid profile reveals elevated cholesterol to 280 mg/dL and high-density lipoprotein cholesterol at 70 mg/dL. Which of the following is the most likely diagnosis?

(A) Choledocholithiasis
(B) Gilbert disease
(C) Carcinoma of the head of the pancreas
(D) Primary biliary cirrhosis (PBC)
(E) Alcoholic cirrhosis

11 Which of the following is the most easily passed by a blood donor?

(A) Hepatitis A
(B) Hepatitis B   ← *easier to transmit*
(C) Hepatitis C
(D) Hepatitis D
(E) Hepatitis E

12 Your patient is a 55-year-old male professor of language at the nearby university. He has been stable in his professional life and as a marital partner and adequately so as a parent. He appears for periodic health profile evaluation. A routine chemistry battery returns with surprise findings of mean cell volume in an otherwise normal hemogram of 97 μm^3 (also 97 fL); gamma-glutamyl transpeptidase 255 U/L (normal is 5 to 40 U/L); serum AST 199 U/L (formerly SGOT, 1 to 36); ALT 101 (formerly SGPT, 1 to 45); and blood urea nitrogen (BUN) 6 mg/dL. Alkaline phosphatase is normal at 75 U/L. Bilirubin levels, conjugated and unconjugated, are normal. What should be your *next* measure?

(A) Order gallbladder ultrasound study
(B) Arrange a liver biopsy
(C) Arrange an esophagogastroduodenoscopy
(D) Order hepatitis profile (tests of antigens and antibodies of hepatitides A, B, and C)
(E) Obtain further information through the medical interview of the patient
   EtOH suggested by labs

13 A 30-year-old white man with a history of ulcerative colitis develops obstructive jaundice, associated with fever. There has been no colicky pain and very little abdominal pain in general. A gallbladder ultrasound study is negative for gallstones. The direct-acting bilirubin level is elevated, as is the alkaline phosphatase level, whereas the indirect-acting bilirubin level is normal. ALT and AST levels are elevated to less than 10% above the upper limits of normal. An empiric course of ciprofloxicin results in rapid subsidence of the fever. Which of the following is the most likely cause of this constellation of findings?

(A) PBC
(B) Primary sclerosing cholangitis (PSC)
(C) Choledocholithiasis
(D) Steatohepatosis
(E) Viral hepatitis

14 A 45-year-old woman presents with fatigue, anorexia, brown urine, and malaise. She denies alcohol intake entirely, illicit drug use, and history of treatment with blood products, and she is on no medications that may cause elevation of hepatocellular enzymes. Examination reveals scleral icterus and mildly tender hepatomegaly. Both AST and ALT levels are elevated to four times normal, and smooth muscle antibody (SMA) and antinuclear antibody (ANA) levels are positive. She has a history of Hashimoto thyroiditis, but no history suggestive of inflammatory bowel disease. Alkaline phosphatase and gamma-glutamyl transpeptidase are both elevated to twice normal limits. A hepatitis profile yields no evidence of hepatitides A, B, C, or E. Which of the following may be the best initial presumptive diagnosis?

(A) PSC
(B) PBC
(C) Viral hepatitis
(D) Choledocholithiasis
(E) Autoimmune hepatitis

15 A 15-year-old girl presents with malaise, fatigue, depression, and clinical evidence of hepatitis in the absence of viral causation. An older sister is awaiting liver transplantation. Which of the following blood studies may be most specifically helpful in establishing the diagnosis?

(A) ANA levels
(B) Anti-SMA levels
(C) Complete blood count
(D) Ceruloplasmin level   *Wilson's = ↓ ceruloplasmin*
(E) Serum iron, total iron-binding capacity, and ferritin levels

Knowledge of incubation periods and portals of entry of the five identified hepatitides is critical for prognosticating and preventing the spread of cases. For Questions 16 through 20, match the numbered hepatitis types with the lettered modes of transmission.

16 Hepatitis A   *Fecal oral, ∅ complications*

17 Hepatitis B   *high sex risk*

18 Hepatitis C   *very high risk of chronic hep ↓ sex risk*

19 Hepatitis D   *Needs Hep B*

20 Hepatitis E   *Fecal oral, 3rd Trimester*

(A) Transmitted by body fluids other than gastrointestinal; carries high risk of chronic hepatitis and high risk of sexual transmission
(B) Transmitted mainly by fecal–oral contamination; fraught with no complications except in third-trimester pregnancy
(C) May be transmitted by percutaneous or nonpercutaneous means; requires presence of hepatitis B to procreate
(D) Transmitted by body fluids other than gastrointestinal; carries very high risk of chronic hepatitis; prominent in transfusion-induced hepatitis but risk of sexual and accidental needle-stick transmission is relatively low
(E) Transmitted mainly by fecal–oral contamination; fraught with no complications

Examination Answers

1. The answer is B. When the pulse rate drops by about 25%, or generally, 55–56 BPM, the therapeutic goal has been reached for reduction of the chances of bleeding from esophageal varices in a case with cirrhosis. Thus, reduction of cardiac output appears to be the determining factor in such prevention. None of the other objectives can be reached through the use of beta-adrenergic blocking agents, and, of course, elevation of blood pressure carries no saving grace.

2. The answer is A. Glucocorticoid toxicity is outranked by the other choices as a cause of steatohepatosis. The main causes are, in descending order, alcoholic liver disease and obesity roughly 28% each; diabetes and hypertriglyceridemia, about 14% each; the remaining 15% to 16% are distributed among the treating drugs, glucocorticoids, amiodarone, diltiazem, tamoxifen, and others; Cushing syndrome, hypopituitarism, obstructive sleep apnea, and so on. Virtually all obese alcoholics have fatty livers. As the metabolic syndrome consists of prediabetes, diabetes, and dyslipidemia (in addition to hypertension), differentiation among those main causes must necessarily be somewhat arbitrary. In any event, the top four sources of steatohepatosis are major health conditions and must be ruled out forthwith after the finding of fatty liver.

3. The answer is C. 10 g (actually 9.8 g or 140 mg/kg) is defined as the single toxic dose of acetaminophen. This is based on the classic estimate of average human size 70 kg person, which is likely outdated, so that the average toxic single dose may be higher. Be that it may, this is astounding considering that the therapeutic dose (single dose as opposed to *daily dosage*) range is 10 to 15 mg/kg, which with five doses or 75 mg/kg amounts to more than 5 g per day in a 70-kg person. Considering that patients with nonlethal illnesses such as chronic low back pain are not infrequently prescribed hydrocodone 5 mg/acetaminophen 500 mg (e.g., Vicodin 5/500) 2 pills 4 times per day, thus may reach the maximum safe dosage daily for extended periods. For smaller people, such as women, the toxic dosage will be lower.

4. The answer is E. HBsAg positive, anti-HBc positive, IgM anti HBc negative, anti-HBs negative denote the carrier with chronic infection. Such a patient is probably a candidate interferon therapy. The other choices have the following meanings: (A) HBsAg negative, anti-HBc negative, anti-HBs negative denotes the unexposed state, a candidate for vaccination; (B) HBsAg negative, anti-HBc positive, anti-HBs negative yields multiple interpretations; (C) HBsAg negative, anti-HBc negative or positive, anti-HBs positive denotes immune status; (D) HBsAg positive, anti-HBc positive, IgM anti-HBc positive, anti-HBs negative denotes the acutely infected state; HBsAg negative, anti-HBc negative, anti-HBs negative signifies susceptibility to hepatitis B because both types of antibody are absent while surface antigen is absent as well. HBsAg negative, anti-HBc negative, anti-HBs positive signifies immunity through HB vaccination (the vaccine functions to produce antibodies to surface antigen but not to core antigen). HBsAg positive, anti-HBc positive, IgM anti-HBc negative, anti-HBs negative signifies chronic infection (core antibodies present, IgM antibodies absent but surface antigen also present). HBsAg positive, anti-HBc positive, IgM anti-HBc negative, anti-HBs negative signifies chronic HB infection.

Finally, not among the choices, HBsAg negative, anti-HBc positive, anti-HBs negative may have four interpretations: (a) patient may be recovering from acute infection; (b) patient may be distantly immune (testing may miss very low levels of anti-HBs); (c) patient may be susceptible but exhibit a false-positive anti-HBs; and (d) there may be undetectable levels of HBsAg and the patient a carrier.

5. The answer is C. HBeAg correlates with a high degree of viral replication. Conversely, HBe antibody correlates with a low rate of replication. HBV DNA also correlates with replication and is used to monitor response to therapy for HPV infection, especially in cases where there has occurred an HBeAg mutant.

6. The answer is D. The pattern test results given show no evidence of hepatocellular disease, absence of HBsAg, and positivity of HBc and HBs antibodies, indicating immunity from past infection. No precautions are indicated regarding hepatitis B. Recombinant alpha-2b is employed in chronic active hepatitis.

7. The answer is B. Alpha-fetal protein is a marker for hepatoma (hepatocellular carcinoma). Carcinoembryonic antigen is best used for follow-up of progress for treated colorectal carcinoma; the *BRCA1* gene is a marker for inherited tendency for breast cancer; human chorionic gonadotropin is a marker found in choriocarcinoma and testicular cancer; prostate-specific antigen is a marker for follow-up of prostate cancer. Not any of these markers are perfectly specific, and thus, they are best applied for following the progress of the cancer once diagnosed and treated.

8. The answer is D. Ultrasound of the liver should not be done until the factors included in the other choices have been investigated as well as several others. The latter include presence of uncontrolled diabetes, obesity, and dyslipidemia. Every drug on which a patient has been placed should be perused for possibilities of elevation of liver enzymes, and the list is too long to address in this work. Chronic hepatitides B and C are common. Hemochromatosis is much more common than appreciated decades ago. If the ALT is twice that of the AST, then alcoholism should be suspected. However, that relationship is neither quite sensitive nor specific.

9. The answer is C. Ultrasound. Conjugated bilirubinemia (direct-acting bilirubin), when in the absence of unconjugated bilirubin, indicates extrahepatic obstructive jaundice. Ultrasound is more likely to elucidate the cause than computed tomography, the latter generally giving more information regarding the parenchyma of the liver and of the pancreas. The hepatitides cause more often a mixed picture of elevations of both conjugated and unconjugated bilirubin. Plain x-rays are seldom helpful in jaundice. ALT and AST levels may be mildly elevated in obstructive jaundice, but neither confirms nor rules out obstruction; if obstruction is present, no anatomic diagnosis will be made from the test.

10. The answer is D. PBC occurs more often in women than men by a ratio of roughly 4 or 5:1. Steatorrhea is typical, as are xanthelasmas and xanthomas. Patients are asymptomatic for years before beginning complaints of pruritus, a common symptom of biliary obstruction. Along the way, first alkaline phosphatase and then conjugated bilirubin become elevated. Antimitochondrial antibodies are positive in 95% of cases, although the test is not adequately specific. Alcoholic cirrhosis is not characterized by the skin manifestations alluded to and is not characterized by the symptoms of biliary obstruction from early on, as is PBC. Choledocholithiasis, although a cause of biliary obstruction, is neither a slowly progressive process nor insidious in onset. The same can be said for carcinoma of the pancreas. The latter is noted for "painless jaundice" with a palpable gallbladder (the Courvoisier sign). Gilbert disease (or syndrome) is a mild condition in which there is an inherited tendency for intermittent elevation of unconjugated bilirubin levels.

11. The answer is B. Hepatitis B is more transmissible than hepatitis C, although hepatitis C is significantly more likely to cause chronic hepatitis, once passed (75%), cirrhosis (20% within 20 years), and hepatocellular carcinoma (1% to 4% per year). Hepatitis A never becomes chronic nor does it result in a carrier state, nor does hepatitis E. Hepatitis D occurs only in concert with hepatitis B.

12. The answer is E. The answer is E. The combination of elevated GGT and normal alkaline phosphatase strongly suggests active drinking. The increased red cell volume

was eye-catching, and alcoholism is associated with macrocytosis, due to nutritional deficiency. The elevation of AST out of proportion to ALT (typically 2:1) is suggestive of alcoholic hepatitis, and a lower than expected BUN may be found in active alcoholism. Examining for the stigmata of cirrhosis is appropriate as well (spider angiomata, palmar erythema, testicular atrophy, distended flank veins, etc.). Gallbladder ultrasound study is not indicated in the absence of abdominal pain and biliary obstruction. Approximately 15% of patients with laboratory findings from constant drinking will develop cirrhosis even though one-third will have fatty liver at one time or another. Other tests and procedures can be deferred to results of further inquiry, and empiric response to alcohol abstention is known.

13. The answer is B. PSC is associated with ulcerative colitis or Crohn colitis in two-thirds of cases, although only 1% to 4% of ulcerative colitis cases have coexisting PSC. As in PBC, pruritus and incidental findings of elevated alkaline phosphatase may precede clinical jaundice. The diagnosis is confirmed by endoscopic retrograde cholangiography, which usually shows evidence of extrahepatic ductal inflammatory injury or liver biopsy. PSC is most commonly found in men more so than women at a ratio of 1.5 to 2:1 between the ages of 20 and 30 years. The diagnosis is also confirmed by histopathology in liver biopsy. PSC is commonly complicated by bacterial ascending cholangitis. PBC is noted for xanthomas and xanthelasmas and is found in women between the ages of 40 and 60 years (see Question 8 and explanation). Choledocholithiasis is unlikely in the absence of colic and gallstones in the gallbladder. Steatohepatosis (fatty liver) is common in many asymptomatic conditions such as diabetes, morbid obesity, and alcoholism and in itself would not cause the symptoms in the vignette. Viral hepatitis is not considered during the acute phase without elevations of AST and ALT that are 50 to 100 times normal.

14. The answer is E. Autoimmune hepatitis is initially a diagnosis of exclusion in a patient who manifests evidence of acute, subacute, or chronic hepatitis without evidence of viral, chemical, infectious, or pharmacological causation. Presence of SMA and ANA as well as other autoimmune diseases (e.g., thyroiditis in this case) lends further circumstantial evidence of autoimmune disease. PSC is less likely because of the absence of colitis.

15. The answer is D. A ceruloplasmin level that is lower than normal may be indicative of Wilson disease. The disease is characterized by copper overload, damaging the liver and kidneys and resulting in central nervous system abnormalities, most commonly depression. SMA and ANA may be connected with autoimmune hepatitis, but the patient is younger than expected for that condition. Iron studies would be appropriate for diagnosis of hemochromatosis, but patients with that disease do not become symptomatic until late middle age for men and later still for women.

16. The answer is E. Hepatitis A is transmitted mainly by fecal–oral contamination; it generally risks no complications.

17. The answer is A. Hepatitis B is transmitted by body fluids other than gastrointestinal; it carries high risk of chronic hepatitis and sexual transmission.

18. The answer is D. Hepatitis C is transmitted by body fluids other than gastrointestinal; it carries a very high risk of chronic hepatitis; it is prominent in transfusion-induced hepatitis, but there is less risk of sexual and accidental needle-stick transmission (4% chance). Approximately 50% of cases progress to chronic hepatitis.

19. The answer is C. Hepatitis D may be transmitted by percutaneous or nonpercutaneous means; it requires presence of hepatitis B to procreate.

20. The answer is B. Hepatitis E is transmitted mainly by fecal–oral contamination; it is fraught with no complications except in third-trimester pregnancy.

References

Giboney PT. Mildly elevated liver transaminase levels in the asymptomatic patient. *Am Fam Physician.* 2005; 71:1105–1110.

Lin KW, Kirchner JT. Hepatitis B. *Am Fam Physician.* 2004; 69: 75–82, 86.

McPhee SJ, Papadakis MA. *Current Medical Diagnosis and Treatment 2010*, 49th ed. New York/Chicago: McGraw-Hill; 2010.

Nidiry JJ. Diseases of the liver. In: Rudy DR, Kurowski K, eds. *Family Medicine: House Officer Series.* Baltimore: Williams & Wilkins; 1997:255–268.

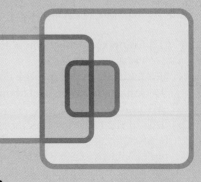

SECTION VII

Urology and Nephrology in Primary Care

chapter 17

Problems of the Urinary Tract

Examination questions: *Unless instructed otherwise, choose the ONE lettered answer or completion that is BEST in each case.*

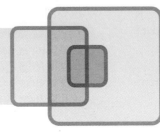 A 60-year-old multifarous, 10-year postmenopausal woman complains of loss of urine while coughing and laughing, increasing over the past several months to the point that she has taken to stop and cross her legs to avoid loss of urine at those times. Pelvic examination shows a first degree urethrocele and involuntary passage of urine when she bears down. Each of the following is acceptable conservative therapy except for which one?

(A) Intermittent catheterization
(B) Urecholine
(C) Imipramine
(D) Metoclopramide
(E) Pseudoephedrine

2 A 35-year-old woman enters your office with complaints of fever, malaise, and vague abdominal discomfort. She denies gastrointestinal symptoms, cough, coryza, and pain in specific areas. A urinalysis reveals positive dip tests for leukocyte esterase, nitrite, and occult blood and a white blood cell (WBC) count of 10 to 15 WBCs/high-power fields. She has never had a urinary tract infection (UTI) in the past. Before examining her, you know with 98% certainty that the patient has which of the following diagnoses?

(A) Cystitis
(B) Ureterolithiasis
(C) Bladder cancer
(D) Pyelonephritis
(E) Trigonitis

3 Which of the following is the organism most likely to be grown and isolated in pyelonephritis?

(A) *Escherichia coli*
(B) *Staphylococcus saprophyticus*
(C) Proteus organisms
(D) Klebsiella organisms
(E) Enterococci

4 In a new case of pyelonephritis in an adult, diagnosed on the basis of clinical, historical, and physical evidence, which of the following should be carried out next?

(A) Intravenous urogram
(B) Culture and sensitivity of the urine
(C) Initiation of a course of a fluoroquinolone antibiotic

(D) Computed tomography scan of the kidneys and upper urinary tracts

(E) Initiation of therapy with double-strength sulfamethoxazole/trimethoprim (e.g., Bactrim)

5 Each of the following conditions or findings would be an indication for hospitalization of an adult with pyelonephritis except which?

(A) Costovertebral angle tenderness
(B) Lack of a responsible other adult in the home
(C) Immunocompromised state (e.g., cancer chemotherapy)
(D) Persistent nausea and vomiting
(E) Discovery of an anatomical basis for the pyelonephritis (e.g., bifid ureter)

6 In which of the following categories of patients is screening for asymptomatic bacteriuria the standard of care?

(A) Sexually active woman
(B) Sexually active woman with history of recurrent UTIs
(C) Adult man with history of prostatitis
(D) Anyone with a history of pyelonephritis
(E) Pregnant woman

7 You are consulted by a 27-year-old woman who has become sexually active over the past 3 years and had five episodes of cystitis within the last year. She has otherwise been in good health and is not taking medication. Which of the following mechanisms is most likely responsible for the recurrences?

(A) A cystocele
(B) Bifid ureters
(C) A bladder diverticulum
(D) Hydronephrosis
(E) Vaginal seeding by coliform bacteria

8 You are viewing a "KUB" (plain abdominal) x-ray film of a 45-year-old woman who has a history of left bifid ureter and pyelonephritis at least once. You see an opacity that fills and outlines the pelvis of the left kidney. What is the basis and content of this calcification?

(A) Uric acid in hyperuricemia
(B) Calcium oxalate from chronic infection
(C) Calcium oxalate from hypercalciuria
(D) Magnesium ammonium phosphate from urease-producing organisms
(E) Cysteine caused by hypercysteinuria

9 Which of the following bacterial uropathogens is most commonly associated with the stone formation referred in Question 8?

(A) *E. coli*
(B) *S. saprophyticus*
(C) *Proteus mirabilis*
(D) Enterococci
(E) *Chlamydia trachomatis*

10 A 24-year-old man complains of dysuria and a slight discharge. He was alarmed when he noticed some blood at the beginning of the urinary stream. A urinalysis from split specimens (beginning, middle, and terminal stream) confirms microscopic and chemical evidence of blood in the beginning stream, less in the midstream, and none in the terminal stream. Which of the following is the likely site of the hematuria?

(A) Anterior urethra
(B) Bladder neck
(C) Bladder
(D) Ureter
(E) Kidney

11 A 55-year-old woman who underwent a uterine suspension operation for stress incontinence developed cystitis the day after surgery, having had a Foley catheter inserted the day before surgery. Which is the most likely causative organism?

(A) *Pseudomonas aeruginosa*
(B) *S. saprophyticus*
(C) *E. coli*
(D) Enterococci
(E) *Staphylococcus epidermidis*

12 A 49-year-old woman notes bloody urine recurring intermittently during the last several weeks. She denies abdominal pain, dysuria, and frequency. Vital signs are normal, including body temperature. Physical examination is not remarkable and included deep palpation in the abdominal flanks and the suprapubic area. The urinalysis shows only red blood cells with WBCs in proportion to what one should expect in the peripheral blood. Which of the following is the best first working diagnosis?

(A) Ureterolithiasis
(B) Hemorrhagic cystitis
(C) Urinary tract carcinoma → *painless hematuria*
(D) Pyelonephritis
(E) Vaginitis

13 Which of the following is correct regarding the presence of leukocyte esterase in a urinalysis dip test?

(A) Positive test indicates definite presence of leukocytes.

(B) Negative test rules out presence of leukocytes.

(C) Positive test indicates presence of organisms that reduce nitrate to nitrite.

(D) Positive test is suggestive of bacteria.

(E) Positive test indicates presence of blood.

14 You are re-evaluating a 3-year-old girl with cystitis whom you are treating for the second time within 6 months. She has been on amoxicillin for 7 days with complete resolution of her symptoms. Which of the following listed studies would be most likely to demonstrate the most common urinary tract abnormality that is associated with a UTI in this age group?

(A) Radionuclide cystogram

(B) Renal ultrasound

(C) Cystoscopy

(D) Intravenous pyelogram

(E) Urodynamic study

15 Each of the following statements is true regarding UTIs in boys and girls, except for which one?

(A) Girls are more prone to UTIs than boys at all ages.

(B) Girls may be allowed to have one bout of uncomplicated lower UTI without an evaluation for anatomic urinary tract abnormalities.

(C) The onset of sexual activity in females may give rise to UTIs in females aside from sexually transmitted disease.

(D) The first UTI in boy is an indication for evaluation for anatomic abnormalities.

(E) Uncircumcised male infants are prone to UTIs.

16 Which of the following is the most powerful risk factor for bladder cancer in today's western society?

(A) Schistosoma haematobium infection

(B) Cigarette smoking

(C) Chemical dyes

(D) Aromatic amines

(E) Alcoholism

Examination Answers

1. The answer is D. Metoclopramide, the one choice that would not be appropriate in the treatment of stress incontinence. The α_1 adrenergic agonists pseudoephedrine and phenylpropanolamine stimulate the bladder neck and proximal urethra, hence sphincter tone. The tricyclics such as imipramine have both α_1 adrenergic agonist effects and anticholinergic activity, the latter reducing bladder tone. Clean intermittent catheterization has a place with both stress incontinence and hypotonic bladder.

2. The answer is D. A patient with fever, pyuria, and suggestions of systemic illness or symptoms more specific for upper tract involvement has a 98% chance of having pyelonephritis. Chances are quite good, but not certain, that upon examination she will manifest definite costovertebral angle tenderness. Cystitis usually presents with symptoms of frequency and dysuria. Urolithiasis manifests colicky lateralizing pain, at least when the stone is moving. Bladder cancer and hypernephroma (renal cell carcinoma) are notorious for painless hematuria with no particular pyuria. Trigonitis is a syndrome encountered in mature females consisting of irritative bladder symptoms that are out of proportion to clinical findings.

3. The answer is A. *E. coli* is the cause of 88% of cases of uncomplicated pyelonephritis (e.g., cases in nonelderly individuals, nonrecurrent cases, cases with the absence of diabetes mellitus, and cases without known anatomical bases for recurrence, without indwelling catheters, and without clinical sepsis). Diabetics tend to have UTIs caused by Klebsiella, Enterobacter, Clostridium, or Candida organisms. Other complicated cases of pyelonephritis also involve Pseudomonas but usually not Candida organisms. Immunosuppressed patients tend to develop subclinical pyelonephritis caused by nonenteric, aerobic Gram-negative rods and Candida organisms.

4. The answer is B. With the suspicion of pyelonephritis, treatment of this serious infection comes first. Before antibacterial therapy can be started, a culture and sensitivity must be obtained to avoid wasting precious time in treating with ineffective anti-infectious agents while risking sterilizing the urine and blood for culture and sensitivity after the fact. The fluoroquinolones are a good first choice while one is awaiting the culture results; sulfamethoxazole/trimethoprim, being bacteriostatic as opposed to bacteriocidal, would be a poor choice with suspected pyelonephritis. The diagnostic studies mentioned are important but should take place after therapy is underway and the infection is abating.

5. The answer is A. Costovertebral angle tenderness in an uncomplicated case is not an indication for hospitalization within itself. However, each of the other factors mentioned are such indications. Others are outpatient treatment failure, sepsis or suspected sepsis, age >60 years, inadequate access to follow-up care, and uncertainty of diagnosis.

6. The answer is E. Pregnant women who are between 12 and 16 weeks gestation, if tested by urine culture (rather than urinalysis), will have significantly fewer UTIs, as well as a lower risk of low birth weight babies and of preterm delivery. In no other category, culture of asymptomatic patients is supported by evidence at this time.

7. The answer is E. Vaginal lactobacillus has been replaced with rectal coliform bacteria. The coliform bacteria now in the vagina and introitus can easily ascend through the urethra into the bladder. The absence of lactobacillus raises vaginal pH and creates a more favorable vaginal and periurethral environment for these bacteria. Only about 1% of adult women (nongeriatric) with recurrent cystitis have an identifiable anatomic abnormality. The conditions that predispose a woman to this development include sexual activity without voiding both before and afterward; entrapping clothing (more often resulting in Candida infection but leading also to coliform vaginal inoculation); wiping from anus forward after voiding instead of from the vaginal opening backward; voiding without adequately spreading the knees (caused by inadequate lowering of tight underwear); and occasionally changing hormone status, as in inauguration of contraceptive medication. Oral contraceptives, for example, increase in vaginal secretions, providing a culture medium for bacteria and contamination of clothing near the anal orifice. All people with recurrent UTIs should take in more water and other fluids than otherwise inclined.

8. The answer is D, magnesium ammonium phosphate from urease-producing organisms. These are called struvite stones, and insofar as they become molded by the calyceal collecting system, they are often referred to as "staghorn" calculi.

9. The answer is C. *P. mirabilis* is associated with struvite stone formation, as are Pseudomonas, Providencia, and, less commonly, Klebsiella, Staphylococcus, and Mycoplasma organisms. These organisms commonly produce a urease, which causes the hydrolysis of urea to ammonia and carbon dioxide. The result is an alkaline urine, which is more conducive to struvite stone formation.

10. The answer is A. The anterior urethra of the penis is likely the cause of the hematuria and, in this case, an infection. This could be either gonorrhea or chlamydia. The split specimen results would be similar in the case of urethral trauma as in vigorous sexual activity. Hematuria found through all three specimens, total hematuria, points toward bladder or kidney for the cause. Terminal hematuria suggests bladder neck, prostate, or trigon involvement.

11. The answer is C, *E. coli*. In complicated UTIs (those acquired in anatomically or functionally abnormal tracts or with suspected resistant organisms), the percentage of cases of cystitis caused by *E. coli* drops to about 35%, but it remains the most prevalent responsible organism.

12. The answer is C. Although in a given clinical setting painless hematuria cancer may not pose even a majority probability of cancer, because of the potentially life-threatening nature of the cancers, painless hematuria must be considered to be urinary tract carcinoma until proven otherwise. The cancers are generally transitional cell carcinomas of the bladder or renal cell carcinoma (in the past often called hypernephroma). Occasionally the lesion may be so small as to be missed grossly. Therefore, studies of urine such as cytology or other chemical evaluation of tumor cell by-products are necessary and must be repeated as long as the cause of painless hematuria, particularly microscopic hematuria, remains unexplained. If hematuria persists and nothing is found grossly, the patient must be monitored every 6 months. Hemorrhagic cystitis is common in women, usually younger than the woman presented in the vignette, and is always characterized by a rapid onset and accompanied by irritative symptoms (frequency and dysuria). Urolithiasis is in the differential diagnosis and must eventually be ruled out but is rarely unaccompanied by lateralized colicky pain. Pyelonephritis rarely occurs without pain or at least flank or costovertebral tenderness (e.g., in chronic cases), and urinalysis would show pyuria rather than microscopic or gross blood.

13. The answer is D. A positive test for leukocyte esterase is suggestive, but not diagnostic, of bacteria. To be sure, the inference is based on the presumed presence of leukocytes (WBCs). Leukocyte esterase is an enzyme elaborated by WBCs. However, its sensitivity is compromised by the false negatives that can be produced by high specific gravity of the urine, glycosuria, presence of urobilinogen, and medications including rifampin and ascorbic acid. Furthermore, false positives are produced by specimen contamination. There is a separate dip test for organisms that reduce nitrate to nitrite. They include many Gram-negative bacteria but not all. The sensitivity of the nitrite test is only 30%.

14. The answer is A, Radionuclide cystogram. Vesicoureteral reflex is the most likely urinary tract abnormality in this age group and setting. A voiding cystourethrogram is the most common initial diagnostic tool but is not used for follow-up because of the radiation exposure. A radionuclide study for reflux involves less radiation exposure and appears to be more sensitive once the fact of reflux is established. Vesicoureteral reflux is most often secondary to UTI in women and as such is reversible with therapy. In both sexes, anatomic abnormalities, such as a short intramural ureteral segment, preclude a functional valve effect. With bladder distention the segment fails to shut off retrograde flow of urine with distention, leading to retrograde spread of infection. Females' incidence and prevalence are significantly greater than males'. However, in males that mechanism accounts for the vast majority of reflux and upper genitourinary tract spread of infection.

15. The answer is A. This statement is wrong. Male infants have a greater incidence of UTIs as a group than female infants do. A significant portion of this excess morbidity, but not enough to account for it alone, is attributed to noncircumcised male infants; thus, Choice E is a correct statement. All other statements are true. Male children over the age of infancy who have a single UTI should be evaluated for anatomic abnormalities. Female children, especially those over the age of 5 years, may be allowed at least one UTI without such evaluation.

16. The answer is B. Cigarette smoking is easily the strongest risk factor for bladder cancer in western society that is found in male:females 2:1. Each of the others mentioned is a risk factor, stronger in different times and places, except that alcohol is not mentioned as a ranking factor.

References

Family Medicine Board Review 2009. May 3–10, 2009. Kansas City, Missouri.

Kurowski K. Urinary tract infections. In: Rudy DR, Kurowski K, eds. *Family Medicine: House Officer Series*. Baltimore, MD: Williams & Wilkins; 1997:269–284.

Ramakrishnan K, Scheid DC. Diagnosis and management of acute pyelonephritis. *Am Fam Physician*. 2005; 71:933–942.

Sharma S, Ksheersagar P, Sharma P. Diagnosis and treatment of bladder cancer. *Am Fam Physician*. 2009; 80(7):717–723.

Stoller ML, Carroll PR. Urology. In: Tierney LM, McPhee SJ, Papadakis MA, eds. *Current Medical Diagnosis and Treatment,* 43rd ed. New York: McGraw-Hill/Appleton & Lange; 2004:899–940.

U.S. Preventive Service Task Force. *Guide to Clinical Preventive Services,* 2nd ed. Washington, DC: Office of Disease Prevention and Health Promotion; 1996.

chapter **18**

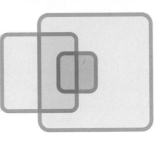

Nephrology

Examination questions: *Unless instructed otherwise, choose the ONE lettered answer or completion that is BEST in each case.*

1 A new patient enters a practice complaining of malaise over a period of 10 days. The chemical profile and hemogram stand out in the finding of a serum creatinine of 3.0 mg/dL and blood urea nitrogen (BUN) 60 mg/dL. In taking a medical history, the doctor is alert to reversible causes of acute renal failure (ARF). Each of the following causes of ARF is reversible except for which one?

(A) Fluid depletion
(B) Toxic medications
(C) Loop diuretics
(D) Arteriolonephrosclerosis
(E) Radiographic contrast media

2 The preceding patient has a blood pressure (BP) of 128/78, takes no long-term medications, has no history of diabetes, and has a random blood sugar of 95 mg/dL. The urinalysis showed a few hyaline casts plus significant number of red blood cells per high-power field (HPF) and a specific gravity of 1.010. In referring to a nephrologist, the primary doctor has in mind a possible renal biopsy. Each of the following could be an indication for renal biopsy except for which one?

(A) Hematuria with glomerular filtration rate (GFR) <30 mL/minute
(B) Proteinuria above 1 to 2 g/24 hours
(C) Chronic renal failure (CRF) with large kidneys
(D) ARF of unknown cause
(E) Creatinine and BUN in uremic levels (see text of previous question) with longstanding diabetes and poorly controlled hypertension

3 Each of the following may retard the rate of progression of chronic renal disease except for which one?

(A) Statin drugs
(B) Low-protein diet
(C) Control of hypertension
(D) Control of diabetes
(E) Metformin 500 mg bid

4 A 25-year-old Caucasian man had experienced an upper respiratory infection in the past 10 days and now complains of dyspnea, cough, and hemoptysis. A routine complete blood count (CBC) shows hemoglobin 8 g/dL, mean cell volume 75 μm^3 (normal 80 to 96 μm^3); urinalysis showing microscopic hematuria with misshapen red cells and red cell casts. Serum creatinine is elevated at 2.8 mg/dL. Sputum examination shows hemosiderin-laden macrophages. Which of the following laboratory studies is most likely to lead to the diagnosis of this condition?

(A) Antineutrophil cytoplasmic antibody (ANCA)
(B) Antiglomerular membrane antibodies
(C) BUN
(D) Antistreptolysin O antibodies (ASO)
(E) Fasting blood sugar (FBS)

5 Your 45-year-old type II diabetic weighs 240 lb (108.72 kg) at a height of 5 ft 10 in. (1.77 m). You have treated him with 500 mg of metformin thrice daily and 10 mg of glyburide twice daily. His glycohemoglobin this week was measured at 8%. A 24-hour urine specimen reveals 250 mg of albumen. Which of the following is the chief significance of this finding?

(A) It constitutes microalbuminuria.
(B) It is a normal finding.
(C) It indicates nephrotic syndrome.
(D) It is presumptive of pyelonephritis.
(E) It indicates an evaluation for cancer.

6 Which of the following pharmaceutical class protects against decline in renal function in both diabetic and hypertensive individuals, independent of direct effects on either blood sugar or BP control?

(A) Nonselective beta-adrenergic blocking agents
(B) Beta-2 selective adrenergic blocking agents
(C) Calcium channel blocking agents
(D) Angiotensin-converting enzyme inhibitors (ACEIs)
(E) Alpha-adrenergic blocking agents

7 Which of the following is the mechanism for development of hyperparathyroidism in renal failure?

(A) Failure to retain calcium in the kidneys

(B) Increased catabolism of osteoid matrix in cancellous bone

(C) Failure of absorption of calcium in the gastrointestinal tract

(D) Faulty conversion of 25-hydroxy vitamin D, or 25(OH)D, to vitamin D_3, or 25(OH)2D

(E) Renal retention of phosphates

8 A 45-year-old African-American man has been treated by you for cardiomyopathy and has had one significant bout of congestive heart failure. He is 50% overweight. Now he has become diabetic. You find on urinalysis an albumen-to-creatinine ratio of 200 mg of albumen to 1 g of creatinine (normal is <17 mg to 250 mg). Which of the following laboratory studies gives the most accurate measure of renal *function*?

(A) BUN

(B) Serum creatinine

(C) Creatinine clearance

(D) Urinalysis

(E) 24-hour measurement of urinary protein and creatinine

9 Renal failure may be caused by diabetes and hypertension in about two-thirds of the cases. Regardless of causation, as renal failure progresses and BUN and creatinine rise in the blood, anemia develops. Which of the following mechanisms accounts for the anemia associated with CRF?

(A) Iron deficiency

(B) Hemolysis

(C) Hypovitaminosis B_{12}

(D) Folic acid deficiency

(E) Decreased production of erythropoietin

10 You are considering ancillary imaging studies on your 46-year-old male patient who has had gross and microscopic hematuria over a 1-week period. A helical computed tomography (CT) scan without contrast shows no evidence of stone. Therefore, other causes for hematuria, including cancer, must be considered. Each of the following constitutes a relative or absolute contraindication for repeating the CT scan with contrast, except for which one?

(A) Multiple myeloma

(B) Diabetes with serum creatinine level >2 mg/dL

(C) CRF with creatinine level >5 mg/dL

(D) Hypovolemia with BUN level of 45 mg/dL (normal level is 10 to 20 mg/dL), creatinine level of 1.5 mg/dL (normal level is ≤1.4 mg/dL)

(E) Suspected renal cell carcinoma *great for contrast study*

11 In an adult patient, if there were a contraindication to the use of contrast materials and a neoplasm were suspected, which of the following would be the most likely choice of ancillary study to rule out neoplasm?

(A) Magnetic resonance imaging

(B) CT scan without contrast

(C) Plain abdominal x-ray

(D) Renal arteriography

(E) Venography

12 Which of the following is the precipitating mechanism of injury that leads to ARF after misguided use of a contrast medium in radiographic imaging?

(A) Ischemia

(B) Direct toxicity

(C) Hypoxia

(D) Autoimmunity

(E) Dehydration

13 A 55-year-old white man enters your practice with a complaint of flank pains that have occurred on either side from time to time. He says that he was treated in another city for hypertension over several years. He says he has had positive tests for blood in his urine in the past but that no cause had ever been found. BUN level is elevated at 40 mg/dL (normal is ≤20 mg/dL) and creatinine is 1.8 mg/dL. A CBC is normal. Examination of the abdomen reveals a mass deep in each flank. Which of the following most likely accounts for the clinical picture presented?

(A) Carcinoma of the bladder

(B) Renal cell carcinoma

(C) Pancreatic cysts

(D) Polycystic kidneys

(E) Colorectal cancer

14 A patient who is new to you is a 46-year-old white woman who complains of headaches over the past 3 days and suspects it may be due to her BP. Her BP is 230/120. Each of the following findings constitutes a diagnosis of malignant hypertension except for which one?

(A) Rising BUN and creatinine levels

(B) Onset of dyspnea and orthopnea in the past 1 to 3 days

(C) A finding of papilledema

(D) Systolic BP >220 mm Hg

(E) Mental confusion

15 A 45-year-old white man has type II diabetes and weighs 245 lb (111 kg) at a height of 5 ft 11 in. (1.8 m), despite your efforts to exhort him to lose weight over the previous 2 years. However, for the past 3 months, he has complained of low-grade fever, abdominal discomfort, and lack of appetite. During this period, he has had a striking weight loss, amounting to 40 lb (18.12 kg). The diabetes has now virtually disappeared so far as clinical evidence exists. However, you cannot explain the weight loss, anorexia, and abdominal pain. Suspecting carcinoma of the pancreas, you ordered a CT scan of the abdomen with and without contrast. The result showed a mass involving the right kidney. Blood studies for liver function, including alkaline phosphatase, and CBC as well as bone scan reveal no abnormalities. Within 3 weeks after right nephrectomy for renal cell carcinoma, the patient's appetite had returned and he began to gain weight. Which of the following most likely explains the foregoing clinical picture?

(A) Metastases from renal cell carcinoma have caused anorexia and abdominal pain.
(B) The mass was misdiagnosed as cancer, allowing full recovery following surgical removal.
(C) Metastases from renal cell carcinoma have become dormant.
(D) The renal cell carcinoma has entered a remission phase.
(E) The patient had suffered from a paraneoplastic syndrome.

16 Each of the following drugs may cause nephropathy, except for which one?

(A) Acetaminophen
(B) Aspirin
(C) Phenacetin
(D) Ibuprofen
(E) Naproxen

17 Which of the following pretreatment medication has been found to reduce the risk of creatinine elevation or renal failure when administered before injection of contrast medium in a case where such a study might be particularly critical?

(A) Acetylsalicylic acid
(B) Sulfasalazine
(C) Acetylcysteine
(D) Amoxicillin
(E) Furosemide

Examination Answers

1. The answer is D. Arteriolonephrosclerosis is the irreversible cause of ARF among the listed choices. Arteriolonephrosclerosis is late stage renal disease attributable to longstanding poorly controlled hypertension. Symptoms of malaise occur in ARF when the BUN rises to 50 to 60 mg/dL, and to be sure, irreversible ARF is a medical emergency to avert irreversible renal failure. In CRF, symptoms do not occur until the BUN approaches 100 mg/dL. Fluid depletion generally first shows a rising BUN out of proportion to the rise in creatinine, that is, the "prerenal" pattern. Normally, the BUN is found to be about 10 times the creatinine level. Obviously, this form of ARF is amenable to rapid fluid therapy. ARF due to toxic medications has been proven to be reversible with withdrawal of the drug in the vast majority of cases. Loop diuretics occasionally cause ARF that resembles and actually is fluid depletion in form. Contrast media are to be avoided stringently in the face of baseline elevated creatinine, but the ARF that may ensue can be avoided and treated by fluid therapy. ACE inhibitors and angiotensin converting enzyme receptor blockers may cause ARF but rarely and easily diagnosable early and reversed.

2. The answer is E. The patient in uremia with small "end-stage kidneys" is not a candidate for renal biopsy. Each of the other choices is an indication for renal biopsy on the basis of possible treatable and reversible causes.

3. The answer is E. Metformin, despite its benefit in control of type 2 diabetes, hence theoretically instrumental in preventing renal failure, is nephrotoxic in the presence of preexisting reduced renal function. Each of the others mentioned in the choices is helpful in the retardation of the advance of CRF.

4. The answer is B. Antiglomerular membrane antibodies (anti-AGB AB). The combination of glomerulonephritis and pulmonary hemorrhage along with anti-AGB AB antibodies defines Goodpasture disease. This a serious and potentially fatal disease whose treatment is best left to those who are experienced in critical care. In 90% of cases, anti-AGB AB antibodies are present. ANCAs are present in about 15%. Iron deficiency anemia is common, reflecting the significance of the blood loss through the lungs. While neither one is particularly specific, Goodpasture is the only acute autoimmune disease that involves both the kidneys and the lungs. Diabetes is not associated statistically. BUN and ASO are entirely nonspecific, albeit sensitive indicators of inflammation with autoimmune components.

5. The answer is A. The 24-hour urine specimen that shows 250 mg of albumen falls within the definition of microalbuminuria for a diabetic, which is 30 to 300 mg of albumen in 24 hours. Other, quick methods of detection of microalbuminuria include a urine spot albumen-specific dipstick finding of ≥3 mg/dL and spot urine albumen-to-creatinine ratio of 17 to 250 mg of albumen to 1 g of creatinine (men) or 25 to 355 mg of albumen to 1 g creatinine (women). Because small amounts of protein may appear in the urine for brief periods, microalbuminuria should be confirmed after a delay of 2 to 3 weeks. If proteinuria persists, the patient should be evaluated for kidney disease, with attention to diabetes, hypertension, and various causes of glomerular disease. Nephrotic syndrome is entirely different, foremost in that the definition of nephrotic syndrome is ≥3 g of total protein (both albumen and globulin) per 24-hour period.

6. The answer is D. ACEIs as well as angiotensin receptor blocking agents (ARBA) protect against renal damage by reducing the GFR per nephron. GFRs per unit number of surviving glomeruli increase as creatinine clearance decreases. An elevated GFR leads to proteinuria. Deterioration of renal function is retarded by control of either BP in hypertensive patients or blood sugar in diabetic patients (see discussion of Question 2). Thus, the other choices, insofar as they are antihypertensive agents, do serve to prevent loss of renal function to the extent that they succeed in control of BP. ACEIs and ARBAs are antihypertensive agents, particularly in patients whose hypertension is driven to a significant degree by the rennin–angiotensin system. Thus, ACEIs and ARBAs protect renal function in hypertensive patients in two ways and in diabetics solely through the effect to reduce the GFR.

7. The answer is E. When creatinine clearance falls to below 60 mL/minute, phosphates are retained and a relative hyperphosphatemia results. The reciprocal relationship between serum phosphates and serum calcium gives rise to hypocalcemia, to which the parathyroid glands respond by increasing the output of parathormone. Negative calcium balance is thus a part of the pathophysiology of CRF and results in a loss of bone density. Failure of calcium absorption occurs secondary to loss of estrogen support in menopause because of the loss of the parathormone-inhibiting effects of estrogen, relevant in Choices C and D but not in renal failure. The postmenopausal state is associated with hyperparathyroidism for a different reason, which in turn contributes to postmenopausal decrease in postmenopausal bone density.

8. The answer is C. Creatinine clearance is the measure of renal function. The stages of kidney disease are defined by creatinine clearance. For example, stage 2 is defined as "kidney damage" (e.g., abnormal urinalysis) with creatinine clearance of 60 to 89 mL/minute/1.73 m^2 (somewhat above 50% of normal renal function for a person under 40 years of age). At this stage, the parathyroid hormone levels begin to rise because of the renal retention of phosphates (as discussed earlier).

Renal failure, stage 3, is defined as creatinine clearance in the range of 30 to 59 mL/minute/1.73 m^2. Calcium absorption declines, leading to further secretion of parathormone; lipoprotein activity declines; left ventricular hypertrophy appears; and anemia develops. Stage 4 kidney disease is defined as creatinine clearance in the range of 15 to 29 mL/minute/1.73 m^2; end-stage disease shows <15 mL/minute/1.73 m^2. A completely accurate creatinine clearance requires a measurement of both 24-hour urine creatinine and serum creatinine levels. Serum creatinine does not begin to rise until renal function has fallen by about 50%. The urinalysis says nothing directly regarding the status of renal function.

9. The answer is E. Decreased production of erythropoietin accounts for the anemia specific to renal failure. Thus, the anemia is normochromic and normocytic. Iron deficiency produces a microcytic, hypochromic anemia, whereas both folic acid and B$_{12}$ deficiency cause a macrocytic anemia. The anemia that accompanies renal failure increases the progression of and the ultimate mortality that is due to end-stage kidney disease. Therefore, a critical part of the treatment of renal failure is the institution of exogenous erythropoietin. As implied in Question 6, hemoglobin should be followed as creatinine clearance falls below 60 mL/minute/1.73 m^2 and hematocrit falls to less than 30% to 35%, whereupon treatment with erythropoietin is started. Recombinant erythropoietin in the form of epoetin alfa is used clinically.

10. The answer is E. In and of itself, renal cell carcinoma is not a contraindication for contrast media in radiographic studies. In fact, because the contrast medium is filtered by the glomeruli and concentrated in the tables, a CT scan with contrast is an excellent modality for diagnosis of cysts and neoplasms. Serum creatinine >5 mg/dL is a contraindication for contrast media because of the danger of precipitating ARF. In diabetics, the tolerance level for serum creatinine is lowered to 2 mg/dL. Even prerenal azotemia (exemplified by the choice showing normal creatinine with elevated BUN) poses a risk for ARF in the presence of contrast medium. Neither glomerular disease nor renal cell carcinoma are contraindications for contrast in the absence of other contraindications.

11. The answer is A. Magnetic resonance imaging is an excellent tool for diagnosing neoplasm when contrast in CT scan or intravenous pyelogram is contraindicated. A CT scan without contrast, as implied in the discussion for

Question 8, is not useful in diagnosing neoplasms; certainly, a plain film is not useful either. Although arteriography and venography may be useful in evaluating masses, both require contrast.

12. The answer is B. Direct toxicity by contrast material in radiographic imaging is the proximate cause of ARF in the clinical setting presented. ARF in this case is due to acute tubular necrosis, the cause of 85% of cases of ARF. However, it is not likely to occur unless other causes of renal damage are present. The latter include any cause of ischemia, hypovolemia, or hypoxia. These are dehydration, preexisting diabetes, hypotension, sepsis, and prolonged anesthesia with vasodilating anesthetic agents. Other causes of direct nephrotoxicity and acute tubular necrosis include the presence of aminoglycosides (gentamicin the most, tobramycin the least potent in that regard); cyclosporine (used to prevent rejection of transplanted organs); various antineoplastic agents (e.g., cisplatin); and organic solvents and heavy metals (e.g., mercury, cadmium, and arsenic). Of cases of ARF, 15% of them are caused not by tubular necrosis but by interstitial nephritis. Causes of the latter are generally autoimmune related. A recently appreciated contrast medium renal toxicity is significantly more complex. It is now known that gadolinium employed as contrast medium in patients with GFR <30 mL/minute/1.73 m^2 can cause nephrogenic systemic fibrosis.

13. The answer is D. Hypertension, history of hematuria, and flank mass together are strongly suggestive of polycystic disease of the kidneys (PCDK). Although any presentation of hematuria of long duration demands evaluation for urinary tract neoplasm, most bladder tumors present with painless intermittent or persistent hematuria, with a small percentage manifesting irritative bladder symptoms (frequency or dysuria). Renal cell carcinoma is notorious for painless hematuria, sometimes over long periods before becoming diagnosable. However, neither of the aforementioned cancers present with bilateral masses. Pancreatic cysts may occur in conjunction with PCDK, as may hepatic and splenic cysts. Of patients with PCDK, 50% have hypertension, often preceding the polycystic manifestations; 50% of cases will progress to end-stage renal disease by the time the patient reaches the age of 60 years. Despite hematuria that may be significant, anemia is unusual because PCDK is associated with the production of erythropoietin.

14. The answer is D. Although a systolic BP >220, a diastolic BP >125, or both constitute a diagnosis of *accelerated* hypertension, which is an urgent medical state, the diagnosis of *malignant hypertension* requires these levels of BP in association with any of the other choices presented in the question. Accelerated hypertension is a medical emergency, requiring BP control to avoid development of malignant hypertension. Malignant hypertension is a more time-urgent emergency that carries 50% mortality if not treated.

15. The answer is E. The patient had suffered from a paraneoplastic syndrome associated with the renal cell carcinoma, for which the tumor is noted. In cases of paraneoplastic syndromes, the patient becomes ill and manifests symptoms related to a humeral manifestation of the primary tumor that causes systemic symptoms, unrelated to metastases. Renal cell carcinoma may be thus associated with symptoms experienced by the patient in the vignette as well as fever alone, erythrocytosis, thrombocytosis, coagulopathy, and amyloidosis.

16. The answer is A. Acetaminophen is the only analgesic among the choices given that it does not cause analgesic nephropathy. Aspirin, ibuprofen, and naproxen are all nonsteroidal anti-inflammatory drugs. In all cases, tubulointerstitial inflammation and papillary necrosis are found on pathologic examination.

17. The answer is C. Acetylcysteine (Mucomyst), 600 mg, orally twice 12 hours before and after a dye load, given before radiocontrast media along with infusion of 0.45% saline solution, has been found to result in a relative risk of elevation of creatinine of 0.11 to 0.18 and an absolute risk reduction of 19%. In a control group given 0.45% saline only, creatinine rose to 0.5 mg/dL in 9 of 42 control subjects.

References

Johnson CA, Levey AS, Corsh J, et al. Clinical practice guidelines for kidney disease in adults. Part I: Definition, disease stages, evaluation, treatment, and risk factors. *Am Fam Physician.* 2004; 70:869–876.

Johnson CA, Levey AS, Corsh J, et al. Clinical practice guidelines for kidney disease in adults. Part II: Glomerular filtration rate, proteinuria, and other markers. *Am Fam Physician.* 2004; 70:1091–1097.

Neeham ED. Management of acute renal failure. *Am Fam Physician.* 2005; 72:1739–1746.

Snively CS, Gutierez C. Chronic kidney disease: Prevention and treatment of complications. *Am Fam Physician.* 2004; 70:1921–1930.

Watnick S, Morrison G. Kidney. In: Tierney LM, McPhee SJ, Papadakis MA, eds. *Current Diagnosis and Treatment.* 43rd ed. New York: McGraw-Hill/Appleton & Lange; 2004:863–898.

chapter 19

Urological Problems Unique to Males

Examination questions: Unless instructed otherwise, choose the ONE lettered answer or completion that is BEST in each case.

1. At what age should a man of average risk for prostate carcinoma begin screening?

   (A) 35 years
   (B) 40 years
   (C) 50 years
   (D) 60 years
   (E) 70 years

2. Each of the following is a method of improving a screening method for carcinoma of the prostate *for the reason given* except for which one?

   (A) Measure bound to free prostate specific antigen (PSA) ratio to improve specificity
   (B) Increase intervals between PSA drawings to reduce cost and inconvenience
   (C) Lower the PSA cut-off to increase specificity
   (D) Determine the rate of increase of PSA to predict aggressiveness of the cancer
   (E) Lower PSA cut-offs for younger blacks to improve sensitivity

3. A 45-year-old white male complains of painless apparent red urine. He is a cigarette smoker with a 30-pack-year history, and he notices increased frequency of voiding and mild irritation. You decide to order a three glass analysis of his urine, that is, the first 3 mL in glass 1; the bulk of the voided urine in glass 2; and only the very last few mL in glass 3. Which of the following patterns of the three-glass urinalysis indicates a bladder source for the hematuria?

   (A) Positive test for blood in the first glass
   (B) Positive test for blood in the second glass
   (C) Positive test for blood in the third glass
   (D) Positive test for blood in all three glasses
   (E) Negative test for blood in all three glasses

4. In treating a 55-year-old man for erectile dysfunction which of the following constitutes an absolute contraindication in taking any of the three phosphodiesterase 5 inhibitors [sildenafil (Viagra), vardenafil (Levitra), and tadalafil (Cialis)].

   (A) A diagnosis of coronary artery disease
   (B) Hypertension
   (C) Diabetes
   (D) Benign prostatic hyperplasia
   (E) Taking nitrates

5. A 14-year-old boy has the rapid onset (<2 hours ago) of severe right testicular pain associated with right flank pain and nausea and vomiting. Upon examination the right testicle is riding higher than the left and is markedly tender within an edematous scrotum. Each of the following may be reasonably included in the differential diagnosis of this case, except for which one?

   (A) Epididymitis
   (B) Testicular trauma
   (C) Torsion of the testicle
   (D) Varicocele
   (E) Testicular cancer

6. Regarding the patient in Question 5, which of the following may yield the quickest office diagnosis?

   (A) Urinalysis
   (B) Complete blood count (include white blood cell count and differential)
   (C) Doppler stethoscope
   (D) Testicular technetium scan
   (E) Intravenous pyelogram

7. Which of the following dispositions is most appropriate for the patient in Question 1, assuming a positive Doppler result?

   (A) Intramuscular ceftriaxone 250 mg followed by 100 mg of oral doxycycline bid for 10 days
   (B) Elective exploration of the scrotum to obtain gross and microscopic evidence to rule out a malignancy
   (C) Emergency exploration to perform bilateral orchiopexy

(D) Sulfamethoxazole/trimethoprim given twice daily for 7 days

(E) Elective general surgery for repair of hernial defect

8 An 80-year-old gentleman complains of testicular pain that had its onset 3 days ago and has built since to prevent sleep the night before this visit. On examination the testicle seems on palpation to be irregular in shape and quite tender. The scrotal contents are difficult to differentiate. The patient's temperature is 100.8°F. The urinalysis demonstrates 20 to 30 white blood cells/high-power field. Which of the following is the most likely diagnosis?

(A) Epididymitis

(B) Testicular trauma

(C) Torsion of the testicle

(D) Orchitis

(E) Testicular cancer

9 A 34-year-old factory worker whose daily activity involves heavy lifting seeks advice for a growing groin mass. He first noted the swelling about 2 months ago after lifting a 75-lb (34-kg) packet of steel rods, and now it has become apparent to him during dressing and undressing. You examine him and find a scrotal mass that transilluminates well. You diagnose an inguinal hernia. Which of the following additional findings renders this clinical situation an emergency?

(A) Inability to reduce the hernia

(B) Finding a direct rather than an indirect inguinal hernia

(C) Associated testicular pain

(D) Tenderness of the hernial sac

(E) History of urinary tract infection

10 A 25-year-old man develops an inflammatory arthritis in his left knee that has been present for 1 week. Upon questioning, he avers that he has had bloody diarrhea that nevertheless had abated by the time of onset of his knee pain, and he complains of blurred vision in the right eye. He denies any history of trauma and any previous history of joint pain or swelling, and there is no family history of connective tissue disease. On examination he exhibits some redness of the right eye and the pupil is smaller than that of the left eye. Which of the following is the most likely etiology for this problem?

(A) Rheumatoid arthritis

(B) Osteoarthritis

(C) Reflux sympathetic dystrophy

(D) Reactive arthritis

(E) Systemic lupus erythematosus

11 You examine a 35-year-old man who presents with a painless enlarged testicle noticed by him over the past 3 months. On examination, the testicle is irregular in shape and does not transilluminate. Alpha-fetoprotein and human chorionic gonadotropin levels are within normal limits (i.e., barely perceptible), as is the lactic dehydrogenase level. You also note developing gynecomastia. You diagnose a testicular tumor. Which of the following types is it *most* likely to be?

(A) Seminoma

(B) Embryonal cell carcinoma

(C) Teratocarcinoma

(D) Choriocarcinoma

(E) Leydig cell carcinoma

12 A 25-year-old man and his 22-year-old wife are seeking consultation to find out why they have been unable to achieve fertility in the marriage after trying for pregnancy for more than 3 years. The wife's pelvic examination showed normal anatomy. The couple has confirmed and timed her ovulations by a temperature graph over the past year and attempted impregnation during the period surrounding ovulation, with no success. You initiate an evaluation to investigate the problem. Which of the following is the most logical first step?

(A) Hysterosalpingogram on the wife

(B) Computed tomography scan of the brain to investigate for pituitary adenoma

(C) Pelvic ultrasound to rule out polycystic ovary syndrome in the wife

(D) Sperm count on the husband

(E) 24-hour urine collection for 5-OH ketosteroids

13 Which of the following is the most common cause of male infertility?

(A) Malnutrition

(B) History of undescended testicle

(C) Varicocele

(D) Adrenal hyperplasia

(E) Klinefelter syndrome

14 A 55-year-old male patient complains of gradually increasing prostatism over the past 6 months. This has taken the form of increasing difficulty in initiating the urinary stream (hesitancy), decreasing size of the stream, and increasing nocturia. There have been times when his symptoms were worse than others. Each of the following statements are correct regarding these developments except for which one?

(A) One cause may be prostatic cancer.

(B) The differential diagnosis includes benign prostatic hyperplasia.

(C) The symptoms may be caused by epididymitis.

(D) The symptoms may be aggravated by ingestion of drugs with anticholinergic side effects.

(E) Prostatitis may be a cause of the symptoms.

15 Each of the following statements is true regarding the Gleason score in prostate cancer except for which one?

(A) The Gleason score includes a measure of the architectural pattern of the primary largest area of cancer in a specimen.

(B) The Gleason score includes a measure of the architectural pattern of the second largest area of cancer in a specimen.

(C) The Gleason score correlates with tumor volume.

(D) The Gleason correlates with staging of the cancer.

(E) An example of a Gleason score is: B2 2 nodules present or no nodule with the lobe indurate.

16 Which of the following medications would be *least* likely to cause erectile dysfunction?

(A) Chlorthiazide diuretics

(B) Cimetidine

(C) Albuterol

(D) Propranolol

(E) Finasteride 4

17 Regarding the PSA, each of the following statements is true except for which one?

(A) The normal limit of 4 ng/mL is a hard-and-fast rule.

(B) A level of 3 ng/mL in a 35-year-old man may be a cause for concern (i.e., without symptoms and a normal digital rectal examination).

(C) A PSA level of 6.5 ng/mL in a 75-year-old man need not be further evaluated.

(D) A minimum proportion of the total PSA should be in the free form as opposed to the bound form.

(E) The yearly rate of rise in PSA levels, regardless of their absolute values, should not exceed 0.7 ng/mL.

Examination Answers

1. The answer is C. 50 years of age in the absence of family history or African race is the time that routine screening of asymptomatic males should begin. In cases of African-American race and family history of prostate cancer in the first degree relatives, screening should begin at the age of 40 years. Screening should be repeated annually once initiated. Screening is recommended by the American Cancer Society, consisting of prostate-specific antigen To be sure the USPSTF does not advocate for screening.

2. The answer is C. Lowering the PSA cut-off to increase specificity is an incorrect statement. Lowering a cut-off for a test whose abnormality is defined as above the cut-off increases sensitivity but decreases specificity. All the other statements are true and for the reasons given. The greater the proportion of free PSA to total PSA the less likely the chances of malignancy for a given level of total PSA. Increasing the intervals between PSA drawings would reduce cost and inconvenience (at the expense of sensitivity). Defining a cut-off for the rate of increase of PSA addresses aggressiveness of the tumor and generally that cut-off is 1 ng/mL/year – above which is considered a criterion for the diagnosis of and a measure of aggressiveness of the cancer. Lowering PSA cut-offs for younger blacks to improve sensitivity makes sense in that African Americans have a higher incidence of carcinoma of the prostate and the cancer appears at younger age. Conversely, increasing the cut-off point defining abnormality in older blacks (as well as older people of all races) improves specificity in the latter groups (reduces chances of false-positive results).

3. The answer is D. Positive test for blood in all three glasses indicates that hematuria emanates from bladder, ureter, or kidney; bladder is the focus because of the smoking history and its risk of bladder cancer. Blood in the first glass indicates a urethral source; in the third glass only, a prostate source. The three glass test is virtually never positive for the second glass.

4. The answer is E. Taking nitrates strictly contraindicated to be taken concomitantly with a nitrate. although nitrates are usually given for coronary insufficiency, that condition per se is not such a contraindication. Studies have ruled out serious side effects by taking any of the phosphodiesterase 5 inhibitors in the face of all the other conditions listed and others. The latter include status post TURP, coronary artery by-pass, depression, prostate cancer, and renal insufficiency, including patients on dialysis.

5. The answer is D. A varicocele is the one choice listed that is not painful. Epididymitis is a well-known cause of acute testicular pain that typically has a slower onset than that portrayed in the vignette. Epididymitis virtually always is associated with pyuria. Trauma should be obvious in the history unless it was associated with head trauma and amnesia for the event. Cancer is typically painless but may be acutely painful and acutely swollen if there occurs hemorrhage into the tumor. The story fits that of testicular torsion in that it occurred in an intra-adolescent boy, and none of the other possibilities has as rapid an onset as torsion. Abdominal pain, nausea, and vomiting are often found in torsion. Thus, although varicocele is ruled out by history and the other choices figure in the differential diagnosis, the most likely diagnosis is torsion of the testicle.

6. The answer is C. A Doppler stethoscope test may be the most readily available test. In torsion, it will demonstrate the audible bruit of arterial blood in the uninvolved side but not on the affected side, except in rare cases. The technetium scan is helpful in confirming the diagnosis and should be the next test to be performed. Complete blood cell count and urinalysis are unremarkable in torsion. The intravenous pyelogram has no application in the diagnosis of any of the choices in the differential diagnosis.

7. The answer is C. Torsion of the testicle must be relieved to restore arterial circulation to the testicle within 6 hours. Otherwise, the testicle is functionally (and cosmetically) lost. Doxycycline is indicated for expectant treatment of infection by *Neisseria gonorrhoeae* and Chlamydia organisms, both of which are frequently implicated in epididymitis. Elective exploration is appropriate for cancer and elective repair for varicocele. Sulfamethoxazole/trimethoprim (Bactrim) is a typical regimen for cystitis and some cases of prostatitis.

8. The answer is A. Epididymitis is well described in the vignette. Although the testicular anatomy may be difficult to differentiate, careful examination usually allows the physician to identify the epididymis and the testicle proper as ovoid and not deformed. Torsion was described and is best identified by the methods alluded to in Questions 5 and 6. However, in torsion, despite confounding edema, one should appreciate that the testicle itself is the source of tenderness and that the epididymis is normal in size and not tender. Orchitis manifests tenderness of the testicle and, in most cases, enlargement but no change in the basic shape of the organ. The signs of ischemia and lack of evidence of obstructed arterial flow usually allow torsion to be ruled out. Testicular cancer manifests an irregular shape of the testicle proper and nearly always is nontender. The exception is the rapidly growing tumor into which hemorrhage occurs.

9. The answer is D. Tenderness of the hernia sac indicates the complication of strangulation of an incarcerated hernia. This surgical emergency requires timely correction to prevent ischemic death of the tissues involved in the hernia, usually a loop of bowel. In the latter case, the specter of bowel obstruction adds a further threat. Inability to reduce the hernia confers urgency and is the precursor of strangulation. Direct inguinal hernias are less likely to become incarcerated than indirect hernias. The latter herniate down the inguinal canal, a defined tight tunnel.

10. The answer is D. Reactive arthritis (formerly called Reiter syndrome in the context of the vignette) is the most common etiology for an acute inflammatory arthritis in a young adult. When following exposure to Yersinia or Shigella organisms, the incidence is equal in male and female patients. When following a sexually transmitted disease, the incidence in men is nine times that in women. The joint fluid is sterile by definition (as opposed to that in septic arthritis). Other components of the classic tetrology of urethritis, conjunctivitis, arthritis, and dermatitis may be present or absent.

11. The answer is E, Leydig cell carcinoma. Leydig cells produce testosterone. Because of the dedifferentiation of these cells and the lack of circulating testosterone, 30% of patients with Leydig cell tumors exhibit gynecomastia. All the remaining tumors mentioned in the choices are germ cell tumors. Although 97% of testicular cancers are germ cell tumors and 5% of them manifest gynecomastia, all except seminomas among them are characterized by the elevations of alpha-fetoprotein or human chorionic gonadotropin; 60% manifest elevated lactic dehydrogenase as well.

12. The answer is D. Performing a sperm count on the husband is the most logical initial step after a thorough history and physical examination, the latter including pelvic examination to rule out anatomic causes of female infertility. Forty percent of the cases of infertility are male related. Polycystic ovary syndrome is unlikely because it appears to be established when the patient is ovulating so that pelvic ultrasound is unnecessary. The other studies are quite expensive compared with the cost of the sperm count.

13. The answer is C. Varicocele is the most common cause of male infertility, accounting for 30% of cases.

14. The answer is C. Prostatism may be caused by or aggravated by all the choices given, except for epididymitis. Epididymitis, though not a cause, may be associated chronologically with prostatitis.

15. The answer is E. B2 is an example of staging of prostate cancer (PrCa), by the Whitmore-Jewett system. A = microscopic presence, found at surgery: A1 focal; A2 diffuse. B = palpable in rectal exam: B1 single nodule, normal lobe; B2 two nodules palpable or the lobe indurated. C = contiguous spread without metastases: C1 minimal, C2 (symptomatic) spread into urethra or bladder. D = metastatic disease: D0 negative bone scan, but increased alkaline phosphatase; D1 pelvic nodes; D2 distant, recurrent after surgery. The Gleason sore is a measure of pathological tumor architecture deduced apparent decreasing differentiation of the PrCa graded as 0–5 based on the pattern of the primary or largest area of cancer in a specimen and 0–5 based on the second largest area of cancer in a specimen. The Gleason score correlates with tumor volume and with staging of the cancer but is not itself a measure of staging. However, the Gleason score has not replaced surgical staging in rendering a prognosis.

16. The answer is C. Among the drugs mentioned, literature for albuterol does not list impotence or erectile dysfunction. As this drug is a beta-2 agonist, some patients will complain of heart pounding if use of the drug is excessive. Such adrenergic effects may interfere with sexual function because of the effect of preoccupation. However, the other medications are well known to cause impotence to varying degrees at therapeutic levels. It behooves physicians to inquire directly of people who take those medications (and many others) about that problem, even if the chief complaint is not related to the symptoms of sexual dysfunction.

17. The answer is A. The incorrect statement is that the upper limit of normal in PSA level is 4 ng/mL in all circumstances. This can be inferred from the other choices (i.e., that the upper limit of normal rises with age and levels <4 can be an indication of cancer in younger men). From the other correct statements, it can be inferred that the free as opposed to bound form of PSA should be present at a minimum of 27% of the total. Less than that is a criterion for biopsy and is used in cases of marginal PSA levels for age. Finally, the yearly rate of rise in PSA levels, regardless of their absolute values, should not exceed 0.7 ng/mL. If it does, further investigation is critical so as not to miss the opportunity for early diagnosis of prostate carcinoma.

References

Hellmann DB, Stone JH. Arthritis and musculoskeletal disorders. In: Tierney LM, McPhee SJ, Papadakis MA, eds. *Current Medical Diagnosis and Treatment*, 45th ed. New York: McGraw-Hill/Appleton & Lange; 2006:807–864.

McPhee SJ, Papadakis MA. *Current Medical Diagnosis and Treatment 2010*, 49th ed. New York, Chicago: Lange/McGraw-Hill; 2010 etc.

Strode SW. Genitourinary problems of the male. In: Rudy DR, Kurowski K, eds. *Family Medicine: House Officer Series*. Baltimore, MD: Williams & Wilkins; 1997:351–369.

Swebber R. Clinical evidence concise (a publication of the *British Medical Journal*). Reprinted in *Am Fam Physician*. 2004; 70:1325–1326.

Tunnila J, Lassen P. Testicular masses. *Am Fam Physician*. 1998; 57:685–692.

Problems Unique to Females in Primary Care

chapter **20**

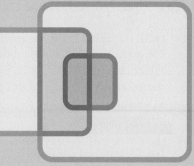

Problems of the Older Woman

Examination questions: Unless instructed otherwise, choose the ONE lettered answer or completion that is BEST in each case.

1 A 68-year-old Caucasian woman who is gravida 3, para 3, 18 years postmenopause, complains of sensation of full bladder in inconvenient situations and consequent frequent inability to make it to bathrooms without losing significant amounts of urine. She has no cardiac conditions. Which of the following measures is the most appropriate therapeutic approach to the problem?

(A) Prescription for oxybutynin (Ditropan) orally
(B) Recommendation for pseudoephedrine orally
(C) Prescription for estrogen replacement therapy
(D) Placement of a pessary
(E) Evaluate for bladder neck obstruction

2 Each of the following may be likely causes of amenorrhea in a 45-year-old woman except which of the following condition?

(A) Hyperthyroidism
(B) Hypothyroidism
(C) Polycystic ovary syndrome (PCOS)
(D) Prolactinoma
(E) Estrogen deficiency

3 A family doctor is treating a 60-year-old woman for osteoporosis with alendronate (Fosamax). As a bisphosphonate, this medication may be associated with each of the following side effects except for which one?

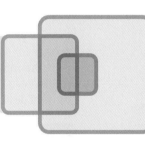

✓(A) Esophagitis
✓(B) Bone and joint pains
✓(C) Osteonecrosis *of jaw*
✓(D) Uveitis
✗(E) Clinical hypoparathyroidism ↑*parathyroid in some cases*

4 A 48-year-old white woman for whom you have cared for 5 years complains of bouts of depression for the first time in her life. This is the first occasion for her to visit you in the past 6 months. These bouts come on rapidly over periods of less than an hour, last for as long as 12 to 24 hours, and rapidly disappear. She denies headaches and difficulty thinking and calculating, although she notes that during the depressive episodes, she finds it difficult to concentrate on problems that require focused attention. She denies any relationship between these episodes and the menstrual

125

cycle. Her apical rhythm is regular and the rate is 84. You proceed to entertain a differential diagnosis of this complaint. Which of the following diagnoses is the least likely as a cause of this patient's problem?

(A) Neurotic depression
(B) Thyrotoxicosis
(C) Premenstrual syndrome
(D) Incipient menopause
(E) Hypoglycemic episodes

5 Regarding the patient in Question 4, the doctor notices skin changes toward thinness and dryness. Which of the following levels of follicle-stimulating hormone (FSH) is confirmatory of menopause as a cause of her depression?

(A) 20 IU
(B) 30 IU
(C) 40 IU
(D) 50 IU
(E) 60 IU

6 Regarding the patient in Question 5, she asks about hormone therapy. Which of the following is correct regarding hormone replacement therapy (whether estrogen alone, i.e., ERT, or estrogen/progesterone replacement therapy, known as HRT) after menopause?

(A) HRT is protective against cardiovascular atherosclerotic disease.
(B) If progesterone is cycled in an overlapping fashion with estrogen cycling, HRT is protective against breast cancer.
(C) Cycled estrogen with progesterone poses a risk of endometrial carcinoma.
(D) Conjugated equine estrogen (CEE) given daily at 0.625 mg is protective against osteoporosis.
(E) HRT with 0.625 mg of CEE given daily protects against senile dementia.

7 What is the approximate lifetime risk of hip fracture in octogenarian women?

(A) 5%
(B) 10%
(C) 20%
(D) 33%
(E) 50%

8 Besides suddenness of onset, the way in which surgical menopause is most likely to differ from physiologic menopause is in which of the following characteristics?

(A) Depression is more of a problem in surgical menopause.
(B) Atrophic vaginitis is more severe in surgical menopause.
(C) Osteoporosis is a greater issue in physiologic menopause.
(D) Heart disease is a greater risk after surgical menopause.
(E) Loss of libido is more likely after surgical menopause.

9 A 65-year-old slightly built white woman who is a cigarette smoker is brought to you by her daughter, who is a nurse. The daughter knows that her mother, as a small-boned person, is at high risk for hip fracture, as well as vertebral and radial fractures, as she grows older. The daughter is aware that hip fracture carries a 20% first-year mortality rate and is concerned that if her mother is not placed on hormone replacement therapy then she may suffer that fate. Despite acknowledging that HRT has lost favor and that few physicians are prescribing it as a routine, she presses for hormone replacement. You attempt to place this information in perspective for the family of this woman. Thus, you point out that the ranking cause of death in postmenopausal females is which of the following?

(A) Coronary artery disease (CAD)
(B) Endometrial carcinoma
(C) Carcinoma of the breast
(D) Hip fracture mortality in the first year after the occurrence
(E) Stroke

10 Regarding the patient osteoporotic, smoking patient, you feel the need to address the smoking issue with the 65-year-old Caucasian woman and her daughter, who is a nurse. Which of the following is the most complete and correct perspective?

(A) Smoking's detrimental effect is 10% as strong as estrogen's beneficial effect and increases the CAD risk by 25%.
(B) Smoking's detrimental effect is 25% as strong as estrogen's beneficial effect and increases the CAD risk by 25%.
(C) Smoking's detrimental effect is equal, negates estrogen's beneficial effect, and increases CAD risk by 50%.
(D) Smoking is twice as detrimental to bone density as estrogen is beneficial.
(E) Smoking is irrelevant to bone density as long as the patient is given HRT, but smoking increases CAD risk.

11 What is the best course of action to take if (mild) uterine bleeding occurs for longer than 6 months after institution of HRT, whether estrogen and progesterone are cycled with 25 days (estrogen) overlapping with 10 days progesterone or each drug taken daily in 30 day cycles? This assumes that hemoglobin and thyroid function have been evaluated.

(A) Discontinue all hormonal therapy
(B) Double the dosage of estrogen
(C) Adjust the dosage of progesterone
(D) Perform dilatation and curettage
(E) Perform endometrial biopsy

In Questions 12 through 16, match the lettered types of hormone replacement regimens to the numbered candidates for hormone therapy, assuming all candidates should take supplemental calcium as well (1 g of calcium carbonate in addition to dietary intake). A choice may be correct more than once or not at all.

12 A 33-year-old white woman who has undergone subtotal (ovary-sparing) hysterectomy.

13 A 40-year-old woman with early but physiologic menopause. She is of northern European heritage, of lean body habitus, and is a one pack per day smoker.

14 A 55-year-old white woman who has undergone physiologic menopause at the normal age. Hip fractures have been suffered by both her mother and her maternal aunt, one of whom died within the first year of the incident. None were cigarette smokers.

15 A 40-year-old woman who has undergone total hysterectomy without history of carcinoma of the breast, cervix, or ovary.

16 A 50-year-old woman, with a history of breast cancer, whose status after total hysterectomy is free of evidence of disease 10 years after mastectomy and irradiation therapy. She has suffered two fractures of distal radii and a wedge fracture of the 10th thoracic vertebra.

(A) CEE 0.625 mg and medroxyprogesterone acetate 2.5 mg daily
(B) CEE 0.625 mg daily
(C) Raloxifene 60 mg daily
(D) Observation and periodic measurement of FSH levels
(E) Alendronate 10 mg daily, taken in the morning with significant amounts of water, 30 minutes before eating

Examination Answers

1. The answer is A. Prescription for oxybutynin (Ditropan) orally, among the choices in the vignette. Anticholinergic medications such as oxybutynin, tolterodine (Detrol), and also propantheline (Probanthine) reduce the hyperirritability of an oversensitive detrusor muscle and sometimes an inherently small bladder. Alpha-adrenergic agonists such as *pseudoephedrine* address *stress incontinence* and loss of urine with coughing, laughing, or otherwise straining down with the abdominal muscles, by strengthening sphincter tone. The underlying problem in stress incontinence is atrophic vaginitis, which can be addressed closer to the root of stress incontinence, in the absence of contraindications, by estrogen therapy systemically or topically. A pessary is another approach for stress incontinence by supplying an obstructive component. Bladder neck obstruction should be addressed as a cause of overflow incontinence, characterized by small spurts of urine. It is uncommon in females in the absence of a neoplasm, whereas in males, prostatism causes overflow incontinence quite commonly.

2. The answer is B. Hypothyroidism is an unlikely cause of amenorrhea. Actually, hypothyroidism is associated with excessive uterine bleeding, as may be iron deficiency. Each of the other choices may be associated with or directly cause amenorrhea. PCOS is associated with androgen excess. Prolactinoma may result in hypogonadotropic hypogonadism.

3. The answer is E. Clinical hypoparathyroidism is not a side effect of bisphosphonates. In fact, parathormone rises during treatment with bisphosphonates in 10% of cases. Esophagitis may occur after ingestion of a bisphosphonate orally if the patient does not remain upright (after taking the medication with 8 oz of water and without eating for 40 minutes thereafter). Bone and joint pains as well as myalgias and fatigue may occur after commencement of the drugs but usually subside within a few days in preparations that can be taken infrequently, such as alendronate, administered on a weekly basis. In those cases, the pains tend to recur with each dose. Osteonecrosis is rare with bisphosphonates, but when it occurs, it tends to involve the jaw, particularly after tooth extraction. Uveitis, conjunctivitis, and scleritis may occur and manifest pain and blurred vision. These remit after discontinuation of the drug.

4. The answer is B. Thyrotoxicosis is unlikely in a young person with a normal heart rate. Neurotic depression is always possible with a depressed effect. However, it is seldom expressed in cataclysmic fashion such as it occurs in

the vignette. Premenstrual syndrome actually fits well with the history, except that women with premenstrual syndrome invariably connect the symptoms with the menstrual cycle. Hypoglycemia, regardless of the root cause, may awaken feelings of failure, guilt, and hence depression. Incipient menopause is certainly possible, given the patient's age, although menstrual periods have usually begun to change toward less frequency or irregularity when the premenopause era presents itself.

5. The answer is C. 40 IU is the level of FSH, above which a diagnosis of ovarian failure is secure. Some might choose A, 20 IU, but such a cut point is more liberal. The latter would allow a lower threshold for commencing hormone replacement therapy. At younger ages than appropriate, usually arbitrarily taken as <40 years, having menopausal symptoms associated with FSH levels ≥40 IU is referred to as ovarian failure.

6. The answer is D. CEE 0.625 mg daily is protective against osteoporosis; 0.3 mg of CEE will relieve the acute symptoms such as hot flashes and the cataclysmic depression in menopause. All the other suggested *benefits* of HRT in the stem question were long considered to be true and valid, but with random prospective studies reported in the last 5 years, they are no longer thought to be so. The breast cancer risk associated with estrogen and progesterone replacement was acknowledged but felt to be minimal at the dosages of HRT being used. Moreover, large prospective controlled trials alluded to, including both the Women's Health Initiative and the Heart and Estrogen/Progestin Replacement Study (HERS), have indicated that cardiovascular brain and heart disease risk appear to be in fact increased with HRT, possibly because of the complication of thromboembolic disease risk. Endometrial carcinoma, although a risk with estrogen replacement unopposed, is, however, relatively prevented by combined estrogen replacement cycled with progesterone. To elaborate, HRT is not cardioprotective, because of the progesterone, and in fact poses an increased risk of atherosclerotic events after 3 to 4 years of HRT.

7. The answer is D. If a woman lives to the age of 80 years, she stands a one in three chances of having a hip fracture. For a man, the odds are one in six. In any event, hip fracture is associated with a 20% first-year mortality rate. Therefore, as people live increasingly long after late midlife, the issue of prevention of osteoporosis becomes critical. This is especially so because hormone replacement therapy has been abandoned because of the risks of breast cancer and cardiovascular atherosclerosis.

8. The answer is E. Loss of libido is more likely after surgical menopause, even with hormone replacement therapy. This is because surgical menopause removes the secondary testosterone source in the case of total hysterectomy, wherein oophorectomy is included. This outcome may occur even after subtotal or ovary-sparing hysterectomy because of the possibility of sacrifice of ovarian blood supply during surgery.

9. The answer is A. CAD is the first ranking cause of death in postmenopausal women, whether on hormone replacement or not. Moreover, CAD deaths are no longer predicted to be reduced (by half) by the application of hormone replacement therapy.

10. The answer is C. Smoking has a detrimental effect equally as strong as estrogen's beneficial effect and increases CAD risk by at least 50%. Thus, stopping smoking alone will have a huge beneficial effect toward prevention of osteoporosis as well as decreasing risk of CAD.

11. The answer is E. Perform endometrial biopsy, generally recommended for persistent bleeding beyond 6 months after institution of HRT, or for postmenopausal bleeding of any sort, because of the risk of endometrial carcinoma. In the case of bleeding after HRT (i.e., estrogen and progesterone combined) has been started, this is actually of low urgency because the progesterone in HRT constitutes a negative risk factor for endometrial carcinoma. Bleeding may persist for up to 6 months after HRT is started. ERT (estrogen without accompanying progesterone) in the presence of an intact uterus would increase the risk for endometrial carcinoma. For that reason, ERT is contraindicated in the presence of an intact uterus.

ANSWERS TO MATCHING QUESTIONS

12. The answer is D, observation and periodic measurement of FSH levels. A 33-year-old white woman who has undergone subtotal or ovary-sparing hysterectomy may be presumed to be in an estrogen-sufficient state until the time such as when she undergoes physiologic ovarian involution. In the absence of menstrual periods and assuming no symptoms, humoral menopause can only be diagnosed by a rise in FSH.

13. The answer is A, CEE 0.625 mg and medroxyprogesterone acetate 2.5 mg daily. This is appropriate for the 40-year-old woman with early but physiologic menopause,

but for no longer than 3 years, to avoid increasing the risk of cardiovascular disease associated with HRT. Smoking cessation is mandatory. All forms of prevention of osteoporosis must be supplemented with oral calcium, at least 1 g per day for women.

14. The answer is A, CEE 0.625 mg and medroxyprogesterone acetate 2.5 mg daily. This is appropriate for the 55-year-old menopausal white woman who is assumed to be at high risk for osteoporosis. This should be continued only for 5 years.

15. The answer is B, CEE 0.625 mg daily. For the 40-year-old woman who has undergone total hysterectomy without history of carcinoma of the breast, cervix, or ovary, the ERT is appropriate. No time limit need be applied to ERT because the increased cardiovascular risk associated with hormone replacement therapy appears to be caused by the progesterone in HRT.

16. The answer is E. Bisphosphonates are recommended for high-risk cases to prevent osteoporosis or as secondary prevention for patients who have already manifested pathologic fractures. Alendronate 10 mg daily, taken in the morning with significant amounts of water, 40 minutes before eating breakfast, is appropriate. As Fosamax, alendronate is also available as 70 mg weekly. A new preparation, ibandronate, as Boniva, is dosed as 2.5 mg daily or 150 mg monthly. The history of breast cancer constitutes a contraindication for ERT or HRT. The patient has suffered two fractures of distal radii and a wedge fracture of the 10th thoracic vertebra. Raloxifene, as an estrogen receptor blocker, might be a good supplemental medication in a patient with history of breast cancer but is not as effective in preventing osteoporosis as are the bisphosphonates.

References

Family Medicine Board Review. Kansas City, Missouri; May 3–10; 2009.

McKay HT. Gynecology. In: Tierney LM, McPhee SJ, Papadakis MA, eds. *Current Diagnosis and Treatment.* 45th ed. New York: McGraw-Hill/Appleton & Lange; 2006:728–762.

McPhee SJ, Papadakis MA. *Current Medical Diagnosis and Treatment 2010,* 49th ed. New York/Chicago: McGraw-Hill/Lange; 2010.

Rudy DR. Problems of the female climacteric. In: Rudy DR, Kurowski K, eds. *Family Medicine: House Officer Series.* Baltimore: Williams & Wilkins; 1997:329–340.

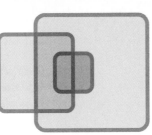

chapter **21**

Gynecology in Mature Adults

1 A 22-year-old single woman complains of a painful labial ulcer and painful inguinal (lymphadenopathy) 4 days after having intercourse with a man she had just met. Which of the following organism is the likely cause of this sexually transmitted disease (STD).

(A) *Treponema pallidum*
(B) *Calymmatobacterium granulomatis*
(C) *Neisseria gonorrhoeae*
(D) *Chlamydia trachomatis*
(E) *Hemophilus ducreyi*

2 A 20-year-old woman calls at 2 AM after a Saturday night the family doctor on call for his group saying she unexpectedly found herself having consensual intercourse and is panicked over the fear of an unwanted pregnancy. She agrees to call in a prescription for the "morning after" pill. Which of the following regimens should accomplish the objective?

(A) Norgestimate 0.180 mg/ethinyl estradiol 0.035 mg two tablets within 24 hours
(B) Levonorgestrel 0.75 mg course of two tablets within 72 hours
(C) Drospirenone/ethinyl estradiol 3.0 mg/0.030 mg three tablets over the next 24 hours
(D) D. Desogestrel/ethinyl estradiol 0.15 mg/0.02 mg two ASAP and one in every 4 hours time four more doses.
(E) Medroxyprogesgterone acetate 10 mg for 10 days

3 A 37-year-old woman in a monogamous marriage complains of a vaginal discharge with a fishy odor. The vaginal pH is 4.8 and clue cells are present on the smear. A culture reveals presence of *Gardnerella vaginalis*. The family doctor diagnoses bacterial vaginosis. Each of the following statements is true except for which one.

(A) This condition may be a cause of premature rupture of membranes in labor.
(B) Bacterial vaginosis may be the cause of premature labor.

(C) The transmission of this condition is sexual.
(D) The condition is associated with postpartum endometritis.
(E) The condition may be a cause of pelvic inflammatory disease (PID).

4 You have treated by telephone a woman whose past experience made her quite credible in self-diagnosing uncomplicated candida vaginitis. Twice you treated her with a single 150 mg dose of fluconazole. Both the times she complained of recurrent symptoms of pruritic curdy discharge within a few days of apparent relief of symptoms. Which of the following is the least likely explanation for the foregoing treatment failures?

(A) Presence of diabetes predisposing to candidiasis
(B) Presence of HIV disease
(C) Infection with candidal species other than albicans
(D) Incorrect diagnosis of candida vaginitis
(E) Presence of immunity compromise due to cancer chemotherapy

5 A 45-year-old woman complains of increasingly irregular menstrual periods, which are becoming lighter and less frequent, seldom appearing sooner than 35 days after the previous one. She complains also of gaining weight over the past 5 years. During the same period, hair has grown on her upper lip and she has developed acne for the first time in her life. She weighs 165 lb (74.8 kg) at a height of 5 ft 4 in. (1.63 m). On examination she manifests central obesity and fading purple striae over the flanks of her abdomen. Which of the following is the best *causal* explanation for these findings?

(A) Type II diabetes mellitus
(B) Hypothyroidism
(C) Metabolic syndrome
(D) Polycystic ovary syndrome (PCOS)
(E) Cushing syndrome

6 Regarding the patient in Question 5, besides an elevation of serum testosterone levels, which of the following laboratory tests, in conjunction with the clinical picture, gives a distinctive pattern for identification of the diagnosis?

(A) White blood cell count
(B) Blood sugar
(C) Serum luteinizing hormone (LH)
(D) Serum electrolytes
(E) Serum creatinine

7 Regarding the patient in Questions 5 and 6, assuming weight loss was effected without success, which of the following should be the first treatment option?

(A) Menstrual regulation with cyclic contraceptive hormonal treatment
(B) Increased physical activity and decreased calorie ingestion Δ phys of PCOS
(C) Prescription of metformin
(D) Prescription of clomiphene
(E) Epilation and electrolysis

8 Each of the following is a relative contraindication for intrauterine device (IUD) insertion except for which one?

(A) Nulliparity
(B) Active STD
(C) History of PID
(D) Presence of an intrauterine pregnancy
(E) Multiparity

9 A 14-year-old nulliparous girl complains of primary dysmenorrhea. She is overweight and attempting to lose weight. Her parents have recently separated, and she has been sporadically involved in drinking fairly heavily and smoking at parties of young people but has not become sexually active. Each of the following aspects of her life situation is a risk factor for dysmenorrhea except for which one?

(A) Drinking alcohol
(B) Smoking
(C) Losing weight
(D) Experiencing family stress
(E) Being nulliparous

10 Which of the following is the only medication approved specifically by the Food and Drug Administration for the treatment of nausea and vomiting of pregnancy?

(A) Prochlorperizine (Compazine)
(B) Promethazine (Phenergan)
(C) Trimethobenzamide (Tigan)
(D) Pyridoxine/doxylamine (Bendectin)
(E) Ondansetron (Zofran)

11 Each of the following conditions occurs at a greater rate than expected in people exposed to diethylstilbestrol (DES) in utero except for which one?

(A) Squamous cell carcinoma of the cervix
(B) T-shaped uterus

(C) Clear cell adenocarcinoma of the vagina
(D) Undescended testicle
(E) Hypoplastic uterus

12 A 21-year-old sexually active woman complains of intense pain in the left vulvar area building over a period of 2 to 3 days. She has not had similar symptoms in the past, and she has not been with her sex partner for several weeks. The pain is of such severity that she has been afraid to attempt intercourse or even to sit down normally. Which of the following is the most likely diagnosis?

(A) Herpes simplex type 2
(B) Craurosis vulvae
(C) Candida vaginitis
(D) Trichomonas vaginitis
(E) Bartholin gland abscess

13 A 65-year-old woman visits you for the first time to complain of vaginal bleeding for the first time since her natural menopause 15 years ago. The bleeding began 2 weeks ago and is mild in flow. Which of the following is the most critical question to be asked in completing the history?

(A) Are there cramps associated with the bleeding?
(B) How many pads per days are needed to keep abreast of the bleeding?
(C) Are you taking hormone therapy of any type?
(D) Have you developed light-headedness upon standing after sitting for prolonged periods of time?
(E) Is there bleeding with intercourse?

14 You have diagnosed chlamydia on "routine" Pap smear with an enzyme-linked test for STDs. The woman confessed that she was concerned about the possible infidelity of her husband. Which of the following may be among the aspects of this infection you must explain to this woman?

(A) The course for the infected female is virtually always benign.
(B) Unless successfully treated she will have significantly increased risk of spontaneous abortion and infertility.
(C) The infection responds to amoxicillin.
(D) Macrosomia may occur in newborn babies of mothers infected during pregnancy.
(E) Symptoms, if she notes them, are likely to include a frankly purulent discharge within 48 hours of exposure.

15 A woman with secondary amenorrhea is given 10 mg medroxyprogesterone acetate by mouth per day for 5 days and monitored for the onset of bleeding following progesterone withdrawal. Which of the causes for amenorrhea listed here will produce a positive response to this challenge (bleeding upon withdrawal)?

(A) Asherman syndrome
(B) Anovulatory cycle
(C) Gonadal agenesis
(D) Ovarian failure
(E) Menopause

16 You are evaluating a 38-year-old woman who stopped having periods 8 months ago. She has normal secondary sexual development and shows no evidence of virilization. Her pelvic exam shows a normal cervix and fundus and no adnexal masses. Her urine beta-human chorionic gonadotropin (hCG) test is negative. Her thyroid-stimulating hormone and serum prolactin levels are normal. She does not have uterine bleeding during the withdrawal phase of a progestin challenge, but does bleed after being on conjugated estrogen (1.25 mg) for 21 days with a progestin agent added on the last 5 days. Follicle-stimulating hormone (FSH) and LH are both elevated. Which of the following is the most likely diagnosis?

(A) Hypothalamic amenorrhea
(B) Asherman syndrome
(C) Premature ovarian failure
(D) Anovulatory cycle
(E) PCOS

17 A 25-year-old woman who is a ballet dancer has felt the need to lose weight to remain competitive. Her height is 5 ft 4 in. (1.63 m) and her weight is 95 lb (43 kg), yet she feels she needs to lose more weight.

Her menstrual periods have become scant and infrequent during the past year. Her last menstrual period was more than 3 months ago. You suspect that she has anorexia. Which of the following is a likely finding?

(A) Normal serum estrogen level
(B) Osteoporosis
(C) Sedentary lifestyle
(D) Healthy dentition
(E) Elevated FSH and LH levels

18 A 28-year-old woman who has never been pregnant missed a menstrual period 4 weeks ago, an unusual circumstance for her. She has been using a barrier method of contraception. Until the past week she noticed nausea, but yesterday she passed much blood and now says she feels better, although she is still bleeding. Her beta-hCG level was 2,500 mIU, but the test was repeated 48 hours later and the level found to be 1,000 mIU. Pelvic examination is negative for adnexal mass and tenderness. Transvaginal pelvic ultrasound reveals intrauterine tissue. You diagnose missed spontaneous abortion. The patient's vital signs are normal and her hemoglobin is within normal limits. She is not seriously concerned and in little pain. Which of the following is the best decision for management in the near future?

(A) Expectant observation
(B) Intravaginal misoprostol, 800 μg
(C) Surgical evacuation of the uterus
(D) Naproxen, 500 mg twice daily if needed to control uterine cramps
(E) Initiation of oral contraceptive medication

Examination Answers

1. The answer is E. *H. ducreyi* is the cause of Chancroid. Chancroid is characterized by *painful ulcers and painful* inguinal *adenopathy*. Special culture is required for *H. ducreyi*. The incubation period is 3 to 5 days. The organism is susceptible to azithromycin, ceftriaxone, ciprofloxin, and erythromycin. *T. pallidum* is the cause of syphilis, which is characterized by a *painless* chancre and *no* regional adenopathy. *C. granulomatis* causes granuloma inguinale, which features a spreading painless ulcer, the pathognomonic cell with Donovan bodies and no adenopathy. *C. trachomatis* causes lymphogranuloma venereum, which causes no ulcer but with impressive *painless* inguinal adenopathy. For this the disease was called by the sailors of old "the blue balls."

2. The answer is B. Levonorgestrel 0.75 mg. The course is one tablet as soon as possible and the second one within 12 hours. If accomplished within 72 hours contraception is achieved in 89% of cases. This has the trade name Plan B. All the other choices except for E are ingredients and combinations found in oral contraceptive pills. Norgestimate 0.180 mg/ethinyl estradiol 0.035 mg is Ortho-cyclen. Drospirenone/ethinyl estradiol 3.0 mg/0.030 mg is part of the cycle in Yasmin 28. Desogestrel/ethinyl estradiol 0.15 mg/0.02 mg is Miracette. (E) Medroxyprogesgterone acetate 10 mg for 10 days is, of course generally prescribed to precipitate menses, effecting "medical D&C" in dysfunctional uterine bleeding. Although protocol demands a negative pregnancy test before this regimen, it can induce abortion after implantation.

3. The answer is C. The *incorrect statement is transmission of this condition is sexual.* Bacterial vaginosis is now not considered an STD. Each of the other statements is correct. The effects on childbirth labor and the postpartum state as well as its causation of PID are surprising and concepts that have crystalized in the past few years. Thus, bacterial vaginosis should be treated for more than relieving the patient of the annoyance. Treatment consists of metronidazole 500 mg bid for 7 days, clindamycin 300 mg twice daily for 7 days or 100 mg clindamycin ovules vaginally nightly for 3 days. That said, clinical PID should be treated for the wide variety of organisms that are known to cause the disease, that is, ceftriaxone 250 mg IM for 1 day; doxycycline 100 mg twice daily for 10 days; metronidazole 500 mg orally twice daily for 14 days.

4. The answer is D. Incorrect diagnosis of candida vaginitis – that is, the least likely cause of treatment failure of the vaginitis in this case. The Pruritic caseous vaginal discharge is virtually pathognomonic. Underlying conditions that prepare a fertile ground for recurrence of Candida (albicans or others) such as diabetes, HIV disease, or immunosuppression by chemotherapy predisposing to candidiasis may account for recurrence and/or emergence of resistant strains of *Candida albicans* or other species. Resistance generally encompasses imadazole antibiotics such as fluconazole. If the infection is invasive, amphotericin-B and echinocandins are the effective treatments. Infection with candidal species other than albicans now accounts for over 50% of blood stream isolates (obviously such a series would be biased toward sicker and more complicated cases).

5. The answer is D. This patient meets the criteria for the diagnosis of PCOS. The Amsterdam consensus states that a patient must have two of the three following conditions to qualify for the diagnosis: anovulation or oligo-ovulation; chemical or clinical signs of androgenization; and sonographic evidence of polycystic ovaries. Elevated testosterone levels are the common pathway of pathophysiology. Besides the androgenizing effect, this results in lack of a dominant developing follicle during the monthly cycle. Therefore, the ovary fills gradually with uncompleted cystic follicles. Androgenic manifestations that may be found with this condition, besides acne and hirsutism, include male-pattern alopecia. Although metabolic insulin resistance and type II diabetes are part of the syndrome, as is central obesity, they are not necessarily accompanied by androgenizing manifestations. Cushing syndrome manifests purple striae along with its other glucosteroid effects, but not androgenization. Hypothyroidism has nothing in common with the patient in the vignette except for sometimes a mild degree of obesity. In hypothyroidism, menstrual periods are increased in flow and frequency, not decreased.

6. The answer is C. A serum LH found at a preovulatory level that is not followed by ovulation within 14 days of the blood drawing is a hallmark of PCOS. The patient with PCOS often goes a long time between periods, 3 months up to a year, so that a random LH level that is elevated to preovulatory levels is suspect immediately. It is as if the hormonal rhythm is "held up" at the preovulatory phase, which is indeed true, caused by androgenic hormone excess. None of the other laboratory tests gives a result distinctive for PCOS. Although blood sugar may be elevated if the patient progresses to type II diabetes, such a finding is not diagnostic of anything except for diabetes. Not listed is serum testosterone, which is typically elevated in PCOS. However, that does not differentiate PCOS from other causes of androgenization, such as adrenal hyperplasia.

7. The answer is B. Increased physical activity and decreased calorie ingestion, that is, weight loss alone, will change the physiology of PCOS in a significant number of patients. Decreased fat stores reduce androgen stores and hence conversion of androgen to estrone, allowing resumption of ovulation. Metformin is an excellent pharmacologic choice as it reduces insulin resistance and aids in weight loss. Metformin is virtually the first choice for drug therapy if weight loss and exercise fail. Metformin facilitates weight loss and may actually result in fertility. Menstrual regulation with cyclic contraceptive hormonal treatment is another common approach and may lead to resumption of ovulation. Clomiphene should be used only in women who are anxious to become pregnant in a short time. Epilation and electrolysis are secondary options for treating the hirsutism directly without affecting the underlying pathophysiology at any point.

8. The answer is E. Multiparity is not a contraindication for insertion of an IUD. Nulliparity certainly is a relative contraindication because it may be physically difficult and usually is very painful at the time of insertion and often remains so until it is removed. Having a present or past STD is a contraindication, unless a matter of 10 or more years has passed. An intrauterine pregnancy will likely be aborted by an IUD. Abortions of normal pregnancy constitute malpractice unless the procedure is done specifically for elective abortion. In the latter case, insertion of an IUD is not an approved procedure. Other contraindications include the presence of liver or breast carcinoma or jaundice specific for hormone-containing IUDs; copper allergy or Wilson disease (specific for copper-containing IUDs); known or suspected pelvic malignancy; and immunodeficiency or immunosuppression.

9. The answer is A. Alcohol drinking, though a risk for numerous other health problems, is not statistically a risk factor for dysmenorrhea. Each of the other choices is associated with dysmenorrhea, although none is proven to be a cause thereof. Obesity per se is not associated with dysmenorrhea but attempts to lose weight are so associated, perhaps because of the confounding issue of poor self-image, itself a risk factor. Nulliparity is well known to be associated with primary dysmenorrhea. Primary dysmenorrhea usually begins with the onset of ovulation, 6 months to 2 years after the menarche, and decreases with age after 20 and with parity.

10. The answer is D. Pyridoxine/doxylamine (Bendectin) or each one prescribed separately is known to safely relieve nausea and vomiting of pregnancy and is approved for that usage. In accord with such approval, its Strength of Recommendation Taxonomy (SORT) classification is A, meaning evidence is case based and adequately studied. Although each of the other drugs mentioned is an antiemetic and utilized for nausea of pregnancy in practice,

they are classified as unproven as to safety in pregnancy and not recommended during nursing. Prochlorperizine is classified as SORT C (i.e., usage is based on clinical custom, usual practice, expert opinion, etc.), as are promethazine and trimethobenzamide. Ondansetron is classified SORT B, based on case evidence but not such that rises to statistical significance.

11. The answer is A. Squamous cell carcinoma of the cervix, according to current data, is caused by a papilloma virus. All the other abnormalities, including undescended testicles, are associated with in utero exposure to DES, which was a common practice to prevent miscarriage between 1938 and 1971. In addition to those mentioned in women are other conditions including cockscomb cervix, cervical collar, cervical pseudopolyp, and vaginal adenosis. Not as well known among clinicians are the abnormalities of male genital development in DES progeny. These include, in addition to undescended testicles, epididymal cysts and sperm and semen abnormalities. There is a resurgence of attention being paid to DES progeny because the female progeny are now postmenopausal and perimenopausal, an epoch of increased susceptibility to the vagaries of hormonal shifts. Both male and female progeny of DES-treated women should be conscientious regarding routine cancer screening for breast, vaginal, and testicular neoplasms.

12. The answer is E, Bartholin gland abscess. Herpes simplex produces a sharp, superficial pain aggravated by sheer force contact (i.e., skin or mucosa sliding over the infected area) but not particularly sensitive to pressure. Craurosis vulvae is a premalignant change secondary to long-standing hormonal deficiency (i.e., the postmenopausal state). Both Candida and Trichomonas are characterized by intense pruritus rather than abscess like pain, though in severe cases, each may produce a superficial soreness not unlike that associated with herpetic pain. Immediate treatment is incision and drainage, which allows virtually instantaneous relief. To avoid recurrence, definitive treatment requires marsupialization after incision and drainage. Bartholin gland cysts occur without abscess formation and, if asymptomatic, merit no therapeutic measures. The organisms involved are usually not sexually transmitted, but culture should be performed and may yield Gonococcus or Chlamydia organisms. If they are present, these should be treated accordingly.

13. The answer is C. Postmenopausal bleeding must be assumed to be caused by endometrial carcinoma until proven otherwise. If a postmenopausal woman has been on hormone replacement therapy (HRT), three possible answers each determine different pathways investigation. If the patient has been on estrogen cycled with progesterone (HRT), the combination is relatively (but not absolutely) protective against endometrial carcinoma, and early in the course of HRT, there may be mild breakthrough bleeding.

If the patient has been taking estrogen replacement or in the past without progesterone and has an intact uterus, the chances of endometrial carcinoma are heightened beyond those inherent in having an intact uterus without hormonal influence. Each of the other questions is relevant but only at a secondary level, after an opinion is formed as to what causes the bleeding. Postural lightheadedness in the present setting is possibly a symptom of relative hypovolemia and therefore anemia caused by blood loss. In the present vignette that is unlikely, given the history of only recent and modest blood loss. Therefore, also unlikely is the relevance of number of pads required. Having associated cramps generally is related to the volume of flow of vaginal bleeding. Bleeding with intercourse is a nonspecific symptom that could relate to vulvar or uterine causes, including cervicitis.

14. The answer is B. Unless this patient is successfully treated, she will have significantly increased risk of spontaneous abortion and infertility. Women who developed active chlamydial infections during pregnancy are at increased risk for premature rupture of membranes, preterm labor with smaller newborns, spontaneous abortion, and intrauterine deaths. *C. trachomatis* may cause severe PID, urethritis, and cervicitis, although both women and men with chlamydial infection may be asymptomatic. The infection responds to doxycycline and azithramycin but to none of the penicillins or cephalosporins. The incubation period is between 5 and 21 days.

15. The answer is B, anovulatory cycle. If the patient has no obstruction to the outflow of menstrual blood and if the endometrium has been sufficiently primed with estrogen, the exposure to and withdrawal of progesterone will induce uterine bleeding. This will not occur in primary or secondary ovarian failure that is due to lack of estrogen priming or if there is an obstruction to uterine outflow such as in Asherman syndrome (uterine obstruction secondary to endometrial scarring, as occurs sometimes after dilatation and curettage). Likewise, gonadal agenesis results in a barren, unprimed endometrium that cannot respond to progesterone withdrawal.

16. The answer is C, premature ovarian failure. The failure to respond to the progestin challenge suggests a problem with estrogen stimulation of the endometrium (from either a pituitary or an ovarian problem), or outflow obstruction in the uterus. Because the patient did bleed after reproduction of the estrogen–progestin cycle, outflow obstruction cannot be responsible and the cause must lie in the ovarian or pituitary axis regulating estrogen, with the result being inadequate serum estrogen level. The increase in FSH and LH shows an appropriate pituitary response to these low estrogen levels, and thus the difficulty must be ovarian failure.

17. The answer is B, osteoporosis. This patient exhibits the criteria to diagnose anorexia nervosa: inappropriate voluntary weight loss, distorted body image, and at least 3 months of amenorrhea in a woman not in the perimenopausal age group. The menstrual abnormality is a form of hypothalamic amenorrhea. It is often a response to physical or psychological stress or to excessive exercise or weight loss. It is associated with osteoporosis. Serum estrogen and LH and FSH levels are decreased or normal in hypothalamic amenorrhea. Many anorectics are also bulimic and compensate by purging or inducing vomiting. The latter activity causes severe dental deterioration.

18. The answer is B. Medical management of missed abortion is highly successful when the situation is uncomplicated and ectopic pregnancy is ruled out. Intravaginal misoprostol, a prostaglandin E analog, allows successful evacuation of the uterine contents. Dilatation and curettage is necessary when there is evidence of infection, bleeding is severe, or if the patient is extremely anxious or presses for such intervention. If the uterus is empty on ultrasonic study and expelled products of conception are confirmed and if none of the aforementioned complications are present, expectant observation only is needed. Symptomatic treatment of cramps is inappropriate, as is initiation of contraception at this time. Naproxen, as an NSAID, is a protaglandin inhibitor, would delay evacuation of the uterus.

References

Bauman KA, Brown DR. Gynecology in primary care. In: Rudy DR, Kurowski K, eds. *Family Medicine: House Officer Series.* Baltimore, MD: Williams & Wilkins; 1997:297–328.

Family Medicine Board Review 2009. Kansas City, Missouri; May 3–10, 2009.

French L. Dysmenorrhea. *Am Fam Physician.* 2005; 71:285–291, 302.

Griebel CP, Halvorsen J, Goleman TB, et al. Management of spontaneous abortion. *Am Fam Physician.* 2005; 72:1243–1250.

Johnson BA. Insertion and removal of intrauterine devices. *Am Fam Physician.* 2005; 71:95–101.

Lozeau A-M. Diagnosis and management of ectopic pregnancy. *Am Fam Physician.*2005; 72:1707–1714, 1719–1720.

McKay HT. Gynecology. In: Tierney LM, McPhee SJ, Papadakis MA, eds. *Current Medical Diagnosis and Treatment,* 45th ed. New York: McGraw-Hill/Appleton & Lange; 2006:728–762.

Owen MK, Clenney TL. Management of vaginitis. *Am Fam Physician.* 2004; 70:2125–2132, 2139–2140.

Sherif K. Polycystic ovary syndrome in primary care. *Female Patient.* 2005; 70:24–28.

Shrager S, Potter BE. Diethylstilbestrol exposure. *Am Fam Physician.* 2004; 69:2395–2400, 2401–2402.

chapter 22

Diseases of the Female Breast

1 A 22-year-old woman has breast cancer and is found to be positive for BRCA1. She prefers to be tested for BRCA. If the 22-year-old woman is positive for BRCA, what is her lifetime risk of breast cancer?

(A) 95%
(B) 85%
(C) 60%
(D) 35%
(E) 20%

2 The 22-year-old woman has tested out positive for BRCA1. What is her lifetime risk of ovarian cancer?

(A) 95%
(B) 85%
(C) 60%
(D) 35%
(E) 20%

3 After breast cancer diagnosis and treatment, each of the following should be the elements of routine follow-up except for which one, assuming there is no evidence of residual local or metastatic cancer?

(A) Physician examination every 6 months
(B) Regular inspections of the ipsilateral arm for edema
(C) Annual bilateral mammograms
(D) Annual magnetic resonance imaging (MRI) survey
(E) Monthly self-examinations

4 A 45-year-old Caucasian woman complains of several weeks of spreading non-painful erythema of the left breast. A course of dicloxacillin had no appreciable effect on the process. Breast examination reveals no palpable mass. Which of the following is the next and best choice of action at this time?

(A) Needle aspiration
(B) Prescribe a different antibiotic
(C) Biopsy
(D) Mammogram
(E) Ultrasound study

5 Which of the following breast complaints warrants the closest and most persistent evaluation?

(A) Bilateral nipple discharge, milky in appearance
(B) Bilateral tenderness with irregular palpable masses, cyclic in course
(C) Purulent discharge, unilateral, with tenderness
(D) Bilateral nipple irritation during nursing
(E) Unilateral sanguineous discharge

6 Nine months later, the patient referred to in Question 1 returns and says that her galactorrhea has not ceased. A pregnancy test is negative. Without any further information, which of the following is the most common pathological cause of galactorrhea?

(A) Prolactinoma
(B) Gigantism
(C) Thyrotoxicosis
(D) Medication
(E) Breast cancer

7 A 32-year-old woman has bilateral nipple discharge that is found to contain fat globules, no red or white cells, and is established to be galactorrhea. She also complains of headaches as well as diminution of her libido and decrease in the flow and frequency of her menses over the last 3 months. Headaches are worse in the mornings. Beta-chorionic gonadotropin level is not elevated, and the remainder of the breast examination is negative. The serum prolactin level is elevated at 250 ng/mL. Serum follicle-stimulating hormone and thyroid-stimulating hormone levels are within normal limits. Which of the following is the logical next step?

(A) Prescribe bromocriptine
(B) Refer for surgery
(C) Prescribe cabergoline
(D) Suggest MRI with contrast
(E) Suggest plain x-rays of the head

8 A 43-year-old woman seeks your opinion for a breast lump that she discovered the previous week. She has no first- or second-degree family history of breast cancer. She had a negative mammogram 2 years ago. The nodule is 2 to 3 cm in diameter. The remainder of the breast examination is essentially normal, but there is a background of granularity to palpation (like small irregularities in the breast tissue). Which of the following is the best next disposition?

(A) Suggest a mammogram
(B) Refer for breast biopsy
(C) Draw prolactin levels
(D) Draw serum calcium and alkaline phosphatase levels
(E) Perform aspiration

9 A 28-year-old woman presents with a single breast nodule that is nontender. There is a second-degree family history of breast cancer in which her aunt (mother's sister) had breast cancer at the age of 48. Which of the following is the best diagnostic test at this time?

(A) Mammogram
(B) Excisional biopsy
(C) Fine-needle biopsy
(D) Serum prolactin level test
(E) Ultrasonic study   U/S

10 Which of the following diagnostic procedures is the best choice for the least expensive method to differentiate *in situ* and invasive carcinoma of the breast and to ascertain the status of estrogen receptor presence in the tumor?

(A) Fine-needle aspiration (FNA) biopsy
(B) Core-needle biopsy (CNB)
(C) Excisional biopsy
(D) Lumpectomy
(E) Mammogram

11 A 35-year-old woman comes to an office setting for a routine breast examination (clinical breast examination, or CBE) by the family doctor. Which of the following findings on this CBE least suggests the possibility of breast cancer in a palpable nodule?

(A) Lack of liquid retrieval on aspiration
(B) Location in the superolateral quadrant
(C) Fixation to underlying tissues
(D) Hardness measured at 60 durometers
(E) Irregular shape

12 Of the following age groups, in which does the largest proportion of breast cancers occur?

(A) Menarche to 25 years
(B) 20 to 40 years
(C) <50 years of age
(D) 50 to 65 years
(E) >65 years

13 A 26-year-woman presents to you with a complaint of a breast lump. Upon examination, the nodule is found to be apparently 1 cm in diameter and tender. It is more tender this week than it was last week and it has been cyclically painful during the premenstrual week the past three months during which she noted the nodule. What is the best course of action at this time?

(A) Suggest mammography this week
(B) Refer for breast biopsy
(C) Observe for 3 months, examining the patient monthly during that time
(D) Perform needle aspiration
(E) Reassure the patient that she is not in the age group to fear cancer of the breast

14 A 28-year-old complains of a breast lump since trauma to the area about 2 weeks ago. What is the best action at the present time?

(A) Suggest mammography this week
(B) Refer for breast biopsy
(C) Observe for 3 months, examining the patient monthly during that time
(D) Perform needle aspiration
(E) Reassure the patient that she is not in the age group to fear cancer of the breast

15 Each of the following may be complications of breast implantations except which one?

(A) Capsule contraction and scarring around the implant
(B) Firmness and distortion of the breast
(C) Rupture of the implant
(D) "Bleeding" of silicone gel through the implant capsule
(E) Precipitation of autoimmune diseases in the recipient

16 In performing a CBE, which of the following is most appropriate in advising your patient regarding this examination?

(A) The sensitivity of the CBE is 90% in the hands of a professional.
(B) Specificity of the CBE is virtually 100%.
(C) If a patient avails herself of the CBE, then she need not perform breast self-examination.
(D) When performed optimally, the CBE is about 70% sensitive.
(E) The patient should make a decision to undergo either CBE or mammography starting at age 40 years.

Examination Answers

1. The answer is B. Eighty-five percent lifetime risk of breast cancer is conveyed by carriage of the BRCA1 or BRCA2. However, only 2.2% of breast cancers are associated with BRCA.

2. The answer is C. Sixty percent lifetime risk of ovarian cancer resides with carriage of the BRCA1 marker. However, BRCA2 that also confers an 85% lifetime risk of breast has a 20% risk of ovarian cancer.

3. The answer is D. Annual MRI survey should not be done in an asymptomatic woman with breast cancer. Computed tomography (CT) and MRI are indicated when symptoms or signs arise suspicious for recurrence or metastases.

4. The answer is C. Biopsy. Infections are generally quite painful in the breast. If it had been painful and the antibiotic had resulted in significant improvement, it would have likely been an infection. The big danger here is the possibility of inflammatory carcinoma, which may be painful, in which case, failure of response to antibiotics would have justified investigation for cancer. Inflammatory carcinoma of the breast is the most malignant type and conveys a poor prognosis.

5. The answer is E. Unilateral sanguineous discharge warrants the closest and most persistent evaluation because it is most likely to be a sign of cancer, most types of which begin as intraductal carcinomas. The chances that bloody nipple discharge is caused by cancer are 1:3. Bilateral nipple discharge, milky in appearance, is galactorrhea, associated with various causes, including pregnancy, mechanical stimulation, pituitary adenoma (prolactinoma), hypothyroidism, and Cushing disease, as well as chronic renal failure. Bilateral tenderness with irregular palpable masses, cyclic in course, is caused by fibrocystic disease and is seen commonly in primary care practice. Purulent discharge with tenderness represents infection, often in a lactating woman.

6. The answer is D. Drugs are the most common pathologic cause of galactorrhea. Galactorrhea may be normal for a brief time in newborns, postpartum women, and pregnant women. The most common drugs associated with galactorrhea are categorized as follows, with certain examples given. First, there are dopamine receptor blocking agents: butyrophenones, metoclopramide, phenothiazines, selective serotonin reuptake inhibitors, tricyclic antidepressants, and thioxanthenes. Second, there are dopamine-depleting agents, such as methyldopa and

reserpine. Third, there are inhibitors of dopamine release: codeine, heroin, and morphine. Fourth, there are histamine receptor blocking agents. Fifth, there are lactotroph-stimulating agents: oral contraceptives and verapamil. Each of the other options may be associated with galactorrhea, but all are unusual except for prolactinoma.

7. The answer is D. MRI with contrast. Prolactin levels above 200 ng/mL should be considered to be caused by prolactinoma until proven otherwise. However, the size of this slowly growing benign tumor and the patient's total symptomatology and attitude toward fertility together determine the therapeutic approach. The best modality for confirming the tumor's size and presence is the MRI, preferably enhanced by gadolinium. Microadenomas may be treated with dopaminergic agents such as bromocriptine. Cabergoline is a longer acting and thus more convenient drug, but it is more expensive. Macroadenomas, especially if suprasellar, may warrant surgical removal, particularly if fertility is a critical issue.

8. The answer is E. Performing aspiration before otherwise legitimate options makes sense in this woman, who is over the age of 40 and not with epidemiologic evidence of high risk. Fluid-filled cysts are most likely to occur in women over the age of 40. If aspiration results in fluid with the disappearance of most of the nodule, the likelihood of cancer as a basis for the mass is very low. To be sure, the patient should be followed for several weeks afterward and a mammogram should be done early, if only as a recommended routine for all women over the age of 40. Nodules in women younger than 40 years of age are more likely to be fibroadenomas and other benign solid tumors. Breast biopsy need not be rushed into in this circumstance, although it should never be withheld unnecessarily. Prolactin levels are reserved for nipple discharge. Calcium and alkaline phosphatase are indicated when metastatic disease is suspected.

9. The answer is E. An ultrasonic study of the breast tissue is appropriate in a young woman, even with a second-degree family history of breast cancer. Sonography is 89% sensitive for breast abnormalities in symptomatic women. Women younger than the mid-30s are likely to have dense breast tissue that renders mammography less accurate (less sensitive and less specific). Aspiration is less likely to be fruitful, as fluid-filled cysts are more common in women who are older than 40 years. Prolactin levels are indicated in galactorrhea or other bilateral nipple discharge. Excisional biopsy should be delayed, pending the results of the noninvasive studies. Fine-needle biopsy may be considered after the results of the ultrasound study, and the revelation of fluid would rule out cancer, making the FNA a fluid aspiration procedure, with the same limitations already mentioned.

10. **The answer is B.** The CNB, done with 14- to 18-gauge needle, is as much as 99% sensitive in palpable lesions and 93% sensitive in nonpalpable nodules for diagnosing breast cancer. A minimum of four cores is required to gain these statistics, which include a higher predictive value than found in FNA. Excisional biopsy is the gold standard but is obviously more expensive and more traumatic than the CNB. Lumpectomy is a therapeutic technique, designed to cure a known cancer under favorable circumstances.

11. **The answer is B.** Although the so-called upper-outer quadrant will contain the most breast cancers, so is that location the quadrant that contains the most breast tissue; hence, residency in the superolateral quadrant in of itself is not a particular danger sign in a nodule. Lack of an aspirant retrieval by tapping does not signal breast cancer, but appearance of fluid aspirant in that situation rules strongly against cancer. The durometer is a measure of hardness; 20 durometers is comparable to a soft to medium grape and 60 durometers approaches the hardness of calcified bone, a sign suggestive of cancer. Irregular shape, as opposed to well-circumscribed roundness, is suggestive of cancer as well.

12. **The answer is E.** Nearly 50% of breast cancers in women in the United States occur in women older than 65 years of age. About one-quarter occur in the age group of 50 to 65 years, leaving about one-quarter for the under 50 age group. The latter, as was implied earlier, tend to contract more aggressive cancers, giving rise to a changing view of screening that calls for more frequent routine mammography (i.e., yearly) in the age group of 40 through 49 years. This point is not heavily emphasized in the chapter by Bowman and Szewczyk (1997), but a telling report on the subject was freshly published as that manuscript was being processed.

13. **The answer is D.** Needle aspiration is the first step choice for the 26-year-old woman with a cyclically tender breast lump. All other choices given in the vignette have relevance at certain times and under certain circumstances. However, the clinical picture is that of fibrocystic disease. If the nodule disappears as fluid is yielded in the procedure in the given setting, cancer can virtually be ruled out, assuming the fluid is clear. Disappearance is defined as nonrecurrence of the cystic nodule after a period of several monthly cycles. If the fluid is bloody,

cytological examination of the fluid should be routine in that circumstance. Any other result requires, at the least, an imaging study.

14. **The answer is C.** Observing for 3 months is acceptable, given the history of trauma, because hematomas can persist for 6 weeks or longer before resolving. A mammogram may be obtained, although inaccuracies are attendant to the patient's age; thus, an ultrasound would be preferable. On the basis of the aforementioned information, the breast biopsy can wait. Needle aspiration is acceptable but need not be done on this visit because hematoma is a logical diagnosis.

15. **The answer is E.** Although there was a flurry of medico legal litigation during the early 1990s surrounding the claim of autoimmune disease associated with breast implants, there was never, either at the time or since, even purported incidence or prevalence attached to that alleged association; there were only patients (deluded or self-serving) and eager lawyers driving the claims through courts and too often succeeding, which gave birth to that wave of economic waste. All the other complications do occur. Capsule contraction and scarring occur in 15% to 25% of cases of silicone implants; implant rupture occurs in 5%.

16. **The answer is D.** Several points are relevant here. Perhaps, the most important is that the doctor should explain both the strengths and the weaknesses of any test to which the patient agrees. This is the foremost procedure so that the patient is provided with the best data through which the patient's health care is in accord with the doctors, but avoiding placing the physician in a defensive medico legal position. Thus, the patient in this case is informed that a negative CBE is not a guarantee against breast cancer in the near future. Furthermore, in the present example, there is an approximately 30% chance that the CBE may miss diagnosing a cancer (i.e., 70% sensitivity). It follows that patient and doctor must avail themselves of other reasonable means of screening for breast cancer, such as mammography yearly beginning at the age of 40 years, after a baseline study at the age of 35 (for women of average expected lifetime risk). Mammography itself has been estimated to be only 70% sensitive. Presumably, the cancers missed are most likely to be the smallest nodules by both methods. Although sensitivity is questionable, breast self-examination appears to confer additional advantages only if performed monthly or more often, even by an initially insecure and unpracticed woman. Specificity of all three methods is obviously imperfect, and negative breast biopsies will necessarily occur.

References

Barton MB, Harris R, Fletcher SW. Does this patient have breast cancer? The screening breast examination: Should it be done? How? *JAMA*. 1999; 282:1270–1280.

Bowman MA, Szewczyk MB. Diseases of the breast. In: Rudy DR, Kurowski K, eds. *Family Medicine: House Officer Series*. Baltimore: Williams & Wilkins; 1997:341–350.

Family Medicine Board Review. Kansas City, Missouri; May 3–9; 2009.

Kerlikowske K, Grady D, Barclay J, et al. Effect of age, breast density, and family history on the sensitivity of first screening mammography. *JAMA*. 1996; 276:33–38.

Klein S. Evaluation of palpable breast masses. *Am Fam Physician*. 2005; 71:1731–1738.

Leung AKC, Pacaud D. Diagnosis and management of galactorrhea. *Am Fam Physician*. 2004; 70:543–550, 553–554.

Lucas JH, Cone DL. Breast cyst aspiration. *Am Fam Physician*. 2003; 68:1983–1986, 1989.

McPhee, SJ, Papadakis, MA. *Current Medical Diagnosis and Treatment 2010*, 49th ed. New York/Chicago: Mc-Graw Hill; 2010.

SECTION IX

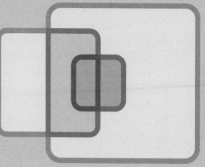

Musculoskeletal and Rheumatological Diseases in Primary Care

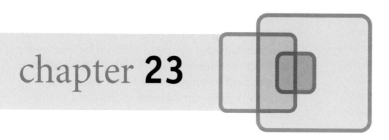

chapter 23

Musculoskeletal Problems of the Upper Extremities

Examination questions: Unless instructed otherwise, choose the ONE lettered answer or completion that is BEST in each case.

1 A 32-year-old female, employed for 2 years in an assembly line, complains to her family doctor of wrist and hand pain increasing over 2 weeks. She has worked with her hands and wrists handling small part and feeding them into an automated machine 100 times per hour, with 30 minutes for lunch break and two 15-minute rest periods. She denies numbness in the extremities. There is no tenderness ventrally over the radius or between the extensor tendons of the thumb. However, on further examination, she complains of pain when the doctor asks her to make a fist and then to ulnar deviate the wrist. This maneuver causes pain in the radial aspect of the wrist. There is tenderness to palpation over the radial styloid near

the base of the metacarpal of the thumb. Which of the following is the diagnosis?

(A) Carpal tunnel syndrome
(B) DeQuervain syndrome
(C) Occult scaphoid fracture
(D) Stress fracture of the distal radius
(E) Reflex sympathetic dystrophy

2 A 25-year-old woman fell onto her outstretched hand and incurred a fracture of the distal radius that appears to be virtually non-displaced. Which of the following would be appropriate for treating this fracture during the acute phase in the family doctor's office?

(A) Volar *splint* extending from the mid forearm to the distal palmar crease.

143

(B) Long arm posterior *splint* extending from the axilla over the 90 degree flexed elbow to the proximal palmar crease

(C) Short arm *cast* extending from the proximal forearm to the distal palmar crease

(D) Long arm *cast* from the mid humerus to the distal palmar crease

(E) Sugar-tong splint from the elbow to the distal palmar crease

3 A 45-year-old man works repetitively lifting 30- to 40-pound boxes of steel auto parts overhead to place them on a conveyer belt. Yesterday during one such move, he tripped and fell forward to catch himself with his full weight on his arms and shoulders while still holding the box. This resulted in an acute severe sharp pain in the left shoulder accompanied by an audible pop. Among other tests the family doctor stands behind the patient with the patient's left arm at his side and elbow flexed 90 degrees. She places her right hand on the left shoulder with modest downward pressure while applying upward pressure on the left elbow that directs the humerus upward into the shoulder joint. There is an audible pop and the feeling of the head of the humerus riding over an apparent brief obstruction. Which of the following is diagnosed by that sign?

(A) Impingement syndrome

(B) Biceps tendonitis

(C) Supraspinatus strain/sprain

(D) Clavicle fracture

(E) Torn superior labrum

4 A 45-year-old man has had intermittent numbness in his (dominant) right hand palmar index and middle fingers for 2 years, particularly in the night. Since experiencing prolonged use of a handheld posthole digging tool a year ago, he has found that the numbness has persisted even by day and involves the thumb and part of the ring finger. He complains also of midventral forearm pain and shoulder pain on the right. He exhibits weakness of thumb opposition with all four fingers but denies and exhibits no hypesthesia of the dorsal aspects of any of the fingers of the right hand. He denies triggering of the digits with flexion of the fingers. Which of the following is the most likely cause of his symptoms?

(A) Median nerve compression

(B) Cervical disc herniation involving C5, C6, and C7

(C) Scalene anticus syndrome

(D) Herpes zoster

(E) Ulnar nerve compression

5 Regarding the patient in Question 1, you perform and find positive the Phalen and Tinel tests. These

are increased numbness in the median nerve distribution within 30 seconds of 90-degree flexion of the wrist (Phalen test) and numbness and paresthesia in the median nerve distribution when tapping with the percussive finger the ventral wrist in the position of the median nerve (Tinel test). You consider conservative management consisting of wrist splinting in the neutral position, to prevent repetitive gripping and wrist flexion, glucocorticoid injection into the carpal tunnel space, or both. What are the chances of alleviation for an indefinite or permanent period?

(A) Excellent

(B) Good

(C) Not good

(D) Poor

(E) Nil

6 A 28-year-old male patient slips and falls onto his outstretched left hand during a winter ice storm. He is complaining of wrist pain, and you examine him. You conclude that the distal radius is neither tender to direct pressure nor painful with the application of longitudinal or torque stress to the distal radius. An x-ray is negative for fracture of the distal radius or distal ulna. You apply a wrist brace and ask the patient to return in 1 week. However, 3 days later the patient is still complaining of wrist pain. On re-examination you note tenderness near the base of the left thumb metacarpal between the extensor tendons. The patient complains that the persistent pain is made worse by clenching his fist. Which of the following is the likely diagnosis?

(A) Fracture of the thumb metacarpal

(B) Colles fracture of the wrist

(C) Soft tissue sprain of the wrist

(D) Carpal navicular fracture

(E) Rupture of the flexor carpi radialis tendon

7 An 18-year-old male high school student got into a fist fight after school and is brought to you the next morning complaining of pain in the right hand where he had struck his adversary with his doubled fist. He has swelling of the hand seen prominently on the dorsal aspect. There is a break in the skin of the dorsal aspect of the hand in the shape of a tooth mark. The fifth digit deviates in an ulnar direction when the fist is closed. Which of the following is the most complete diagnosis:

(A) Contusion of the right hand

(B) Closed fracture of the fifth proximal phalanx

(C) Open fracture of the fifth metacarpal

(D) Closed fracture of the fifth metacarpal

(E) Infected open fracture of the fifth metacarpal

8 A 35-year-old house painter who was a catcher in baseball on his high school and industrial league teams complains of right shoulder pain that has become increasingly annoying over the past 3 weeks. His pain interferes with his work because it is engendered by the motion of abduction and by forward placement of his dominant right arm. Which of the following maneuver would be useful in determining whether this man has the impingement syndrome?

(A) Testing the proximal biceps insertion for tenderness

(B) Patient actively supinating the forearm against resistance

(C) Passive inversion of the shoulder while the arm is forward, held in the horizontal

(D) Testing for pain with active extension of the elbow against resistance

(E) Observe patient's performance of digit to thumb apposition

9 A 35-year-old man, while playing touch football at a family reunion, fell on his abducted right shoulder with his right arm in abduction behind his back. He heard a "pop." The patient is fully alert but in pain, holding his right arm with his left; the arm is held in slight abduction and external rotation. On examination his right acromion is prominent, a depression is noted in the superior portion of the deltoid, and his right humeral head is palpated anterior to the acromion. Which of the following fractures is commonly associated with this dislocation?

(A) Fracture of distal third of clavicle

(B) Posterolateral humeral head

(C) Posterior rim of glenoid

(D) Transverse fracture of upper third of humerus

(E) Coracoid process fracture

10 A 21-year-old wide receiver on a prominent college football team, in catching a pass, makes a twisting leap and lands directly on his right shoulder. Immediately he is in pain, holding his right arm with his left hand. There is no glenohumeral tenderness, and there is full range of motion. The right acromion manifests prominence that is reduced by downward pressure on the clavicle. There is tenderness and ecchymosis around the acromioclavicular (AC) joint. Distal motion, pulses, and sensory examinations are normal. Which of the following examinations or ancillary studies would you obtain?

(A) Anteroposterior (AP) and lateral and modified axillary view of left shoulder

(B) Magnetic resonance image (MRI) of the left shoulder

(C) AP views of both AC joints with the patient holding 10-lb (4.5-kg) weights in each hand

(D) Right clavicle x-ray

(E) Arthrogram of left AC joint

11 A 35-year-old male mechanic sustained a small puncture wound on the volar surface of his left index finger while working on an engine. Three days later he complains of increasing pain in the digit. You find the finger to be swollen to about half above its normal diameter and being held in a semi-flexed position. There is pain with passive extension of the finger, and the hand otherwise presents no remarkable change. Active flexion and extension are intact though painful. Which of the following is the most likely diagnosis?

(A) Cellulitis of the hand

(B) Palmar space infection

(C) Flexor tendon rupture of the index finger

(D) Tenosynovitis of the flexor tendon

(E) Stoving injury involving the joint capsule of the proximal interphalangeal (PIP) joint

12 A 32-year-old former competitive athlete complains of 3 weeks of right elbow pain, coming on 2 weeks after he had decided to take up tennis. There has been no trauma to the elbow. He first noted his pain when performing his backhand stroke on the tennis court. Later he began to complain of pain upon shaking hands, turning a screwdriver, and now even when he turns a doorknob. He denies any other musculoskeletal symptoms. He is afebrile, and there is no elbow joint swelling or discoloration. There is tenderness over the lateral epicondyle of the proximal forearm. Which of the following therapeutic approaches would be inappropriate?

(A) Addressing the ball with increased wrist and elbow extension during the backhand stroke

(B) Hand grip exercises with a rubber ball

(C) Forearm splinting

(D) Paralesional injection of a glucocorticoid solution

(E) Cold applications to the elbow

13 A 35-year-old woman has an accident in the kitchen with a paring knife. As she is brought to your office, you note a laceration of the skin across the dorsum of the PIP joint of the middle finger of the left hand. You note also that the PIP joint is in partial flexion while the distal interphalangeal (DIP) joint is in extension. Which of the following injuries causes this result?

(A) Collateral ligament injury

(B) Transection of the flexor tendon of the middle finger

(C) Laceration of the central slip of the extensor tendon

(D) PIP dislocation

(E) Stoving injury to the end of the middle finger

14 A 16-year-old male catcher on the high school baseball team had a foul tip strike his left (non-gloved) hand and arrives with pain the next day to your office. There is tenderness and ecchymosis over the dorsal aspect of the DIP joint of the thumb. The patient can fully flex the joint, but he has lost 20 degrees of extension, compared with the normal hyperextension seen in the thumb. No fracture is revealed on x-rays. What is the most likely treatment of the patient?

(A) Surgical repair of injured extensor mechanism

(B) Continuous splinting in extension for 6 weeks

(C) Continuous splinting in 20 degrees of flexion for 6 weeks

(D) Arthrodesis (fixation of the joint) in hyperextension of the thumb PIP joint

(E) Only NSAIDs because the x-ray shows no fracture

15 A patient has incurred a fracture of the middle phalanx of left ring finger that extends into the DIP joint, involving 50% of the articular surface. Which of the following treatment plans is most appropriate?

(A) Open reduction and internal fixation

(B) Splint the finger in 25 degrees of flexion for six weeks

(C) Buddy tape the finger to the adjacent middle finger for 6 weeks

(D) Immobilization for 2 weeks followed by active range of motion

(E) Physical therapy forthwith to retain range of motion

Examination Answers

1. The answer is B. DeQuervain syndrome, also called DeQuervain tenosynovitis. The maneuver that produces the pain with ulnar deviation while "making a fist" is called Finkelsteins maneuver. Treatment is conservative with physical therapy modalities in the vast majority of cases. Carpal tunnel syndrome exhibits the typical median nerve distribution of numbness and weakness of thumb to finger opposition. Scaphoid fracture seldom if ever occurs without a clear cut history of fall onto the outstretched hand and manifests tenderness in the anatomic snuffbox as well as the scaphoid tuberosity. Stress fracture of the distal radius is a non-entity but in traumatic fracture this injury too results from falling onto the outstretched hand. Reflex sympathetic dystrophy presents with marked palor, rubor, pain, and regional sweating.

2. The answer is C. A short arm *cast* as described proximal and distal to the fracture. A Volar *splint* extending from the mid forearm to the distal palmar crease is too short and allows too much movement at the fracture, that is, forearm pronation and supination. The long arm posterior *splint* extending from the axilla to the proximal palmar crease may be used but is overly long for the Colles or distal radius fracture and thus immobilizes more length than necessary while not adequately immobilizing the distal radius fracture, especially if the latter were unstable. The long arm *cast* may be applicable in cases initially treated with the long posterior splint but are not appropriate for the distal radius alone. It may be utilized in children who often have combined radius and humerus fractures. The sugar-tong splint from the elbow is no more immobilizing for the distal radius than the posterior splint.

3. The answer is E. Torn superior labrum is diagnosed by the described maneuver, called the "anterior slide test." The tear diagnosed by the slide test is common and is called the superior labrum anterior to posterior lesion, or SLAP lesion. Impingement syndrome, usually associated with rotator cuff injury, is diagnosed by the Hawkins test (pain with passive inversion of the shoulder while flexed forward to 90 degrees) among other tests that involve flexion and internal rotation of the shoulder. Biceps tendonitis is best diagnosed by the Yergason's test, pain with supination of the forearm against resistance while the elbow is flexed and the upper arm at the side. Supraspinatus injury is diagnosed by the finding of pain and/or weakness in the ability to hold the outstretched arm at 90 degrees abduction with the thumb pointed downward, resistance being supplied by the examiner or, when severe, gravity alone, sometimes called the "empty bucket test." Clavicle fracture is shown by obvious deformity (caused by a direct blow or by falling laterally against the shoulder.

4. The answer is A. This patient has, of course, classic carpal tunnel syndrome, compression of the median nerve, secondary to relative contraction of the flexor retinaculum of the wrist that contains the tendons, blood supply, and median nerve. It occurs commonly and is aggravated by repetitive hand gripping. Involvement of three cervical disc levels is unlikely. More important, however, is that this patient does not exhibit dermatomal distribution of the sensory symptoms, because the dorsa of the thumb, index, middle, and (half) of the ring fingers are not involved proximal to the PIP joints. The scalene anticus syndrome is a variant of thoracic outlet syndrome wherein the scalene anticus muscle in the thoracic outlet contracts and causes compression of the peripheral roots of C7, C8, or both, thus involving a distribution that approximates the ulnar nerve (sensation to the ring and fifth fingers). Herpes zoster, or "shingles," causes mostly superficial pain rather than hypesthesia and is associated with a painful varicelloid rash in a dermatomal distribution. Ulnar nerve lesions cause fourth (ulnar half) and fifth finger sensory involvement and weakness of lumbrical and interosseous musculature of the hand (abduction or spreading) of the fingers, not opposition movements.

5. The answer is D. The chance of indefinite alleviation with conservative management is 6.8%. See the table that follows here.

TABLE 23–1 Predicting the Outcome of Conservative Treatment for Carpal Tunnel Syndrome

1. Have symptoms been present for more than 10 months?	Yes____	No____
2. Does the patient have constant paresthesias?	Yes____	No____
3. Does the patient have tenosynovitis (triggering of the digits)?	Yes____	No____
4. Is the Phalen maneuver positive within less than 30 seconds?	Yes____	No____
5. Is the patient older than 50 years of age?	Yes____	No____

Source: Used with permission from Viera (2003).
Notes: Score 1 point for each yes answer and 0 for each no answer. The scoring key for success rate is as follows: 0 points, 65%; 1 point, 41.4%; 2 points, 16.7%; 3 points, 6.8%; 4 or 5 points, 0%.

6. The answer is D. Fracture of the carpal navicular (also called the scaphoid) occurs with falls onto an outstretched hand, acutely showing tenderness in the "anatomic snuffbox," which is that space between the extensor tendons of the thumb at the base of the metacarpal. Tenderness at this locus is 90% sensitive for scaphoid fracture but only 40% specific. Thus, diagnosis must be confirmed by x-ray with specific focus for the scaphoid bone. Regardless of x-ray findings on the first few days, given the snuffbox and scaphoid tubercle tenderness, a short arm thumb spica should be applied and the patient brought back for reexamination and repeat x-ray in 2 weeks. Chronically, failure to diagnose may lead to aseptic necrosis and osteoarthritis. Missing this fracture has been the subject of litigation for failure to diagnose.

7. The answer is E. The ulnar deviation of the fifth digit is typical of a fifth metacarpal or "boxer's" fracture. The fact that there is skin break defines it as an open or "compound" fracture. The assumed human bite to which the skin break is ascribed defines the wound as infected, as would a lower animal bite. Thus, the fracture should be immobilized in good alignment, often by a hand surgeon and antibiotics prescribed to cover a human bite. Amoxicillin-clavulanate (Augmentin) is the first choice in nonpenicillin allergic patients.

8. The answer is C. Passive inversion of the shoulder while the arm is forward, held in the horizontal by the examiner – this is the Hawkins maneuver and when it causes pain in the shoulder it signifies impingement syndrome. Pain of the impingement syndrome is also particularly increased by active abduction at the shoulder. Radiographs are usually normal, but MRI will reveal any swollen tendon producing impingement and can identify tears in the rotator cuff. The pain of rotator cuff tendonitis usually has an insidious onset and is poorly localized – it is treated in the vast majority by physical therapy. Pain in the biceps proximal insertion is elicited by supination against resistance and is called the Yergason maneuver. Tenderness also occurs in the proximal insertion in biceps tendonitis. Neither biceps nor elbow extensor strength is an issue in impingement syndrome since abduction of the shoulder is involved. Thumb-finger apposition tests the motor function of the median nerve as commonly done in probing for carpal tunnel syndrome.

9. The answer is B. A right anterior glenohumeral dislocation is associated posterolateral humeral head fracture. The dislocation tends to occur anteriorly, and it is the anterior rim of the glenoid that may take off the posterolateral part of the humeral head.

10. The answer is C, AP views of both AC joints with the patient holding 10-lb (4.5-kg) weights in each hand. Clin-

ically the case seems to involve a grade III or IV sprain of the right AC joint (suggested by the high-riding right clavicle). Hanging weights bring out the separation between the clavicle and acromion if the joint capsule is torn and comparison with the contralateral side is made. MRI or arthrogram could also show the capsule tears, but they are more expensive and unnecessary in deciding treatment. For this purpose, the right clavicle will be adequately viewed on the AC joint films.

11. The answer is D. Tenosynovitis of the hand is a surgical urgency calling for interruption and control of the infection and surgical drainage and decompression when indicated to save function of the affected digit. Cellulitis of the hand produces diffuse swelling of the whole hand; palmar space infection causes swelling of either the thenar or midpalmar space. Flexor tendon rupture, assuming no infectious involvement, is not noted for the degree of swelling found in the vignette and active flexion would not be demonstrable at all. A stoving injury of the PIP joint is caused by a blow to the end of an extended finger wherein the impact is transmitted axially to the joint capsule of, usually, the PIP joint. It produces fusiform swelling centered on the joint itself, not the whole finger.

12. The answer is B. Hand grip exercise would aggravate the problem, which is a type of overuse syndrome, lateral epicondylitis. It is commonly called tennis elbow; lateral epicondylitis is caused in tennis by an amateurish tendency to stroke the backhand with the heavy tennis racquet as if it were a table tennis paddle. However, it may develop through any repetitive supination or gripping action (handgrip calls upon the wrist extensors to stabilize the wrist against flexion in doubling the fist as well). The brachioradialis muscle attaching to the epicondyle operates at a great mechanical disadvantage. Forearm splinting prevents the wrist extension and supination. A glucocorticoid mixed with a local anesthetic injected into the region of the epicondyle, but not directly into it, may give dramatic relief. Relief may be lasting, provided the underlying mechanical cause is dealt with. Cold applications may give relief during the acute phase.

13. The answer is C, laceration of the central slip of the extensor tendon. The configuration of the boutonniere deformity is flexion of the PIP and extension of the DIP joint. The DIP attachment of the extensor tendon is a convergence of two lateral slips that course to the two sides of the PIP and thus are spared in an injury to the dorsal midline of the proximal phalanx and the PIP joint. However, the central slip is involved by that injury. Activation of the extensor tendon apparatus without the functional presence of the central slip allows the lateral strands of the tendon to slip sideways and relatively ventrally, allowing their action to take a "shortcut" to the DIP, resulting in paradoxical flexion of the PIP while extending the DIP.

14. The answer is B, continuous splinting in extension for 6 weeks. This is an example of a partial avulsion of the extensor tendon, in this case brought about by the careening baseball's striking the patient's flexed thumb and violently stressing the PIP into hyperflexion. In a similar case involving one of the fingers, the result is referred to as a mallet finger. Prolonged splinting (6 to 8 weeks) in extension is necessary for the extensor mechanism to heal. Delayed treatment can result in the situation in which the patient is unable to extend the finger at DIP joint without surgical intervention. Surgical repair has not produced satisfactory results; splinting in flexion is counterproductive; arthrodesis is virtually never resorted to; and NSAIDs as a sole treatment is inadequate.

15. The answer is A, open reduction and internal fixation of the fracture. Closed treatment in a fracture involving more than 30% of the articular surface is highly likely to develop degenerative arthritic change. All the other choices offer less aggressive treatment than open reduction.

References

Boyd AS, Benjamin HI, Asplund C. Splints and castings: Indications and methods. *Am Fam Physician.* 2007; 75:342–348.

Churgay C. Diagnosis and treatment of biceps tendinitis and tendinosis. *Am Fam Physician.* 2009; 80:(5):470–476.

Daniels JM, Zook EG, Lynch JM. Hand and wrist injuries: Part I. Emergent evaluation. *Am Fam Physician.* 2004; 69:1941–1948.

Daniels JM, Zook EG, Lynch JM. Hand and wrist injuries: Part II. Non-emergent evaluation. *Am Fam Physician.* 2004; 69:1949–1956.

Dixit S, DiFiori JP, Mines B. Management of patellofemoral pain syndrome. *Am Fam Physician.* 2007; 75:194–202, 204.

Myers A. Common Problems of the Upper Extremities. In: Rudy DR, Kurowski K, eds. Family Medicine: House Officer Series. Baltimore, MD: Williams & Wilkins; 1997:383–398.

Phillips TG, Reibach AM, Slomiany WP. Diagnosis and management of scaphoid fractures. *Am Fam Physician.* 2004; 70:879–884.

Viera AJ. Management of carpal tunnel syndrome. *Am Fam Physician.* 2003; 68:265–272.

chapter 24

Musculoskeletal Problems of the Neck and Back

Examination questions: Unless instructed otherwise, choose the ONE lettered answer or completion that is BEST in each case.

1 A 36-year-old male assembly line worker complains that 2 days ago, while hefting a bucket of metal parts that slipped from his right hand while still grasping the other handle, experiences sudden pain in the left side of his neck that radiates into the left lateral upper arm into the thumb, associated with paresthesias in the thumb. Strength testing shows that his left wrist extension is 3/5. Which of the following is the nerve root involved?

(A) C5
(B) C6
(C) C7
(D) C8
(E) T1

2 Which of the following maneuvers or signs elicits or signifies pain of cervical radiculopathy?

(A) Hawkins maneuver
(B) Yergason maneuver
(C) Empty bucket test
(D) Spurling maneuver
(E) Babinski sign

3 A 45-year-old man with back pain complains of medial forefoot numbness and weakness of extension of the great toe. Knee jerk and ankle jerk deep tendon reflexes are normal and matching those of the other extremity. Which of the following nerve roots is involved in this radiculopathy?

(A) L3
(B) L4
(C) L5
(D) S1
(E) S2

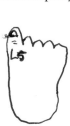

4 A 25-year-old woman comes to you for neck pain that had its onset 6 hours after she was "rear-ended" in her automobile. In addition to her pain, she complains that her head feels "heavy" on her shoulders. She denies radiation of the pain into her arms. She was seen at an emergency room soon after the accident because of the insistence of the emergency medical technicians, and x-rays of the cervical spine were negative for fracture and dislocation. Besides the finding of normal strength and deep tendon reflexes of the upper extremities, you find you can elicit tactile crepitus when you move the larynx against the cervical vertebral column. Which of the following expresses best the significance of the last finding in this situation?

(A) It rules out fracture of a vertebral body.
(B) It assures you that there is no retrolaryngeal neoplasm.
(C) It assures you that there is no Ludwig angina.
(D) This finding raises the likelihood of a laryngeal fracture.
(E) It rules against the presence of a hematoma between the larynx and the cervical vertebrae.

5 A 65-year-old man complains that he has deep hip and buttock pain on both sides, worse the longer he walks and when dorsiflexing the spine. The pain is immediately alleviated when he sits down. Deep tendon reflexes of the lower extremities and straight-leg raising (SLR) tests are normal and symmetrical. Which is the most likely diagnosis?

(A) Herniated disc at L5, S1
(B) Lumbosacral strain
(C) Cauda equina syndrome
(D) Lumbar spinal stenosis
(E) Prostatitis

6 A 35-year-old woman complains of tingling and numbness of the little finger on the left hand. On examination, you corroborate hypesthesia of the 5th finger and also all of the ring finger, and you also find left-side weakness of flexion of fingers and wrist. The patient is able to spread the fingers adequately. Which of the following diagnoses is likely to account for these symptoms?

(A) Ulnar nerve injury
(B) Carpal tunnel syndrome
(C) C6 nerve root compression
(D) C7 nerve root compression
(E) C8 nerve root compression

7 You have a 38-year-old female patient who complains of lower back pain with no radiation with its onset 2 days ago after she did some heavy lifting. She is afebrile. There is some limitation to full flexion and rotation. There is no spinal or paravertebral tenderness. Motor and sensory examinations of her legs are normal. On the SLR test, you can raise each of her legs (with her knees in extension) 80 degrees off the table without any radicular pain. Her pain is made worse when she bends forward at the waist or twists at the waist. The patellar and Achilles deep tendon reflexes are 2+ and symmetrical bilaterally. When she arises from the examining table, she turns onto one side, throws her legs over the table side, and arises from her flank down position with the help of her arms. Which of the following therapies or evaluations would you recommend?

(A) Order a magnetic resonance imaging (MRI) of her lumbar spine after plain x-rays of the lumbar spine
(B) Complete the physical examination and then order strict bed rest at home for 1 week
(C) Order a nerve conduction velocity (NCV) test, electromyogram (EMG), and alkaline phosphatase isoenzyme testing (hepatic vs. bone origin)
(D) Order physical therapy sessions consisting of traction, massage, and diathermy 3 times per week for 2 weeks
(E) Prescribe nonsteroidal anti-inflammatory drugs (NSAIDs) for 5 to 7 days

8 A patient comes to you with the exact same story as the one in Question 5 except for two differences. Instead of 38 years old she is 55 years old, and the pain, instead of starting at a definite known time 2 days before she consulted you, has been present for several weeks. She is unable to tell you what day or even what week the pain began. What she says is that the pain had been bothering her mostly at night for a number

of weeks during which she had difficulty finding a position comfortable for sleeping. For the last 2 to 3 weeks, she notices the pain by daytime as well. Her pain is not influenced by position and she can bend forward at the waist and twist at the waist without aggravating the pain. Her SLR test is negative, and the knee jerks and ankle jerks are 2+ and symmetrical bilaterally. Which of the following therapies or evaluations would you recommend first?

(A) Complete the physical examination, order an MRI of her lumbar spine, and draw alkaline phosphatase isoenzymes
(B) Complete the physical examination and then order strict bed rest at home for 1 week
(C) Order NCV test and EMG
(D) Order physical therapy sessions consisting of traction, massage, and diathermy 3 times per week for 2 weeks
(E) Prescribe NSAIDs for 5 to 7 days

9 A car driven by a 35-year-old woman was struck from behind. She notes the onset of pain several hours later and by morning has significant neck pain with movement in any direction. Which of the following mechanisms is most likely the cause of her symptoms?

(A) Hyperextension of neck
(B) Subluxation of the body of C3 on C4
(C) Contusion to the neck
(D) Extreme rotation of the cervical spine
(E) Fracture of a cervical vertebra

10 You suspect a 55-year-old man has cervical radiculopathy. On examination, you note that there is diminished sensation over the right radial aspects of the thumb and index finger. The triceps reflex is normal and compares with the left triceps, but the biceps reflex is diminished as are the strengths of right elbow flexion and supination, as compared with the left side. The patient is right-handed. Which of the following listed cervical roots do you believe is most affected in this patient's radiculopathy?

(A) C4
(B) C5
(C) C6
(D) C7
(E) T1

11 Regarding the patient in Question 10, he reports 1 week later that his pain is no better after heat, massage, NSAIDs, and cervical traction. You consider seeking the opinion of a neurosurgeon. Which of the following studies would be the most helpful to provide the specialist with a useful database before he or she sees the patient?

(A) Plain x-rays of the cervical spine
(B) EMG of the upper extremities
(C) NCV test of the upper extremities
(D) MRI of the cervical spine → herniated discs
(E) Erythrocyte sedimentation rate

12 A 24-year-old man has complained of back pain and stiffness sometimes radiating into his right groin for the past 4 years. In the past 2 months, he has noticed limitation of motion of twisting. There has been no trauma. He was treated for iritis by you 3 years ago and again in another city while on vacation last year. The back pain increases with spine rotation. On physical examination, he is afebrile with tenderness of the right sacroiliac joint and with loss of lumbar lordosis and a slight increase in the thoracic kyphosis. A sedimentation rate is 50 mm/hour and a test for rheumatoid factor is negative. You find on routine examination aphthous buccal ulcerations, whereupon the patient is reminded of this annoyance that has been present for several weeks. Which of the following is correct in the diagnosis, treatment, and prognosis of this condition?

(A) Of afflicted patients, 85% are positive for human leukocyte antigen (HLA) B-27.
(B) The majority of patients with this condition are female.
(C) Most patients experience resolution of their pain within 4 to 6 weeks.
(D) Proximal interphalangeal and metacarpophalangeal joints are involved with morning stiffness and afternoon gelling.
(E) Radiographs of the peripheral joints will show symmetrical involvement manifesting erosions and demineralization.

13 A 54-year-old man complains of neck, shoulder, and left arm pains that are aggravated by certain neck movements. You suspect herniated nucleus pulposus of a cervical disc. Which of the following is the most appropriate regarding such cervical radiculopathy?

(A) Hand and arm muscle atrophy can be observed in chronic cases.
(B) Acutely, an EMG will show signs of denervation.
(C) There is usually a history of recent blunt neck trauma.
(D) Numbness of the 5th finger and the medial aspect of the adjacent ("ring") finger are typical symptoms.
(E) The Spurling test is highly sensitive and specific in confirming the diagnosis.

14 You are asked to be a consultant for a company that is employed in manufacturing small parts for the automotive industry. The chief of human resources is concerned about the rate of disability among both floor workers and office staff, as defined by days of absence from the job because of health reasons. Without knowing anything specific about the types of illness reported by the employees, which of the following is most likely the leading cause of disability in the employees under the age of 50?

(A) Upper respiratory tract infections
(B) Depression
(C) HIV infection
(D) Heart disease
(E) Lower back pain

15 A 45-year-old woman, otherwise healthy, complains of pain in the left hip area (located in a diffuse area inferior to the iliac crest), present for the past 3 weeks. The pain radiates down the left anterior thigh. She complains of pain while walking with an extended stride. You examine her and find you can evert the left hip without inducing aggravation of the pain. Deep tendon reflexes are symmetrical at about 2+ in the lower extremities, in both the Achilles and the patellar tendons. The SLR test is negative bilaterally. You find tenderness to fairly firm palpation with two fingers distal to the iliac crest over the prominence of the "hip bone." Which of the following is the likely diagnosis?

(A) Hip fracture
(B) Aseptic necrosis of the left femur
(C) Trochanteric bursitis
(D) Herniated nucleus pulposus at the L3-L4 level
(E) Colon diverticulitis

16 Regarding the patient in Question 15, which of the following is the most logical diagnostic or therapeutic approach?

(A) Order 25 to 35 lb (11.3 to 16 kg) of pelvic traction for 30 minutes, repeated every 3 hours, daily
(B) Order 5 days of modified bed rest in the supine Williams position
(C) Order an MRI of the lumbosacral spine
(D) Make a paralesional injection of a glucocorticoid and a local anesthetic agent
(E) Refer the patient for a neurosurgical opinion

Examination Answers

1. The answer is B. C6 supplies sensory fibers to the thumb and motor innervation to the biceps and wrist extensors. C5 through C8 compressions all cause neck pain (C4 and T1 do not). C4 pain radiates into the trapezius and sensory coverage is in the upper shoulder and cape area. C5 radiculopathy radiates into the neck, shoulder, and lateral arm with motor fibers to the deltoid and elbow flexors; the biceps reflex might be depressed and sensory loss in the lateral arm. C7 compression radiates into the lateral and middle finger. C8 supplies motion to the digital flexors triceps and wrist flexors with sensory involvement dorsal forearm and the long finger. C8 compression radiates to the medial forearm and ulnar digits (4th and 5th). T1 involves motor function of the finger intrinsic muscles of the hand and sensory involvement of the ulnar forearm.

2. The answer is D. The Spurling maneuver is axial compression of the cervical spine (by the examiner pressing downward on the patient's head while extending the neck and turning to one side, then the other). The maneuver precipitates closure of any narrowed foramina in the cervical spine and causes radicular pain. Eponyms used here must be forgiven because the listed ones are among many that inflate the common orthopedic glossary. The Hawkins maneuver brings out the pain of rotator cuff impingement through eliciting pain with passive inversion of the shoulder while the elbow is flexed 90 degrees and the shoulder forward flexed 90 degrees; Yergason maneuver uncovers biceps weakness by eliciting pain with forced pronation and supination of the forearm, typically against the examiner's gripped hand; the "empty bucket" sign brings out supraspinatus weakness by showing weakness in holding the upper extremities at 90 degrees abduction with the thumbs pointed downward. The Babinski sign needs no introduction.

3. The answer is C. L5, among the three most often radiculopathy involved lumbar roots in the lumbar area (L4, L% and S1), L5 is the one root that can be implicated in advanced lumbar pathology and not affect either the quadriceps or the Achilles deep tendon reflexes. L3 is not commonly involved in radiculopathy and S2 virtually never.

4. The answer is E. The presence of retrolaryngeal crepitus against the vertebral column is a normal finding. In this situation, it rules against a hematoma resulting from the cervical ligament strain, from which this patient suffers. "Whiplash" by auto accident through rear-ending is the most common cause of neck pain in young people. The

best way of ruling out vertebral body fracture is, of course, by x-ray. Although retrolaryngeal crepitus disappears in the presence of a neoplasm in that space, it is not the reason for affecting the maneuver in this circumstance. Ludwig angina is cellulitis of the submaxillary and hence sublingual and submandibular spaces. It does not occur on the retrolaryngeal space. This maneuver is not needed to rule against a laryngeal fracture. The latter would be manifested by crepitation and tenderness in the thyroid cartilage.

5. The answer is D. This story is typical of spinal stenosis. The majority of patients are over 60 years of age, although there are uncommon congenital versions. The cause is any combination of degenerative changes about the lumbar spinal cord: osteophytic spurs, herniated disc(s), or hypertrophied ligamentum flavum. This syndrome may lead to weakness of the proximal lower extremities. Only 25% of patients with this syndrome exhibit decreased deep tendon reflexes, and 10% have positive SLR tests. Eighty percent of cases will respond to laminectomy, at least for an indefinite period.

6. The answer is E. Sensory deficit of the 4th and 5th finger is typical of a C8 root syndrome, as are weakness of flexion of the fingers and wrist. The fact that the hypesthesia involves all of the ring finger as opposed to only the ulnar half favors C8 rather than ulnar nerve compression, as does the intact lumbrical and interosseous muscle function. Carpal tunnel syndrome causes median nerve symptomatology, that is, sensory deficit of the palmar aspects of the thumb and fingers through the radial half of the ring finger, as well as dorsal aspects of those fingers distal to the proximal interphalangeal joints. Carpal tunnel syndrome also causes a motor deficit consisting of weakness of thumb–finger apposition. The C6 syndrome is associated with hypesthesia and anesthesia of the palmar and dorsal aspects of the thumb and pointing finger; C7 lesions cause sensory involvement of the middle finger and the narrow corresponding aspects of the distal ventral forearm and a longer streak of the dorsal forearm.

7. The answer is E. Without more chronicity than is found in this case and in the absence of radicular symptoms and signs, one should treat the case as lumbosacral strain, with NSAIDs given for a period of about 1 week. Bed rest in a case such as this is to be recommended only until the patient feels she can begin to move and is not to be overemphasized. There is no hurry for x-rays and certainly no hurry for an MRI. It takes 3 or 4 weeks for the NCV test and EMG to show denervation changes in acute compression radiculopathies, even when there are positive symptoms and signs of radiculopathy such as sensory or motor changes (e.g., changes in deep tendon reflexes, dermotomal numbness, and weakness of heel or toe walking). Physical therapy modalities would be employed only after more conservative measures fail over a period of at least 2 weeks.

8. The answer is A. This patient is in the age group for breast cancer; there are no symptoms or signs of radiculopathy, and there are no signs of any musculoskeletal condition whatever. Completion of the physical examination is, in this case, for the specific purpose of searching for a breast lesion (after review of her family history for breast cancer and inquiry as to whether she has had timely mammograms as recommended for the patient 40 years of age and older). Although the MRI could await the results of the plain x-rays, it might as well be ordered immediately, along with alkaline phosphatase testing. The latter is sensitive for bone metastases. Electrical studies are not indicated in the absence of suggestions of radiculopathy. NSAIDs may be helpful but are not relevant to the main thrust of ruling out cancer.

9. The answer is A. Hyperextension of neck, commonly referred to as whiplash injury. The hyperextension is most typically produced by the victim's being in a motor vehicle that is rear-ended by another vehicle. Cervical vertebral body subluxation or fracture would cause most certainly neurological symptoms. The greatest risk for either of these injuries would be a sharp hyperextension such as occurs with a sharp blow to the head from the front as opposed to the hyperextension that occurs with the whiplash mechanism. Extreme rotation of the neck also is fraught with serious sequelae but does not commonly occur in the whiplash mechanism. Contusion of the neck itself requires a direct blow to the soft tissues of the neck, something that would not occur in a rear-end strike unless there were objects loose in the cab of the car. In this and any of the alternative examples given, the pain would not be expected to be delayed as it is in the cervical ligament strain employed in the whiplash mechanism.

10. The answer is C. The affected cervical nerve root is C6. This is a result of a herniation of C6 to C7 or, less often and certainly more possible in a person over the age of 50 years, an osteophytic spur. The classic picture of a C6 lesion shows sensory symptoms of the radial forearm, the index finger, and thumb, and motor involvement of the biceps and wrist extension. Patients are treated conservatively at first, by NSAIDs, warm applications, massage, physical therapy, and possibly cervical traction with 5 to 15 lb (2.3 to 6.8 kg).

11. The answer is D. An MRI is useful as a diagnostic tool for herniated discs but should rarely be used for neck (or back) pain in the absence of radicular symptoms because the test is too sensitive. The more sensitive a test's criteria for positivity, the less specific. Many patients will have positive findings of intervertebral discs showing discernible degrees of herniation that will never become surgical cases. Thus, consulting a neurosurgeon implies not only radicular symptoms (radiation of pain in the distribution of the involved root, sensory symptoms in the appropriate dermatomes, motor symptoms appropriate to the foregoing findings, or any combination thereof) but also the possibility of the case becoming appropriate for surgical correction. Electrical studies are helpful for pinpointing symptoms but do not generally become positive until the symptoms have been present for 3 weeks. Plain films, although included virtually always in evaluation of neck pain, tend to be too sensitive and not specific enough. Sedimentation rate is useful in evaluating a patient for inflammatory arthritis, which would not be considered in this case because of the rapidity of onset and the precipitating activity.

12. The answer is A. This is an example of ankylosing spondylitis. These patients are HLA B-27 positive in 85% of cases. Men are affected more often, more severely, and earlier than women. Peripheral joint involvement occurs transiently in about 50% of cases, and hips, shoulders, and knees permanently in about 25%. Involvement is not symmetrical and does not manifest erosion and demineralization as occurs in rheumatoid arthritis.

13. The answer is A. Hand and arm atrophy are common advanced signs of herniated nuclear pulposus of a cervical disc. It takes 3 or 4 weeks for the EMG to show denervation changes in acute compression radiculopathies. The Spurling test is positive when there is aggravation of the patient's radicular pain or sensory changes when the neck is rotated toward the side of the pain (while in extension) with pressure applied to the head. Although this test is highly specific, it is poorly sensitive. Patients do not usually report a history of recent blunt trauma to the neck, but they may report noticing their symptoms after activities that stress the cervical musculature, including sneezing or violent maneuvers of snuffling during upper respiratory infections. Numbness of the 5th and the medial half of the ring finger are typical symptoms of ulnar nerve dysfunction. Although radiculopathy involving C8 causes hypesthesia of the 4th and 5th fingers, the syndrome is dermatomal and does not spare the lateral half of the ring finger.

14. The answer is E. Lower back pain. Even in patients older than 50 years of age, it ranks second only to heart disease as cause of disability. Although upper respiratory tract infection competes with all other causes of disability in incidence of illness, the number of days of absence caused by back pain in the under-50 age group exceeds that caused by upper respiratory tract infection and, certainly, HIV infection.

15. The answer is C. The pain in the lateral hip area, radiation down the ipsilateral thigh, and tenderness over the greater trochanter are typical. Aseptic necrosis of the femoral head and fracture both would have been very painful upon eversion of the hip. Colon diverticulitis most often occurs in the sigmoid colon and results in deep tenderness in the left lower quadrant of the abdomen. Hip fracture would prevent the patient from walking into the office; a herniated disc would have resulted in a positive SLR test.

16. The answer is D. Injection of a glucocorticoid mixed with a local anesthetic agent into the area of tenderness would be appropriate and effective in the great majority of cases. Such injections are best directed to within a centimeter of, but not into, the most tender point. Pelvic traction was in the past employed in lumbar disc herniation but never had a place in the management of this condition. MRI of the lumbar spine would, at some point, be appropriate in lumbar disc disease, not in trochanteric bursitis. Neurosurgical opinion would not be sought in trochanteric bursitis.

References

Boyd RJ. Evaluation of neck pain. In: Coroll AH, May LA, Mulley AG, eds. *Primary Care Medicine*. Philadelphia: JB Lippincott Co; 1995.

Hellmann DB, Stone JH. Arthritis and musculoskeletal disorders. In: Tierney LM, McPhee SJ, Papadakis MA, eds. *Current Medical Diagnosis and Treatment*. 43rd ed. New York: McGraw-Hill/Appleton & Lange; 2004:778–832.

Maropis CG. Musculoskeletal problems of the neck and back. In: Rudy DR, Kurowski K, eds. *Family Medicine: House Officer Series*. Baltimore: Williams & Wilkins; 1997:371–382.

McPhee SJ, Papadakis MA. *Current Medical Diagnosis and Treatment 2010*, 49th ed. New York/Chicago: McGraw-Hill (Lange); 2010.

chapter 25

Musculoskeletal Problems of the Lower Extremities

Examination questions: Unless instructed otherwise, choose the ONE lettered answer or completion that is BEST in each case.

1 Each of the following is an accepted indication for plain x-rays of the knee following injury except for which case description?

(A) Patient older than 55 years old
(B) Tenderness of the fibula
(C) Patient hears and feels a "pop" as he pivots with a heavy box
(D) Tenderness of the patella
(E) Patient unable to flex knee to 90 degrees

2 A 28-year-old factory worker pivoted on the left leg while transferring a 75-pound item from one bench to another and experienced immediate left knee pain followed shortly by swelling. Upon examination the physician finds a positive "sag test." Which of the following is the equivalent to that test?

(A) McMurray test
(B) Lachman test
(C) Anterior drawer test
(D) Posterior drawer test
(E) Valgus stress test

3 A 35-year-old woman complains of knee pain and manifests tenderness over the medial retinaculum of the patella. Which of the following would most corroborate a diagnosis of patellofemoral pain syndrome?

(A) Pain and tenderness over the patella proper
(B) The "J sign" on examination
(C) Swelling over the patella without palpable effusion
(D) Tenderness over the quadriceps tendon
(E) Knee pain without local findings but with tenderness over the lateral epicondyle

4 A 24-year-old male graduate student and committed amateur athlete comes to see you 1 day after suffering an inversion injury (ankle turned violently inwardly) of the left ankle in pick-up basketball. He was able to bear weight painfully and applied ice last evening with a resultant reduction of moderate swelling. On examination the patient has a "goose egg" type of swelling just inferior to the lateral malleolus, with a negative anterior drawer test; passive inversion of the ankle allows 10 degrees as it does on the right (non-injured) side. There is no tenderness of the tip or posterior edge of the left lateral malleolus and no tenderness of the posterior edge of the medial malleolus. Which of the following initial dispositions is the most logical?

(A) Use supportive dressing (e.g., double layers of sheet wadding or similar material before applying two 4-in. or 10-cm elastic support bandages) followed by a magnetic resonance image (MRI) of the left ankle.
(B) Order stat x-rays of the left ankle and same-day referral to an orthopedic surgeon.
(C) Order stat x-rays, as well as crutches for ambulation for 3 weeks.
(D) Use supportive dressing or an air cast, order crutches until weight bearing takes place without pain, and suggest continued ice application for 1 day more. Have the patient return for follow-up in 1 week.
(E) Encourage immediate weight bearing by the patient and have him return if not improved in 3 days.

5 The patient in the previous question did well on your management but returns to you 1 year later after another inversion injury of the left ankle. On this occasion, he was unable to bear weight at the site of the accident. Examination within the first 2 hours showed a large fusiform swelling centered anteriorly on the lateral malleolus. When you grasp the ankle and pull the foot forward, there is definite forward motion compared with the response to the same maneuver on the right. Which of the following dispositions constitutes the wisest course?

(A) Use supportive dressing (e.g., double layers of sheet wadding or similar material before applying two 4-in. or 10-cm elastic support bandages) followed by MRI of the left ankle.

(B) Order stat x-rays of the left ankle, supportive dressing, crutches, and referral to an orthopedic surgeon.

(C) Order stat x-rays, as well as crutches for ambulation for 3 weeks.

(D) Use supportive dressing or an air cast, order crutches until weight bearing takes place without pain, and suggest continued ice application for 1 day more. Have the patient return for follow-up in 1 week.

(E) Encourage immediate weight bearing by the patient and have him return if not improved in 3 days.

6 A 35-year-old woman comes to you with the complaint of left heel pain, which had its onset over several days with no history of trauma. It is worst during the woman's first steps in the morning or after she has been sitting for prolonged periods or standing for significant periods of time. You ask her to walk without shoes in the back hallway of your office suite. You note that she exhibits valgus deformities at both ankles when walking slowly or standing. The os calcis is tender to compression but exhibits no erythema. There is neither hypesthesia of the overlying skin of the heel nor the medial tract from the heel to the proximal sole. Which of the following is the most likely cause of this patient's complaint?

(A) Achilles tendonitis
(B) Retroachilles bursitis
(C) Tarsal tunnel syndrome
(D) Plantar fasciitis
(E) Osteomyelitis

7 An 18-year-old high school football player complains of left hip pain after being tackled. The pain increases with rotation and lateral bending of the trunk. He denies radiation of the pain into the lower extremities. He bears weight well and examination finds increased pain neither with eversion of the left hip nor with active flexion at the waist. Which of the following is the probable diagnosis?

(A) Contusion of the iliac crest
(B) Inflammation of the greater trochanter of the hip
(C) Inflammation of the lesser trochanter of the hip
(D) Fracture of the left hip
(E) Contusion of the pubic ramus

8 A 19-year-old male high school football player is brought to you 2 hours after the sudden onset of severe right anterior thigh pain during an explosive sprint in an early-season practice game. From a sitting position on the examining table, he is able to extend the knee painfully. He exhibits visible swelling of the thigh with ecchymosis but no depression or unnatural concavity of the thigh contour. Which of the following is the *least* appropriate in the initial management of a grade II muscle strain of the quadriceps?

(A) Stretching of the affected muscles to decrease shortening
(B) Resistance training to rebuild muscle strength
(C) Ice and compression with an elastic wrap
(D) Crutch walking until patient can ambulate without limping
(E) Avoidance of strenuous physical activity

9 An 18-year-old high school football player was tackled from the right side by a linebacker who hit low with his shoulder thrusting against the lateral aspect of the knee. This occurred just as your patient was planting his right foot to pivot for turning left. The event occurred 8 days earlier, and he has been trying to walk on the leg despite pain and swelling. Which of the following would you expect to find on examination (assume swelling has decreased enough to allow adequate examination), in addition to a positive anterior drawer test, if your patient tore his anterior cruciate ligament 8 days earlier?

(A) Prepatellar swelling
(B) Abnormal degree of varus deformity with varus pressure on the leg below the knee
(C) Tenderness of the patella
(D) Tenderness over the anterior aspect of the knee
(E) An abnormal valgus deformity with valgus pressure applied below the knee

10 Which of the following symptoms or signs would be among those characteristic of that knee injury?

(A) Positive posterior drawer sign
(B) Immediate intense pain
(C) A knee-locking sensation
(D) Pain and tenderness in the patella
(E) A palpable spongy sensation overlying the patella

11 A 17-year-old boy has grown from 66 in. (1.68 m) to 71 in. (1.8 m) within the past 18 months. He now complains of pain in the posteromedial aspect of the distal one third of his right tibia since initiation of track training in the past 7 days. On examination he exhibits pes planus and tenderness in the area of described pain. The 128-Hz tuning fork applied to his medial malleolus gives a normal result. Which of the following is the most likely diagnosis of this condition?

(A) Tibial stress syndrome

(B) Stress fracture of the tibia

(C) Fracture of the fibula

(D) Grade 3 anterior ankle sprain

(E) Venous insufficiency of the long saphenous system

12 A 30-year-old athlete noted an instantaneous pain in the proximal posterior medial aspect of the right calf while long-distance running earlier that day. He is afebrile. He limps on his right leg. There is swelling and ecchymosis and tenderness in an area approximately 5 cm in diameter in the proximal posterior medial aspect of the calf as well as ecchymosis in the lower leg and heel. He cannot stand on his toes on the right because of pain precipitated in the calf. Which of the following diagnoses is most likely?

(A) Achilles tendonitis

(B) Achilles tendon rupture

(C) Shin splints

(D) Tibial stress fracture

(E) Gastrocnemius tear

13 A 40-year-old former athlete had been playing football during the annual family reunion. He noted sudden pain in the left lower calf area and is brought to you complaining of posterior distal leg pain. With the patient supine and with his knee flexed, you squeeze the midportion of his calf and do not observe any plantar flexion of the foot. Which of the following diagnoses is most strongly suggested by these findings?

(A) Shin splints

(B) Ruptured Baker cyst

(C) Deep venous thrombosis

(D) Tibial stress fracture

(E) Achilles tendon rupture

14 An 18-year-old white female collegiate track competitor has complained of pain in the left midportion of the tibia over the past 2 weeks during her training, increasingly severe and longer lasting after running sessions. In evaluation of this condition, you utilize the test of the vibrating 128-Hz tuning fork, for sensation when the stem is placed upon the ipsilateral medial malleolus. The patient complains of pain in the area of complaint. Which of the following is true regarding the condition from which this patient suffers?

(A) Normal x-rays rule out stress fractures as a potential cause of a patient's symptoms.

(B) Some limited running or jumping is permitted after 2 weeks of treatment.

(C) This is the most common of stress fractures.

(D) It is caused by a blow to the lower leg.

(E) Swimming is forbidden for the first 4 weeks of treatment.

15 A 35-year-old male army infantry reservist returns from 2 weeks of annual field training that consisted of daily marches increasing in distance from 5 miles (8 km) the first day to 40 miles (64 km) the last day. He complains of pain in the left foot that began 3 days before the end of the tour and increased in severity with the distance walked. The pain lasted longer each evening. Which of the following parts of the bony anatomy of the foot deserves special attention on the plain x-ray?

(A) First metatarsal

(B) Talus

(C) Navicular

(D) Calcaneus

(E) Fifth metatarsal

16 A running back on a high school football team falls backward while being tackled. He lands with one defender on his chest and another on his right foot, which is thus subjected to forced plantar flexion. As team physician you examine the player in the locker room in the supine position and perform the "bounce test," pressing downward on the forefoot. The patient reacts with pain. If the player has a fracture, which of the following sites for it is most likely?

(A) Navicular

(B) Fibula avulsion

(C) Talus

(D) Calcaneus

(E) First metatarsal

17 For several years, your 65-year-old male patient has complained of deep pelvic area pain following strenuous physical activity. Lately he finds that this pain comes on whenever he walks any distance beyond 1 mile (1.6 km). If he stops and sits down for as little as 1 minute, the pain subsides and he can resume walking for another 10 minutes or so. The pain tends to radiate into both posterior proximal thighs, not reaching below the knees. He denies bowel or bladder symptoms of dysfunction. Occasionally he notices weakness and tends to buckle in the left leg before getting relief from sitting and resting. Deep tendon reflexes, results of the straight-leg raising test, and pulses of the lower extremities are all within normal limits. Which of the following is the most logical diagnosis to explain this patient's symptoms?

(A) Lumbar spinal stenosis

(B) Herniated nucleus pulposus at the L5 to S1 level

(C) Osteoarthritis of the lumbar spine

(D) Prostatitis

(E) Lumbosacral strain

Examination Answers

1. The answer is C. Patient hears and feels a "pop" as he pivots with a heavy box, that is, a non-impact injury, does not warrant a plain x-ray unless the criteria of the Ottawa knee rules: patient older than 55 years; tenderness of the patella or of the fibula or inability to flex the knee more than 90 degrees; TTP fibula (at the knee) or confined to the patella; inability to flex knee ≥90 degrees. To the above indications should be added that plain x-rays in an urgent setting should be taken if there was an impact injury of any kind involved. Falls in which the patient lands on straightened legs, especially in patients at risk for osteoporosis, must alert the physician to tibial plateau fracture.

2. The answer is D. Posterior drawer test is the same as the sag test if it is performed with the patient supine. In the sag test the knee is flexed 90 degrees while the examiner pushes the proximal tibia posteriorly and notes the position of the anterior tibial plateau with respect to anterior extent of the femoral condyles. That distance should be 10 mm and should be compared to that of the other side. If the clearance is significantly less, there appears a sag that produces a concavity in the quadriceps tendon below the patella, signifying a posterior cruciate ligament rupture. The anterior drawer test is more or less the opposite in performance and signifies an anterior cruciate tear. The valgus stress test employs application of a valgus stress while stabilizing the knee. A valgus deformity signifies a medial collateral ligament tear; the varus stress test is the opposite. In an apologia for eponyms, they are the daily verbal trade of orthopedic surgeons whom the primary care physicians must consult. The McMurray test is for meniscal injury, and the Lachman is a variant of the anterior drawer test.

3. The answer is B. The "J sign" is observable lateral tracking of the patella as it moves superiorly during extension of the knee. The pain is caused by the patella repetitively riding laterally over the ridge that is the lateral border of the groove through which the patella rides, more commonly found in those with greater valgus carrying angles at the knee, mostly females. Causes are anatomical (excessive valgus angle at the knee, more likely in females), dysfunctionally weak vastus medialis and excessively tight vastus lateralis. Treatment is physical therapy in the vast majority of cases with surgery being a rarity. Pain and tenderness over the patella proper may occur with patella stress fracture. Swelling over the patella without palpable effusion in the joint is prepatellar bursitis. Tenderness over the quadriceps tendon occurs in quadriceps tendinopathy. Knee pain without local findings (i.e.,

referred) but with tenderness over the lateral epicondyle is iliotibial band syndrome or in the past called trochanteric bursitis.

4. The answer is D. On the basis of the moderate swelling and lack of evidence of grade III sprain, this patient had a grade II inversion ankle sprain. This patient has no indications for a plain x-ray, not to mention an MRI. This is based on the patient's ability to bear weight immediately, a negative anterior drawer test, and a negative inversion test; both tests, if positive, would not allow weight bearing according to most experts. Weight bearing in this scenario does not mean the ability to push off normally on the toes in walking but to stand on the axis of the ankle. Indications for plain x-rays of the ankle, in the interest of cost effectiveness, are based on the Ottawa rules: tenderness of the posterior edge of the lateral malleolus (in an inversion injury or medial malleolus in an eversion injury), or inability to bear weight immediately, or in the emergency care situation. To send the patient out bearing full weight would be foolhardy, risky (because of the possibility of aggravating an unappreciated grade III sprain or a fracture), and probably unenforceable. The use of supportive dressing or an air cast can never go wrong. Grade I or II sprains should be 90% well in 10 days and completely well and ready for full athletic activity in 3 weeks.

5. The answer is B. This patient has a grade III sprain, based on the positive anterior drawer test, and thus a complete rupture of the talotibial ligament. Therefore, as a devoted athlete under the age of 40, he becomes a surgical candidate. Stat x-rays are indicated based on the Ottawa criteria that include inability to bear weight, virtually always present in the case of grade III sprains. Failure to appreciate the extent of this injury results in sending the patient forth with an unstable ankle. The latter may lead to further injury. That said, however, the outcomes of repair in the acute phase are very little different from those of repair of chronic ankle instability.

6. The answer is D, plantar fasciitis. This patient, by her ankle valgus deformity (eversion), shows that she has pes planus. That condition is one of the causes of plantar fasciitis through the process of increasing tension on the plantar fascia. Others are pes cavus, decreased subtalar joint mobility, and tight Achilles tendon. The other choices are possible causes of heel pain as well. Retroachilles bursitis is caused by a loose-fitting shoe band at the heel that allows repetitive motion of the skin overlying the bursa. (Quick relief is achieved by cutting a slit in the shoe at the area of friction.) Achilles tendonitis is made worse by running, jumping, and quick turning on the ball of the foot and is aggravated by dorsiflexion. Tarsal tunnel syndrome causes numbness or pain of the heel radiating medially into the sole of the foot. Osteomyelitis would be apparent by the signs of inflammation and infection.

7. The answer is A. The patient has a contusion of the iliac crest, commonly referred to as a "hip pointer." These are usually produced by a direct blow to the iliac crest, such as by a football helmet as the patient is being tackled. Seldom does the player lose playing time beyond a few minutes or a quarter, after cold applications and increased local padding. Hip fracture is ruled out by failure of eversion to elicit the pain. Trochanteric bursitis pain radiates anteriorly down the ipsilateral thigh and is characterized by local tenderness at the greater trochanter. The lesser trochanter is "not in play" for injury except in the presence of a hip fracture, in which case one of the two common types is the intertrochanteric fracture. The patient would neither be bearing weight with hip fracture nor would he painlessly do so in the face of a pubic ramus fracture.

8. The answer is B. The patient has a grade 2 strain of the quadriceps. Resistance training to rebuild muscle strength should not be initiated until swelling and pain have resolved and full range of motion has been restored, usually within about 10 to 14 days. Grade 1 strains show no specific physical findings and little functional impairment. Grade 3 strains involve a complete tear of any of the quadriceps muscles and require ice and compression initially followed by crutch assistance for ambulation until the patient can walk limp free. This would not occur for at least 6 weeks.

9. The answer is E. Valgus deformity with pressure applied is indicative of an associated torn medial collateral ligament, an injury that often accompanies an anterior cruciate ligament tear. These patients may have medial or lateral joint line tenderness secondary to menisci or collateral ligament injury, but no anterior aspect tenderness. The Lachman test is a variant of the anterior drawer test, which is the confirming test for anterior cruciate tear, and as such would be positive. These injuries usually produce a large knee effusion. The effusion would have decreased in size by 8 days later, but it would still be present.

10. The answer is C. As an acute change, a locking sensation is fairly specific for a ruptured meniscus; in addition patients virtually always exhibit tenderness to palpation of the anteriomedial joint space of the knee. Of interest is that immediate pain is not characteristic of meniscal tear. A posterior drawer sign is diagnostic of a posterior cruciate ligament tear. Patellar pain occurs with direct injury to

the patella, either a contusion or a fracture from a direct blow. Anterior knee sponginess is a description of prepatellar effusion, found in prepatellar bursitis (housemaid's knee).

11. The answer is A. The patient has tibial stress syndrome, also known as shin splints. Although precipitated by running exercise, patients who have pes planus or have recently come through rapid growth are more susceptible. Stress fractures may have a similar history (without the association with the foregoing risk factors). If followed for longer periods, unlike with medial tibial stress syndrome, tibial stress fractures result in increasing pain precipitated by decreasingly strenuous activity. Testing for vibration sense upon the tibia results in pain in the case of tibial stress fracture. Neither fibula fractures nor anterior ankle sprain would manifest tibial tenderness and pain. Long saphenous venous insufficiency could cause soft tissue congestion with visible venous ectasia or soft tissue tenderness.

12. The answer is E, torn medial head of the gastrocnemius. The tenderness and swelling are proximal in gastrocnemius tears, whereas in Achilles tendon injuries the pain and tenderness are distal. Swelling and ecchymosis are not typical of shin splints or stress fractures. Ecchymosis distal to the injury site is typical of gastrocnemius tears and actually nonspecific for any injury in a dependent portion of a limb that results in internal bleeding, such as any sprain or other soft tissue renting.

13. The answer is E. The question describes the Thompson test. If the Achilles tendon were intact, squeezing the calf between the examining thumb and fingers would produce plantar flexion. Often, with this injury one can appreciate a notch or depression in a segment of the Achilles tendon. The Homan test (poorly sensitive for deep venous thrombosis) involves forced dorsiflexion of the foot with a positive test elicited if the patient complains of calf pain. See the explanation for Question 9 for a discussion of shin splints and tibial stress fracture. A Baker cyst is a popliteal extension of the joint capsule of the knee. When this cyst ruptures, diffuse calf swelling ensues. However, it is not characterized by focal tenderness, and extravasation of blood is not of defining significance.

14. The answer is C. Tibial stress fracture is the most common of stress fractures, except in the military population, in whom metatarsal ("march") fracture has the highest incidence of stress fracture. Tibial stress fracture occurs most commonly in white female athletes. This is directly related to associated amenorrhea in female track athletes and baseline bone density in white as compared with black athletes. Plain x-rays do not always rule out stress

NMS Q&A Family Medicine

fractures, and bone scans may be necessary. There is no one blow that causes stress fracture; it is the results of cyclic repetitive axial impact. Cortical thickening on x-ray may be seen in advanced stages of stress fractures. Running and jumping are forbidden for at least 6 weeks, but swimming is allowed as early as tolerated.

15. The answer is E, fifth metatarsal. Metatarsal stress fractures are the most common stress fracture among military personnel. Metaphyseal fifth metacarpal stress fractures carry a higher risk of conversion to a complete fracture and nonunion. For that reason, unlike with other metatarsal fractures, a fifth metatarsal fracture has to be managed more aggressively, including short-leg-cast application, complete non-weight-bearing status, or open reduction and internal fixation.

16. The answer is C, posterior process of the talus. Rapid plantar flexion of the ankle (the bounce test), reproducing the original mechanism of injury, will produce pain in the posterior talus.

17. The answer is A. This is a story typical of lumbar spinal stenosis: lumbosacral and deep pelvic pain, more often than not symmetrical, coming on during walking upright and relived by the sedentary position or otherwise flexing at the hips for less than a minute. It occurs most often in a person's seventh decade and later. The cause tends to be a mixture of osteophytic spur formation and varying degrees of herniated discs (nuclei pulposi), effectively narrowing the spinal canal. Claudication is often suspected but palpability of the pulses rules it out. Although a herniated disc can contribute to the syndrome, it seldom occurs with this presentation; knee buckling, as mentioned in the vignette, implies the L4 to L5 root, not the L5 to S1. Prostatitis should be considered in the differential diagnosis of deep pelvic pain, but back pain referral in that situation is sacral, and the pain of prostatitis has no relationship to posture or activity. Lumbosacral strain does not radiate from the low back.

References

Aldridge T. Diagnosing heel pain in adults. *Am Fam Physician.* 2004; 70:332–338.

Family Medicine Board Review 2009. Kansas City, Missouri; May 3–10, 2009.

Sickles RT. Mechanical problems of the lower extremities. In: Rudy DR, Kurowski K, eds. *Family Medicine: House Officer Series.* Baltimore, MD: Williams & Wilkins; 1997:399–412.

Terrell TR, Leski MJ. Sports medicine. In: Rakel RE, ed. *Textbook of Family Practice*, 6th ed. Philadelphia: WB Saunders; 2002:845–890.

Wexler RW. The injured ankle. *Am Fam Physician* 1998; 57: 474–480.

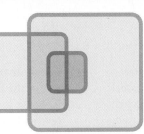

chapter **26**

Rheumatology in Primary Care

Examination questions: Unless instructed otherwise, choose the ONE lettered answer or completion that is BEST in each case.

1 Each of the following complications or associated conditions decreases the 10-year survival projection for a patient with systemic lupus erythematosus (from 85% to 55%) except for which one?

(A) Nephrotic syndrome
(B) Elevated serum albumen
(C) Proliferative glomerular changes
(D) Serum creatinine >1.4 mg/dL
(E) Hypertension

2 A 60-year-old woman who takes hydrochlorothiazide and triamterene in combination for hypertension complains of acute onset of pain in the left great toe metatarsophalangeal (MTP) joint that is surrounded by angry red erythema for a diameter of 4 to 5 cm. The family doctor diagnoses gout and considers prescribing a uric acid lowering agent. Each of the following is an indication for instituting such agents except for which one?

(A) Presence of tophi
(B) Erosive arthritis on x-ray
(C) Uric kidney stones
(D) Uric acid level >7.5 mg/dL
(E) Three attacks of gout/year

3 It is now believed that early diagnosis, hence early treatment, of rheumatoid arthritis (RA), permits not only earlier alleviation of symptoms and prevention of later complications but also prolongation of survival. Which of the following would secure a diagnosis of RA?

(A) Presence of a positive rheumatoid factor by serum test
(B) Sedimentation rate over 60 mm/hour, combined with positive rheumatoid factor
(C) Choice B combined with morning stiffness of arthralgic joints
(D) One hour of morning stiffness; 3 swollen joints; joint erosions on XR; rheumatoid nodules
(E) More than 6 weeks of symptoms; hand involvement, symmetric involvement

4 A 35-year-old woman consults you for pain in the left knee region that appears to be associated with an effusion. No other musculoskeletal pain is present and there is no history of trauma. Each of the following is among the first group of measures to take in diagnosing this patient, except which one?

(A) Take a complete history and perform a relevant physical examination
(B) Determine whether the pain emanates from the knee joint
(C) Obtain plain x-ray films of the joint
(D) Perform arthrocentesis
(E) Order a magnetic resonance imaging of the knee

5 Regarding the patient in Question 4, you determine that she has an effusion in the left knee joint, which is warm to the touch. The pain had its onset only over the past 3 weeks. The bouts of this pain have had no relationship to atmospheric changes. There has been no history of trauma, whether acute or chronic. Which of the following is the most likely cause of the monoarthritis in this patient?

(A) RA
(B) Gout
(C) Staphylococcal septic arthritis
(D) Gonococcal arthritis
(E) Osteoarthritis

6 Regarding the patient in Questions 4 and 5, aspiration yields no crystals and shows a white blood cell (WBC) count of 35,000/mm³. To your surprise, a culture of the joint fluid yields growth of Gram-negative rods. Which of the following items might explain this departure from the flora expected in this situation?

(A) Positive human immunodeficiency virus (HIV) titer
(B) Positive antinuclear antibody
(C) A uric acid level of 11 mg/mL
(D) A transferrin saturation level of 60%
(E) A reexamination shows erythema migrans

163

7 For a patient with diagnosed RA, you consider starting a disease modifying drug (DMARD) based on the belief that early use of DMARD results in delayed progression of bone erosion compared to delayed treatment. Each of the following is an example of a DMARD except which one?

(A) Azathioprine < Methotrexate 2e
(B) Hydroxychloroquine < Antimalarials
(C) Auranofin < Intramuscular gold 2e
(D) Cox-2 inhibiting NSAIDs
(E) Etanercept

8 A 45–year-old man has complained of low back pain, worse in the morning and occasionally during the nights, gradually increasing over the past 3 months. Three days ago, he began to have discomfort in the left eye, which upon entering the office appears red and the patient is squinting in the lights of the examining room. There are no gastrointestinal complaints nor skin lesions. Stain of the cornea with fluorescein is negative for disruption of the epithelium. The pupil in the left (affected) eye is smaller than that of the right. You draw blood tests and find that the patient's human leukocyte antigen (HLA) is type B27. Which of the following tests or signs is likely to be positive/present?

(A) Plantar reflex
(B) Murphy sign
(C) Schirmer test
(D) Rovsing sign
(E) Schober test

9 A 48-year-old man who has been diagnosed with ankylosing spondylitis now complains of left foot pain. In what part of the foot is the most likely locale for this pain to appear?

(A) Retrocalcaneal
(B) First metatarsal
(C) Between the first and second metarsals
(D) Across the dorsum of the forefoot
(E) Supracalcaneal

10 You are examining a 12-year-old male patient with a history of arthralgias. Upon examination, you note that the skin is easily stretched and has a dry, rubbery feel. The patient's mother asks him to demonstrate that he can place his hand flat on the examining table, then lift it, and rotate it painlessly 360 degrees and place it back flat on the table. Which of the following is the most likely diagnosis?

(A) Congenital dislocation of the shoulder
(B) Ehlers–Danlos syndrome
(C) Polymyositis
(D) Fibromyalgia
(E) RA

11 A 45-year-old white woman complains of pain on the sole of the foot. It has been present for several weeks, is worse in the mornings for several minutes, and tends to subside when the patient walks significant distances; it is aggravated by walking upstairs. Which of the following is the likely diagnosis?

(A) Calcaneal epiphysitis
(B) Lumbar radiculopathy
(C) Osteomalacia
(D) Claudication of the foot
(E) Plantar fasciitis

12 Which of the following statements regarding fibromyalgia (fibrositis) is correct?

(A) In its pure form, NSAIDs are often of benefit.
(B) Affected patients usually have decreased delta-wave sleep on sleep studies.
(C) Affected patients have evidence of neuropathy on nerve conduction studies that is consistent with the paresthesias they report.
(D) Sedimentation rates and C-reactive protein levels are elevated.
(E) Patients demonstrate diffuse joint effusion.

13 A 60-year-old man complains of right hip pain, which has progressed over the past 5 years. There have been no recent falls or trauma. He used to play halfback in football during his high school and college days. He is afebrile and has no visible joint deformities on examination. You note poor right hip abduction and slight pain to palpation. You believe he may have osteoarthritis of his right hip. Which of the following statements regarding osteoarthritis is correct?

(A) Women tend to have fewer joints involved than men.
(B) Patients typically complain of 1 to 2 hours of morning stiffness.
(C) It is more likely to be seen if significant trauma has occurred to the affected joint.
(D) There is usually pain only on active range of motion of the involved joint.
(E) It is always symptomatic with pain, crepitus, and stiffness.

14 After being started on hydrochlorothiazide, a 60-year-old man complains of bouts of intense pain at the great toe MTP joint, and you suspect gout. Which of the following would have to be true for you to confirm this diagnosis with certainty?

(A) The pain is located in the first MTP joint.
(B) The patient has an elevated serum uric acid level.
(C) The patient has an erythematous, painful joint associated with a fever and serum leukocytosis.

(D) A 24-hour urine uric acid level is <800 mg/dL.

(E) Aspirated joint fluid shows negatively birefringent, needle-shaped crystals within WBCs when viewed with a polarizing microscope.

15 Which of the following is correct with respect to calcium pyrophosphate deposition disease (CPDD, also known as pseudogout)?

(A) Its incidence is increased with advanced patient age.

(B) The crystals are easier to detect in this disease than in gout.

(C) It may be associated with hypoparathyroidism.

(D) It typically affects only the weight-bearing joints.

(E) Attacks are always monoarticular.

For Questions 16 through 20, match the numbered soft tissue causes of heel pain with the lettered descriptions of clinical presentations.

16 Fat pad atrophy

17 Heel contusion

18 Plantar fascia rupture

19 Posterior tibial tendonitis

20 Retrocalcaneal bursitis

(A) Pain is retrocalcaneal.

(B) Pain is in the inside of the foot and the ankle.

(C) There is an intense tearing sensation on the bottom of the foot.

(D) There is a history of trauma.

(E) Pain is in the area of a thinned plantar aspect of the heel.

Examination Answers

1. The answer is B. Elevated serum *albumen* is not a poor prognostic sign. In fact, low albumen is one of the factors that presage a poor prognosis. Each of the other choices is associated with poor survival prognosis; other poor prognostic signs besides those given include anemia and refractoriness to therapy.

2. The answer is D. Uric acid level >7.5 mg/dL, although present at some point (75% of the time in a given patient) in 95% of cases, in itself it *is not* an indication for uric acid lowering agents. Each of the other factors is such an indication (number of attacks/2 years or more).

3. The answer is D. One hour of morning stiffness; three swollen joints; joint erosions on XR; rheumatoid nodules. Specifically, the diagnosis can be made by presence of any four of seven criteria – those of choice D and the three in choice E: more than 6 weeks of symptoms; hand involvement, symmetric involvement. Early diagnosis of RA prevents suffering, deformity, progression, and it also prolongs life and improves quality of life. The mechanism for prolonging life in large part is preventing stroke and heart disease by decreasing inflammation and thereby stabilizing plaques rendering them less likely to rupture and occlude vessels.

4. The answer is E. At the point at which this patient enters the system, the patient presents with a monoarthralgia that may or may not be a monoarthritis. Monoarthritis is defined as arthritis existing in one joint for more than a few days. The first priorities are to obtain a complete history and physical examination to ascertain that the pain indeed originates in the (knee) joint. If a determination is made that monoarthritis exists, then plain x-rays and joint aspiration should be obtained, along with basic laboratory studies (complete blood cell count, sedimentation rate, and uric acid level), before a magnetic resonance imaging study is ordered. Many patients complain of pain in the *regions* of joints whose pains are not truly arthralgias.

5. The answer is D. Gonococcal arthritis is the most common form of nontraumatic monoarthritis. It is three times as common in women as in men. RA may pass briefly through a monoarticular phase but generally affects joints in a symmetrical fashion. Nongonococcal arthritis is most often caused by *Staphylococcus aureus* and is much more destructive to the joint than is gonococcal arthritis. It is also monoarticular in 80% of cases

and most often affects the knee. Osteoarthritis of severity to produce an effusion would be unusual in a young woman without significant history of trauma.

6. The answer is A. Monoarticular *septic* arthritis (as opposed to traumatic arthritis or gout, among others) in which Gram-negative or anaerobic bacteria, Lyme disease, or tuberculosis organisms grow from joint fluid, must be investigated for the possibility of immunodeficiency.

7. The answer is D. Cox-2 NSAIDs are not disease modifying, although they are anti-inflammatory as well as analgesic. Each of the other drugs or categories is disease modifying. Other DMARDs besides those mentioned include leflunomide, methotrexate, azathioprine, penicillamine, and sulfasalazine as well as other tumor necrosis factor (TNF) antagonists besides etanercept and other antimalarials besides hydroxychloroquine.

8. The answer is E. The Schober test. This is a test of mobility of the spine, performed by marking the spinous process of L5 and marking at a point 10 cm above the L5 spine. The patient is directed to bend forward, and normally, the two marks are observed to move apart by 5 cm or more. Although the test is nonspecific, when back pain exists in the presence of spine immobility and extra-articular manifestations, the Schober test may clinch the diagnosis of ankylosing spondylitis. The differential diagnosis includes, besides ankylosing spondylitis, reactive arthritis (Reiter syndrome) as well as psoriatic arthritis. The eponym *Schober test* in this case is more convenient than a descriptive term; therefore, the student will expect to hear mention of the Schober test in practice and training. An upper motor neuron sign such as the Babinski is hardly likely in the vignette presented. The Murphy and Rovsing signs are relevant in the surgical diagnosis of abdominal pain, and the Schirmer test is for adequacy of lacrimal response in the eye.

9. The answer is A. The retrocalcaneal would be the location of pain in the foot area associated with ankylosing spondylitis. Two common sites of inflammation of the attachment of tendon to bone (enthesitis) in ankylosing spondylitis are the Achilles tendon at the calcaneus and plantar fascia at the calcaneus. Enthesitis occurs also with Reiter syndrome and psoriatic arthritis, but not with spondyloarthropathy related to inflammatory bowel disease.

10. The answer is B. To test for Ehlers–Danlos syndrome, one should assess for passive hyperextension at the knee, elbow, and MCP joints. There are no characteristic joint deformities or effusions in patients with Ehlers–Danlos syndrome, although many affected patients can develop a secondary osteoarthritis. In fact, the greatest morbidity over time is osteoarthritis.

11. The answer is E. Plantar fasciitis is well described in this vignette. Ten percent of the U.S. population suffers from this malady at some time in their lives. Calcaneal epiphysitis causes heel pain in adolescents but no plantar pain. Lumbar radiculopathy causes referred pain that radiates from the lumbar area to the foot when it is referred to that extent. Referred pain is not aggravated by local factors. Osteomalacia is a systemic disease that causes bone pain in multiple sites and total body weakness. The pain of claudication is made worse by exercise and, when involving the lower extremities, generally is felt in the calf, more than the foot proper. Plantar fasciitis is worst after inactivity, usually improving with usage.

12. The answer is B. Fibromyalgia is a diagnosis of exclusion. The two themes that appear consistently are multiple musculoskeletal pains without weakness and sleep dysfunction. Patients affected with fibromyalgia usually have decreased delta-wave sleep on sleep studies. There is no physical or laboratory evidence of joint inflammation in these patients and no documentable neuropathies, even though patients frequently complain of paresthesias. NSAIDs are only useful if the patient has some superimposed osteoarthritis or other NSAID-responsive condition.

13. The answer is C. Osteoarthritis is more likely to be seen if significant trauma has occurred to the affected joint. Osteoarthritis is frequently asymptomatic for years. The typical stiffness of osteoarthritis lasts less than 5 minutes. Women are more likely to have more severe disease than men, with increased numbness of joints involved and deformities. Both passive and active range of motion produces pain in the involved joint. Besides osteophytic spurs, hence the name osteoarthritis, x-ray findings may include asymmetrical joint spaces. Osteoarthritis may exist without symptoms. However, such cases have a way of popping into view with precipitating trauma, which may be relatively mild in and of itself.

14. The answer is E. In gout, aspirated joint fluid shows negatively birefringent, needle-shaped crystals within WBCs when viewed with a polarizing microscope. It is true that the vast majority of patients who present with isolated acute first MTP joint pain will have gout. However, such a description of pain is not 100% specific for gout. Many patients have hyperuricemia (from overproduction or underexcretion) and yet never have attacks of gouty arthritis. Septic joints are also erythematous with fever and serum leukocytosis.

15. The answer is A. Its incidence is increased with advanced patient age. CPDD, especially in its idiopathic form, is seen more with increasing age. CPDD is also associated with hyperparathyroidism, gout, hypothyroidism, and hemochromatosis. It is more likely to be polyarticular than gout is, and it does not have a predilection for the weight-bearing joints.

MATCHING THE NUMBERED CAUSES WITH THE LETTERED DESCRIPTIONS

16. Fat pad atrophy: **The answer is E,** pain in the area of a thinned plantar aspect of the heel.

17. Heel contusion: **The answer is D,** history of trauma.

18. Plantar fascia rupture: **The answer is C,** intense tearing sensation on the bottom of the foot.

19. Posterior tibial tendonitis: **The answer is B,** pain in the inside of the foot and ankle.

20. Retrocalcaneal bursitis: **The answer is A,** the pain is retrocalcaneal.

References

Chokkalingam S, Velasquez C, Mody A, et al. Diagnosing monoarthritis in adults: A practical approach for the family physician. *Am Fam Physician.* 2003; 68:83–90.

Cole C, Seto C, Gazewood J. Plantar fasciitis: Evidence based review of diagnosis and therapy. *Am Fam Physician.* 2005; 72:2237–2242, 2247–2248.

Derk CT, Vivino FB. A primary care approach to Sjogren's syndrome. *Postgrad Med.* 2004; 116:48–65.

Emery P, Suarez-Almazor, ME. Rheumatoid arthritis. *Am Fam Physician.* 2003; 68:1821–1823.

Family Medicine Board Review. Kansas City, Missouri; May 3–10; 2009.

Seigel LB, Gall EP. Approach to the patient with rheumatic disease. In: Rudy DR, Kurowski K, eds. *Family Medicine: House Officer Series.* Baltimore: Williams & Wilkins; 1997:413–438.

chapter 27

Musculoskeletal Problems in Children

Examination questions: Unless instructed otherwise, choose the ONE lettered answer or completion that is BEST in each case.

1 You are caring for an adolescent whose routine chest x-ray shows a curvature in the thoracic spine. Which of the following is *not* consistent with probably idiopathic scoliosis.

(A) Right dorsal thoracic ribcage is more prominent than the left
(B) Female patient
(C) Family history of idiopathic scoliosis
(D) Right thoracic curve
(E) Left thoracic curve

2 A 5-month-old boy is brought to the family doctor by the parents who complain of the baby constantly lying with the head turned onto the left side, that is, the head turning right in his crib when lying face down or turned onto the right asleep on his back. Each of the following is a true statement regarding this condition except for which one?

(A) The condition likely a result of right sternocleidomastoid (SCM) pathology.
(B) There may be congenital deformity of the cervical spine.
(C) There may be a palpable nodular prominence of the left SCM muscle.
(D) Failure to treat will result in facial distortion.
(E) There may be associated hip congenital hip dysplasia.

3 A 7-year-old boy is brought to your office by his parents with complaint of pain in the right knee whose onset was gradual over the past 3 weeks. It is worsened by athletic play and by kneeling on a hard surface. On examination, there is seen to be a tender swelling inferior to the patella. Which of the following statements is true regarding this condition?

(A) Quadriceps exercises are a mainstay of treatment during the acute phase.
(B) There usually is associated knee joint effusion.

(C) This condition is an expression of juvenile rheumatoid arthritis (JRA).
(D) The condition usually remits after fusion of the tibial tubercle with the diaphysis.
(E) The condition is caused by premature closure of the tibial tuberosity with the diaphysis.

4 A 6-year-old boy has developed a limp over a period of 5 days. He appears to be ill and has had a fever with temperatures rising to 102°F. During examination, eversion of the left hip elicits pain. Which of the following is the least logical next step in the disposition in this case?

(A) Open surgical exploration
(B) Determination of complete blood cell (CBC) count and sedimentation rate
(C) Needle aspiration of the left hip joint
(D) Plain x-rays of the left hip
(E) Arthroscopy

5 A 7-year-old boy began limping after exercise several months ago. The parents questioned him at first and he denied pain. Later the boy began complaining of pain in the right hip and at times the right thigh and knee. Over the past week, the pain has been disabling. Vital signs are normal; on examination, the boy is unable to actively abduct and internally rotate as a result of muscle spasm. A CBC count is normal. A plain x-ray shows a "moth eaten" appearance of the femoral epiphysis, flattening of the head, and irregular contours of the acetabulum. Which of the following is the likely diagnosis?

(A) Slipped femoral capital epiphysis
(B) Legg–Calvé–Perthes disease
(C) Septic arthritis of the right hip
(D) Toxic synovitis
(E) Osteomyelitis of the right femur

6 A 14-year-old boy, who is in the early stages of sexual development, complains of left knee pain, developing over a course of 2 weeks. He walks with a limp. On examination his weight is 184 lb (83.4 kg) at a height of 5 ft, 5 in. (1.65 m). He holds his left hip in about 5 degrees of flexion and is unable to fully extend the hip to 180 degrees. He has no constitutional symptoms or signs. The result of a CBC is unremarkable. A plain posteroanterior x-ray film of the left hip is unremarkable. Which of the following is the most logical next step in obtaining a diagnosis?

(A) Order a lateral view x-ray of the left hip
(B) Order serum level tests of calcium and alkaline phosphatase
(C) Perform left hip joint aspiration
(D) Order a magnetic resonance image of the left hip
(E) Consult a surgeon for arthroscopic exploration of the left hip

7 While examining a female newborn, you perform a Barlow maneuver (attempting to dislocate the newborn's femoral heads interiorly from the acetabulum with your forefinger, while grasping the thigh with your thumb placed on the medial proximal thigh). You sense a clear movement interiorly of the femoral head on the baby's left hip. Each of the following statements is true regarding the condition in the patient in the vignette except for which one?

(A) Female infants are affected more than male infants.
(B) For optimal outcome the condition must be diagnosed and treated before the child reaches the age of 6 months.
(C) There may be a history of this condition in the baby's family.
(D) If the baby is not diagnosed before the age of walking, the baby's gait becomes waddling and the perineum broadened.
(E) The presence of intoeing effectively rules out developmental dislocation of the hip.

8 A 5-year-old girl has complained for 5 months of pain in her left wrist and right second and third metacarpophalangeal joints. This week she complains

of photophobia in the left eye. Examination shows the left pupil to be constricted, compared with the right eye. An antinuclear antibody level is elevated. Which of the following is the most likely and most precise diagnosis, given the clinical picture?

(A) Rheumatic fever
(B) JRA or Still disease
(C) Reiter syndrome
(D) Pauciarticular JRA
(E) Rheumatoid arthritis

9 Parents frequently are concerned with "intoeing" in infants. It may be safe to say that parents bring it to their doctors' attention more than the other way around. Being armed with data regarding this complaint makes it much quicker and easier for physicians to manage the families as well as the patients. Which of the following is not true in regard to intoeing?

(A) Metatarsus adductus may be the cause.
(B) Internal tibial torsion may be the cause.
(C) Excessive femoral anteversion may be the cause.
(D) Developmental hip dislocation may be associated with it.
(E) The majority of cases require surgical correction if they have not resolved by the time the child reaches the age of 8 years.

10 A father brings to you a 6-year-old boy who fell onto his outstretched hand while playing at recess in grade school. The boy complains of pain and the extremity manifests swelling in an area just proximal to the wrist. An x-ray done stat in the office building comes back to reveal a buckling of the distal radius, visible in both anteroposterior and lateral views. Which of the following is the best treatment strategy?

(A) Open reduction
(B) Short-arm cast for 6 weeks
(C) Closed reduction followed by casting for 3 weeks
(D) Long-arm cast for 3 weeks
(E) Observation only

![Examination Answers icon] *Examination Answers*

1. The answer is E. Left thoracic curve is not consistent with idiopathic scoliosis; that is, right thoracic curvature is common. A prominent right posterior ribcage is the anatomic equivalent of the right thoracic curvature as the curvature in scoliosis is due to the rotation of the thoracic spine counter-clockwise from above. Femaleness is more common than males, at least insofar as symptomatic cases go. Family history is common.

2. The answer is A. The condition likely is a result of the *left, not the right* SCM pathology, that is, due to shortening and spasm of the left SCM. The deformity generally is caused by a fibrous transformation in the left SCM in this case, which, when it contracts, turns the head in the opposite direction. This is apparently caused by congenital cervical spine deformity. It is generally successfully treated conservatively through stretching exercises. If not treated, due to the immaturity of the bones involved with their developing growth plates, facial asymmetry will result. In 20% of the cases, there may exist congenital hip dysplasia.

3. The answer is D. The condition is called Osgood–Schlatter disease and is caused by traction apophysitis of the tibial tubercle. The tibial tubercle becomes enlarged (the apophysis) in a preadolescent boy (more often than a girl) and the unclosed connection to the diaphysis becomes inflamed as a result of microtrauma and traction on the tubercle by the quadriceps apparatus at its attachment; thus, the condition is called a "traction" apophysitis. Quadriceps exercises would likely aggravate the condition in the acute phase, but activity level in general is guided by the symptoms associated; that is, activity is curtailed when it aggravates symptoms. The condition usually remits when the tubercle fuses with the diaphysis, when the child is between the ages of 9 and 15 years. The knee joint is not involved; therefore, there is no joint effusion. Osgood–Schlatter disease is not related to JRA. Because the disease is a result of trauma to an unclosed ossification system, it cannot be a sequela of a lack of closure of tubercle with diaphysis.

4. The answer is A. Open exploration of the hip joint need not be the first move. The differential diagnosis of acute hip pain in a child includes septic arthritis and toxic synovitis, as well as Legg–Calvé–Perthes disease. The most critical in terms of early diagnosis to prevent joint destruction is septic arthritis of the hip. All three would present with pain upon hip eversion. The patient with septic arthritis is ill. The first step is aspiration of the joint along with a determination of CBC and sedimentation rate. The

joint fluid is cultured and examined for white blood cells and glucose. In septic arthritis, but not toxic synovitis, there is a leukocytosis and neutrophilia with a left shift. The most common organism involved is *Staphylococcus aureus*. Plain x-rays will pick up osteomyelitis, Legg–Calvé–Perthes disease, and slipped femoral capital epiphysis. While culture and sensitivity are awaited, an empiric choice of antibiotic is started. Only if there is no response within 48 hours need there be an arthroscopic approach to the joint. Open exploration appears to be increasingly less frequently employed.

5. The answer is B. Legg–Calvé–Perthes disease is avascular necrosis of the femoral head. It occurs more often in boys than girls at a ratio of 5:1. Early referral for orthopedic correction is crucial.

6. The answer is A. This boy's hip pain fits the clinical setting of slipped femoral capital epiphysis; he is an obese adolescent boy with late and underdeveloped sexual maturation. The posteroanterior view of the hip may fail to show the displacement of the femoral head posteriorly with respect to the femoral neck. Thus, a lateral view x-ray of the left hip would pick up that abnormality. Calcium and alkaline phosphatase levels are of value in investigating possibilities of destructive lesions of the bone, among other things, but they are not relevant in slipped femoral capital epiphysis. Joint aspiration would not be justified as an early diagnostic step, in the absence of constitutional symptoms and signs. A magnetic resonance image would make the diagnosis but is unnecessarily expensive. Although the problem is treated surgically, an early exploration is not necessary to achieve diagnosis.

7. The answer is E. The described maneuver, the Barlow maneuver, has elicited the diagnosis of developmental or congenital dysplasia or dislocation of the hip (DDH or CDD). DDH may be a cause of intoeing. The opposite maneuver that of reduction of the hip dislocation is called the Ortolani maneuver. If the hip joint is dislocated at the initial examination, the Ortolani maneuver may provide the primary diagnostic sign. Examination for asymmetry of skin folds in the thighs posteriorly was taught on pediatric rotations of old. However, such asymmetry is present in 40% of all (i.e., normal) newborns and thus is not helpful. Female patients are affected more than male patients by a ratio of 6:1. The left hip alone is affected in 60% of the time, and in 20% of cases the affliction is bilateral. A positive family history exists in 20%, and this serves as a guiding principle for sonographic screening, when present. The sooner the diagnosis is made, the better the ultimate outcome after correction, the best results occurring if the diagnosis is made no later than 6 weeks after the infant's birth. The waddling gait seen in uncorrected cases is associated with a broadened perineum because of the lateral displacement of the femoral head(s).

8. The answer is D. The onset of fewer than four joints involved in arthritis, within the first 6 months of arthritic pain, is called pauciarticular JRA and carries an increased risk for iritis. A positive antinuclear antibody titer increases the risk. These patients are rheumatoid factor negative. This type of pauciarticular JRA is the foremost cause of blindness in children. These patients need periodic slit-lamp examination by an ophthalmologist. A second type of pauciarticular JRA affects boys between the ages of 8 and 10 years. These boys are antinuclear antibody and rheumatoid factor negative but manifest a high prevalence of human leukocyte antigen, type HLA-B27.

9. The answer is E. The statement that "the majority of cases require surgical correction if not resolved by time the child reaches the age of 8 years" is not true in regard to intoeing, though 95% of intoeing cases resolve spontaneously by that ages. The most common cause of intoeing is excessive femoral anteversion, and it has its onset between the ages of 2 and 3 years. It causes cosmetic and sometimes functional gait changes and may lead to osteoarthritis. As its name would indicate, the intoeing that is due to femoral anteversion is associated with a turning in of the patellae as well as the feet, because the problem exists at the hips. Although most cases will have resolved by the time the child reaches the age of 8, those that do not usually accommodate, unless the condition is severe. Osteotomy, the only treatment available, is fraught with complications and thus is extended to

only a minority of cases that have persisted. Although three other conditions listed may be causes of intoeing and each has its own pathophysiology and therapeutic approach, each seldom requires surgery. Rarely, cases of developmental hip dislocation occur in association with metatarsus adductus and chances of surgery would depend on timeliness of diagnosis. Metatarsus adductus virtually always resolves by the age of 1 year or later in childhood, and internal tibial torsion responds poorly to any surgical approach. Tibial torsion has usually ceased to be noticeable by the time the child reaches the age of 16 months. If it has not, it may be ameliorated by mechanical devices.

10. The answer is D, long-arm cast for 3 weeks. The fracture described is a torus or "green stick" fracture, seen in preadolescent children. It is well named and refers to the fact that the bone is soft, not brittle, at these ages. Virtually by definition, reduction of any type is unnecessary because there is no separation of fragments and seldom angulation. The immobilization should be standard for the fracture, generally following the rule to include a joint both proximal and distal to the fracture within the cast. However, this immobilization need be only for 3 weeks instead of the usual 6 weeks for most fractures.

References

Eilert RE. Orthopedics. In: Hay WW, Levin MJ, Sondheimer JM, et al., eds. *Current Pediatric Diagnosis and Treatment*, 17th ed. New York: McGraw-Hill; 2005:810–828.

Family Medicine Board Review 2009. Kansas City, Missouri; May 3–10, 2009.

Wenacur R, Tucker JB. Musculoskeletal problems in children. In: Rudy DR, Kurowski K, eds. *Family Medicine: House Officer Series*. Baltimore, MD: Williams & Wilkins; 1997:439–446.

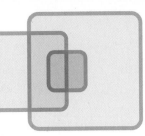

chapter **28**

Connective Tissue Diseases

Examination questions: *Unless instructed otherwise, choose the ONE lettered answer or completion that is BEST in each case.*

1 A 28-year-old woman has had deep vein thrombosis in the past 3 years and is in the emergency department with a diagnosis of pulmonary embolism. Laboratory studies over the following 2 days revealed normal levels of Proteins C and S and antithrombin III. Further testing showed a positive lupus erythematosus (LE) preparation. Serologic test for syphilis is falsely positive. There is no rash; renal function is normal. Which of the following might be the most helpful laboratory test at this point?

(A) Complete blood cell (CBC)
(B) Sedimentation rate
(C) Anticardiolipin antibody level
(D) Prothrombin time
(E) Hemoglobin A1C

2 A 34-year-old Caucasian woman has complained of color change of her right index finger during cold or dampness exposure, particularly during times of fatigue. The changes consist of whiteness of the skin of the finger well demarcated at the proximal interphalangeal joint. The change is associated with a subjective and objective feeling of coldness of the digit. The phenomenon lasts about an hour and recovers with a red or purple color until another half hour later. More recently, she complains of difficulty swallowing. Which of the following is the likely diagnosis?

(A) Sjögren disease
(B) Systemic lupus erythematosus (SLE)
(C) Scleroderma
(D) Dermatomyositis
(E) Raynauds disease

3 A 72-year-old man begins to notice jaw pains on the right side while chewing. On examination, a bruit is heard over the left subclavicular area of anterior chest. The sedimentation rate is 75 mm/hour. Each of the following statements is important in close observation of this situation except for which one?

(A) There is a 50% chance of this patient having shoulder and pelvic girdle stiffness.

(B) There is a risk of unilateral blindness as a sequel.
(C) There may be fever as high as 40°C (104°F).
(D) There is likely a complaint of muscular weakness.
(E) A course of glucocorticoid may be critical.

4 A 34-year-old man notices a rash on the lower extremities, present for 4 days. He had contracted a viral upper respiratory infection (URI) approximately 10 days before. The patient lives in an urban setting and had not sojourned in the wilderness for several years. Upon examination, the rash is found to be erythematous papules that do not blanch with digital pressure. He complains also of arthralgias involving the knees and ankles and has noted bloody urine. Each of the following statements regarding this condition may be true except for which one?

(A) It has a 90% chance of being self-limited.
(B) Renal biopsy will show glomerulonephritis with crescent formation.
(C) If the condition becomes chronic, it would be treated with immunosuppressive agents.
(D) This is an autoimmune disorder.
(E) Cases becoming chronic are more likely to be in children than adults.

5 A 45-year-old woman who has been diagnosed with conjunctivitis twice over the past year and has been frequently complaining of pruritus now complains of a foreign body sensation in the left eye. Examination discloses corneal ulceration. Her office record also shows that she has complained of various muscular pains over the past year. Which of the following is the most logical first test you might order?

(A) Schirmer test
(B) Antinuclear antibody (ANA) test
(C) CBC count
(D) Serum uric acid
(E) Slit-lamp examination

6 A 25-year-old African-American woman living in the Midwest complains of fever, fatigue, malaise, and weight loss over the past 3 months. Lately, she has started to have a dry cough. She has never smoked cigarettes. A CBC is unremarkable. A chest x-ray shows bilateral lymphadenopathy and two noncavitating nodules. Which of the following is least likely in the differential diagnosis?

(A) Pulmonary tuberculosis
(B) Histoplasmosis
(C) Hypersensitivity pneumonitis
(D) Pneumococcal pneumonia
(E) Sarcoidosis

7 The patient in Question 6 began to feel significantly better and has been followed for several more weeks. A tuberculosis skin test, repeated after 2 weeks, was negative. The serum calcium is elevated slightly, and in a bronchial lavage specimen, the ratio of CD4 to CD8 lymphocytes is 4.0. Now she complains of painful red nodules on her lower legs. Which of the following is the most likely diagnosis?

(A) Pulmonary tuberculosis
(B) Histoplasmosis
(C) Hypersensitivity pneumonitis
(D) Acquired immunodeficiency syndrome (AIDS)
(E) Sarcoidosis

8 A 35-year-old African-American woman has complained of weight loss and fatigue for several weeks. In advising her on the phone as to measures to take before her appointment with you the following week, you asked her to keep a record of her temperature 4 times per day. She arrives for the appointment with the record. She also notes diffusely thinning hair. The temperature graph shows that her temperature has sometimes been as high as 101°F. However, the high points of the daily graphs appear at various times in the early hours of the morning or late mornings, not in the afternoons or evenings. She complains also of arthralgia involving her metacarpophalangeal joints of the first and second fingers bilaterally, with 30 to 60 minutes of stiffness in the morning. A urinalysis yields microscopic hematuria and red cell casts. Which of the following diagnoses is most likely, given the combination of clinical findings?

(A) Chronic glomerulonephritis
(B) Alopecia areata
(C) LE
(D) Chronic pyelonephritis
(E) Pulmonary tuberculosis

9 A 35-year-old white woman has had two bouts of pleurisy and a bout of pericarditis, none associated with infection, within 3 months. In addition, she manifests a hemolytic anemia with reticulocytosis and leukopenia (3,500 white blood cells/mm³) on two occasions. You suspect a connective tissue disease and order an ANA test. The result is positive for the homogeneous pattern. Which of the following is the best conclusion to draw from that result?

(A) The patient has SLE.
(B) The patient could have a connective tissue disease or drug-induced SLE.
(C) The patient has had undiagnosed pneumonia.
(D) The patient should be evaluated for mesothelioma.
(E) The patient has a blood dyscrasia.

10 Each of the following is characteristic of scleroderma, except for which one?

(A) Polyarthralgia
(B) Raynaud phenomenon
(C) Intestinal malabsorption
(D) Positive test for Sm antibodies
(E) Pulmonary hypertension

11 A 45-year-old woman complains of difficulty initiating swallowing and increasingly early onset of fatigue of her legs as she climbs stairs and in her arms as she lifts baskets of laundry. She notices skin changes that you see consist of violaceous coloration about the eyes and in the periungual areas that also are manifested over the shoulders and anterior chest. You notice also clubbing of her nails and that she has a cough that she relates to her smoking. Which of the following accounts for her systemic symptoms and rash?

(A) Photosensitivity eruption
(B) Contact dermatitis
(C) Polymyositis
(D) Dermatomyositis
(E) SLE

12 Regarding the patient in Question 11, which of the following most likely accounts for the nail clubbing?

(A) Chronic obstructive pulmonary disease
(B) Reversal of left-to-right shunt through an interventricular septal defect (the Eisenmenger syndrome)
(C) Hepatic cirrhosis
(D) Congenital variant
(E) Lung cancer

13 A 25-year-old man complains of prolonged upper respiratory congestion. You have treated him for sinusitis twice and for otitis media over the past year, although these are the first such occasions he has had these problems in his adult life. This week, he complains of redness of the eyes with vascular ectasia that does not move over the sclera the way one notes the conjunctival movement with changes in gaze. Blood pressure levels are normal. You consult by telephone your favorite rheumatologist, who suggests ordering a number of antibody levels. Their results are as follows: ANA, anti-Sm, SS-A, SS-B, and anticentromere, all negative; rheumatoid factor and antineutrophil cytoplasmic antibody (ANCA) positive. Which of the following is the most likely condition to account for the symptomatology?

(A) Wegener granulomatosis
(B) SLE
(C) Dermatomyositis
(D) Systemic sclerosis
(E) Rheumatoid arthritis

For Questions 14 through 18, match the numbered clinical characteristics with the lettered diseases.

14 Formation of sialoliths (salivary duct stones)

15 Nephrocalcinosis

16 Proximal muscle weakness and difficulty in initiation of swallowing

17 Pleural and pericardial effusions

18 Heliotrope rash about the eyes

(A) Sarcoidosis
(B) Sjögren syndrome
(C) Polymyositis
(D) SLE
(E) Dermatomyositis

Examination Answers

1. The answer is C. Anticardiolipin antibodies are as close to specific as it gets in the murky field of autoimmune diseases, which virtually are all defined arbitrarily. The diagnosis is anti-phospholipid antibody disease. The most significant reason to be aware of this syndrome is the high risk of both intravenous and intra-arterial thromboses. The disease is basically a subset of LE.

2. The answer is C. Scleroderma is the likely diagnosis. This resembles the limited type, comprising 20% of cases and involves hardening of the skin only of the face and hands along with esophageal dysfunction. The limited form may also include calcinosis cutis, Raynaud phenomenon (the digit changes in this patient's description), sclerodactyly, and telangiectasias.

The diffuse type is far more severe and involves hardening of the skin of the trunk and proximal extremities. Unique but not universal in this disease are tendon friction rubs over the forearms and the shins. Treatment is specific to the systems involved, for example, H+ pump blockers for the esophageal dysfunction, the CREST syndrome.

3. The answer is D. The unlikely statement regarding this patient is *there is likely a complaint of muscular weakness.* Jaw pain with chewing equates to jaw claudication, which constitutes a metaphor for giant cell arteritis (GCA). There is a 50% chance of coexistent polymyalgia rheumatica (PMR). PMR is characterized by stiffness but, unlike in polymyositis and polyarteritis nodosa, stiffness does not confer weakness. GCA appears to be self-limited but not without the danger of irreversible blindness. The disease nearly always appears after the age of 50 years; the mean of incidence of GCA is 72 years (the reason for that choice in the vignette). GCA is the cause of 15% of fevers of unknown origin, and the temperature may run as high as 104°F. Unilateral blindness may occur secondary to ischemic neuropathy within the distribution of the ophthalmic artery. The only proven treatment, among the many studied, is a course of a glucocorticoid, usually prednisone, which is continued at a dosage of 60 mg daily for about a month before tapering. GCA's classical presentation is temporal arteritis, which presents often with ipsilateral headaches and a nodular palpable temporal artery. Similarly, PMR, when diagnosed clinically by the complaints of muscle stiffness as in the vignette, yields to the same prednisone course and serves to prevent the possibility of GCA and blindness. GCA may evolve into PMR and PMR into GCA.

4. The answer is E. Although the disease is more common in children, cases that evolve into chronic states are *more likely to be in adults.* The vignette describes Henoch–Schönlein purpura. The condition is an autoimmune disease, albeit self-limited in 90% of cases and more so in children. Non-blanching palpable red papules are by definition petechiae. The differential diagnosis might include Rocky Mountain spotted fever, and in certain presentations, meningococcemia. If in doubt, spinal fluid must be examined.

5. The answer is A. This patient may well have sicca syndrome and Sjögren syndrome. Her myositis could be one of the many extraglandular manifestations of Sjögren syndrome. It is commonly known by physicians that patients with this syndrome complain of dryness of the eyes, mouth, and other mucosae (sicca syndrome). Dryness of the eye also makes the patient more susceptible to corneal ulcerations and bacterial conjunctivitis. The Schirmer test is simple and available to any primary care office. It consists of laying fluorescein-impregnated filter paper on the lower lid to measure how much the migration of the wetness caused by tears advances in a given period. Each of the other choices has a place in the evaluation of autoimmune diseases or eye problems but involves expense and, in the case of slit-lamp examination, consultation with an ophthalmologist.

6. The answer is D. Pneumococcal pneumonia is the least likely in a patient with a subacute course such as that presented in the vignette. Each of the other choices is reasonable to consider. Depending on the clinical setting, in addition, berylliosis, aspergillosis, coccidioidomycosis, Wegener granulomatosis, and several other conditions could be considered.

7. The answer is E. Sarcoidosis is more common in African-Americans and South Asian Indians. Its onset most commonly occurs when a person is between the ages of 20 and 30 years, and it somewhat more likely in women than in men. Of cases, 90% manifest pulmonary involvement, 50% as bilateral hilar adenopathy, 15% as parenchymal infiltrates, and 25% with both types of involvement of the lungs. Skin lesions occur in 25%, and erythema nodosa ranks among the most common, with the other rashes including nonspecific macules, papules, patches, and plaques, and a rash called lupus pernio. The appearance of erythema nodosa portends a more favorable prognosis. Hypercalcemia occurs in about 5% of cases, and the CD4:CD8 ratio is greater than 3:4 in bronchial fluid and other involved organs, as opposed to the normal ratio of 2:1. The etiology remains, despite many theories, unknown, although a possible infectious basis has been postulated. The disease may involve virtually any organ with granulomatous lesions.

8. The answer is C. SLE occurs in African-American women 4 times as frequently as in white women and 23 times as frequently as in white men. The febrile course that does not follow the normal diurnal variation occurs in inflammatory processes not involving response to infection. Eventually, some two-thirds of patients have arthralgia or arthritis. Nearly 3 of 4 have skin manifestations, of which alopecia is fairly common; of course, the facial butterfly rash, not shown in this patient, is a hallmark of the disease. Renal involvement is found in 16% to 38% of cases. Pulmonary tuberculosis would manifest not only pulmonary symptoms but also a febrile course with normal diurnal variation. Although each of the other choices may be characterized by at least one of the clinical findings in the vignette, none except lupus would manifest all of them.

9. The answer is B. The patient could have a connective tissue disease or drug-induced SLE. The homogeneous ANA pattern is the most common positive form. It is sensitive but not specific for SLE. The rim pattern of ANA positivity is more specific for SLE. The homogeneous pattern may be seen in drug-induced lupus, such as that with hydralazine, isoniazid, and chlorpromazine. The patient has 2 of 11 criteria for clinical diagnosis of lupus. To justify a clinical diagnosis of SLE, there must be 4 of the 11 following criteria: discoid rash; malar rash; photosensitivity; oral ulcers; arthritis; serositis; renal disorder; neurologic disorder; hematological disorder; immunologic disorder; and ANA in the absence of drug-induced positivity.

10. The answer is D. Positive test for Sm antibodies does not occur in either diffuse scleroderma or limited scleroderma. The Sm, SS-A, and SS-B antibodies are specific for SLE. Each of the other listed manifestations is present in scleroderma in fairly high prevalence sooner or later in the course of the disease. Arthralgia is common, as is Raynaud syndrome, neither of which is specific for scleroderma. Pulmonary hypertension occurs as a result of the development of pulmonary fibrosis. Malabsorption occurs secondary to atrophy and fibrosis of the intestinal mucosa.

11. The answer is D. Dermatomyositis, of course, is the disease that causes the "heliotrope" violaceous eyes and the similar discoloration of the periungual areas. On occasion, the facial rash involvement mimics the malar rash of SLE. However, SLE does not present a rash that involves

the other areas listed in the vignette. DMS may manifest scaly patches over the Proximal interphalangeal (PIP) and metacarpophalangeal (MCP) joints that are highly suggestive of DMS. The myositic aspects of the disease cause proximal muscle weakness and weakness in the voluntary initiation of swallowing. Although dermatomyositis has muscle symptoms similar to those of polymyositis, biopsy shows recognizable histologic differences. In brief, dermatomyositis manifests perivascular lymphocytic infiltrates, whereas polymyositis is characterized by lymphocytic infiltration of the endomysium, the delicate reticular fibrils that surround each muscle fiber.

12. The answer is E. Dermatomyositis is associated with a malignancy in 25% of cases. The most common are lung, breast, ovary, and stomach cancer. Given the clubbing of the nails and the smoking history, lung cancer is far more likely in the presence of dermatomyositis than chronic obstructive pulmonary disease. Each of the other choices presented is or can be associated with nail clubbing but is not likely to appear in the scenario presented in the vignette.

13. The answer is A. Wegener granulomatosis is characterized by multiple-organ involvement, like so many of the other connective tissue diseases. However, it is important to be able to differentiate this disease from the others because if untreated it is generally fatal within a relatively few years. Of the array of antibody levels usually measured whenever testing for connective tissue diseases, the ANCA level is elevated in virtually only Wegener granulomatosis (except for <1% of SLE). ANCA levels are also elevated in Crohn disease. In Wegener granulomatosis, the antibody is present in 93% to 97% and not present in polyarteritis nodosa, some of whose histologic features it resembles. Polyarteritis nodosa, present in only 30 people per million, 10% of whom have hepatitis B, is not a primary care entity for practical purposes.

ANSWERS TO THE MATCHING QUESTIONS

14. Formation of sialoliths (salivary duct stones): **The answer is B,** Sjögren syndrome.

15. Nephrocalcinosis: **The answer is A,** sarcoidosis.

16. Proximal muscle weakness and difficulty in initiation of swallowing: **The answer is C,** polymyositis.

17. Pleural and pericardial effusions: **The answer is D,** SLE.

18. Heliotrope rash about the eye: **The answer is E,** dermatomyositis.

References

Family Medicine Review. Kansas City, Missouri; May 3–10; 2009.

Gill JM, Quisel AM, Rocca PV, et al. Diagnosis of systemic lupus erythematosus. *Am Fam Physician.* 2003; 68:2179–2186.

Hellmann DB, Stone JH. Arthritis and musculoskeletal disorders. In: Tierney LM, McPhee DJ, Papadakis MA, eds. *Current Medical Diagnosis and Treatment.* 45th ed. New York: McGraw-Hill/Appleton & Lange; 2006:807–864.

McPhee SJ, Papadakis MA. *Current Medical Diagnosis and Treatment 2010,* 49th ed. New York/Chicago: McGraw-Hill/Lange; 2010.

Wu JJ, Schiff KR. Sarcoidosis. *Am Fam Physician.* 2004; 70:312–322.

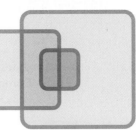

chapter 29

Sports Medicine

Examination questions: *Unless instructed otherwise, choose the ONE lettered answer or completion that is BEST in each case. Many items found in Tests 23 and 24 pertain to sports medicine as well.*

1 Which of the following maneuvers tests the infraspinatis muscle?

(A) Empty bucket test
(B) With the arm held passively horizontal and the elbow flexed 90 degrees to point directly upward the shoulder is rotated internally to bring the forearm into the horizontal position (Hawkins test)
(C) The drop arm test (patient lowers the arm actively slowly from 160 abduction)
(D) Active internal rotation of the shoulder against resistance
(E) Active external rotation of the arm against resistance

2 A 35-year-old runner complains of pain and paresthesias on the medial plantar surface of the right ankle and heel, aggravated by toeing in (ventriflexion and pronation movement) during the donning of his track shoes. There is no specific area of tenderness to palpation. Which of the following is the likely diagnosis?

(A) Plantar fasciitis
(B) Tarsal tunnel syndrome
(C) Stress fracture second metatarsal (MT)
(D) herniated nucleus pulposus (HNP) L5 root
(E) Peripheral neuropathy

3 Which of the following is the most effective management of exercise-induced asthma?

(A) Inhaled glucosteroids
(B) Inhaled anticholinergic agonists
(C) 48 hours of prednisone in advance
(D) Inhaled Beta adrenergic drug
(E) Administration of oxygen prior to an athletic event

4 A 35-year-old athletic man complains of pain and tenderness at a point just distal to the right lateral condyle. The man is right-side dominant. He was active in "major" sports in his youth but has only recently taken up tennis. His condition may be caused or aggravated by each of the following activities, except for which one?

(A) Grasping and turning a doorknob
(B) Driving a screw with a manual screwdriver
(C) Vigorous hand shaking
(D) Using the overhead tennis serve
(E) Employing wrist extension in the tennis backhand stroke

5 An 18-year-old male senior high school athlete has been training hard early in the spring track season. He complains of pain in the left knee region when he runs over a quarter of a mile (0.4 km), and he wishes to have relief so that he may pursue his goal of repeating his performance as district champion in his long-distance event. The pain had a gradual onset and there has been no identifying moment of injury. There is neither morning stiffness nor "gelling" with afternoon inactivity. Each of the following conditions could be a serious consideration as the cause of the symptoms, except for which one?

(A) Iliotibial band syndrome
(B) Rheumatoid arthritis
(C) Anserine bursitis
(D) Popliteal tendonitis
(E) Patellar tendonitis

6 A 15-year-old boy is going out for football for the first time. His pubescence is accelerating and he has grown 3 in. (7.6 cm) in the past year. You are performing a preparticipation sports physical examination. The aortic second sound is louder than the pulmonic second sound, but the P_2 sound is of normal intensity. You hear a systolic "diamond shaped" murmur along the left sternal border. There is neither precordial heave nor thrill. You ask the patient to perform a Valsalva maneuver and find that the murmur is enhanced. You then ask the patient to squat and then auscultate again, only to find that the murmur disappears. He has no complaint of shortness of breath. He manifests no cyanosis or peripheral edema. Which of the following is the likely diagnosis?

(A) Patent ductus arteriosus
(B) Ventricular septal defect
(C) Hypertrophic cardiomyopathy
(D) Pulmonic stenosis (PS)
(E) Congestive heart failure

7 A routine preparticipation physical examination uncovers a systolic cardiac murmur that was loudest at the upper left sternal border and is heard in the neck and posterior lung fields. Which of the following would be the most important disposition to help determine whether this athlete should proceed to participate in high-exertion competitive sports?

(A) Twelve-lead electrocardiogram
(B) Echocardiogram
(C) Right heart catheterization
(D) Computed tomography scan of the chest
(E) Magnetic resonance image of the chest

8 Regarding athletics, what is the main objective of being a physician to athletes and making a preparticipation (medical) evaluation?

(A) To diagnose hypertrophic subaortic stenosis in high-energy-output athletics
(B) To diagnose exercise-induced asthma and significant cardiac conditions that pose a threat to an exertional athlete or one in a sport of high contact
(C) To identify medical threats to an exertional athlete and to recommend techniques of training that would tend to maximize success in athletics
(D) To identify conditions that will place the athlete at risk of exacerbation of an existing illness or injury or at risk of incurring a new problem
(E) To cover the practitioner against liability lest he or she approve for athletic participation an athlete with a condition that might lead to sudden death

9 Which of the following tests is the one in current use to diagnose (illicit) anabolic steroid use in athletics?

(A) Testosterone-to-epitestosterone ratio
(B) Androstendione level
(C) Testosterone level
(D) Estrogen level
(E) Follicle-stimulating hormone level

10 A 20-year-old star receiver for a Big Ten football team with a reputation for heroic catches leaps into the air and outward nearly 90 degrees to his right to effect a reception. His body is rotated so that the right shoulder is positioned straight downward. After catching the pass he falls onto his right shoulder and immediately is seen to writhe in pain in the shoulder area. He misses the next two games because of the pain. There is no sensory component. Hand strength, including intrinsic muscles, as well as elbow flexion and extension are within normal limits. There is an irregularity to the contour of the right shoulder near the humeral head. An x-ray shows no bone fracture but does reveal an abnormality. The patient is able, upon examination, to abduct, albeit associated with pain, to 150 degrees. Which of the following is the most likely diagnosis?

(A) Rotator cuff partial tear
(B) Rotator cuff complete tear
(C) Fracture of the clavicle
(D) Separation of the acromioclavicular joint
(E) Herniated disc at C4

For Questions 11 through 13, match the numbered grade of concussion with the defined clinical picture, represented by capital letters. LOC = loss of consciousness. More than one answer may be correct.

11 Grade 1 concussion

12 Grade 2 concussion

13 Grade 3 concussion

(A) Dazed without LOC, vertigo or amnesia for the event
(B) Confusion with amnesia <15 minutes, no LOC
(C) Confusion with amnesia and LOC <5 minutes, amnesia <24 hours
(D) LOC 20 minutes, confusion 10 minutes, amnesia for 2 minutes prior to the event
(E) LOC >5 minutes or amnesia lasting >24 hours

Examination Answers

1. The answer is E. Active external rotation of the arm against resistance tests the infraspinatus. This will be painful and possibly weak in response. The empty bucket test challenges the supraspinatus whereby the arms are held 90 degrees in shoulder abduction with the thumbs pointed downward. Inability to hold the position with mild downward pressure or gravity alone constitutes a positive test. The arm held passively horizontal (by the examiner) with the elbow flexed 90 degrees as the forearm points directly upward, the shoulder is internally rotated to bring the forearm into the horizontal position is the Hawkins test and pain occurs with impingement syndrome. (Failing) the drop arm test occurs in rotator cuff tear, that is, involves more than just the suprspinatus component. Inability to actively internally rotate the shoulder to where the hand in behind the back and then to push-off the examiner's hand (push-off test) tests the subscapularis.

2. The answer is B, Tarsal tunnel syndrome. Causes of tarsal tunnel syndrome include entrapment of the posterior tibial nerve within the tarsal tunnel by varicosity of the posterior tibial vein; tenosynovitis of the flexor tendon causing interstitial fluid accumulation within the entrapped area; and trauma causing interstitial blood accumulation or hematoma. Pronation of the foot causes the symptoms. There is no specific area of tenderness to palpation. Plantar fasciitis causes plantar pain that remits daily after an hour or so walking. Stress fractures are tender locally (i.e., in this case over the second metatarsal). Radiculopathy such as the L5 example would not cause pain with movements of the foot. Peripheral neuropathy causes symptoms in the distribution of an identified peripheral nerve without localization of tenderness commensurate with the area of pain.

3. The answer is D. An inhaled beta adrenergic drug administered before an athletic session is the much preferred method. By definition the asthmatic attacks are quick in onset and remitting between bouts of physical exercise with time periods analogous to those encountered in rescue treatment. Choices A, B, and C are too long in onset and in their prolonged action. Oxygen has no direct effect on reactive airway disease, though in acute, more severe dyspnea oxygen obviously is beneficial to the global well being of the patient.

4. The answer is D. This patient has, of course, lateral epicondylitis, inflammation of the point of the supinator apparatus at the condyle. It is also called "tennis elbow." The latter term refers to the condition's frequent causa-

tion by improper backhand motion, invoking wrist extension and supination instead of the whole arm and shoulder in the tennis backhand. In the correct technique, the wrist is splinted in the neutral position and the elbow extension is minimized. The professional-style serving motion puts a stress on the medial epicondyle. This inflammatory syndrome is also referred to as "golfer's elbow," as many players' golf swings employ that medial elbow stress as well. The screwdriver, hand shaking, and doorknob motions all invoke the supinator and wrist extension apparatus.

5. The answer is B. The absence of morning stiffness and afternoon gelling rules out rheumatoid arthritis in this patient who has been training hard and whose onset of pain has been gradual and precipitated by running. The other conditions are each subtly different from one another but may all be lumped into the category of overuse syndromes involving the knee. And despite athletes' desires to the contrary, they all require, first and foremost, a period of rest. Iliotibial band syndrome and popliteal tendonitis both cause pain in the lateral aspect of the knee. Patellar tendonitis causes pain in the area of insertion of the quadriceps into the patella (i.e., the pain is located at the superior aspect of the patella). Anserine bursitis results in pain at the location of the anserine bursa, in the inferior and medial aspect of the knee.

6. The answer is C. Hypertrophic cardiomyopathy results in a choking of the aortic outflow tract, more marked when venous return is diminished as when the subject stands erect, and conversely alleviated when venous return is enhanced as when squatting. The latter displaces blood to the upper body, increasing right-sided return and subsequent left-sided return. Patent ductus arteriosus is seldom discovered and corrected later than infancy, and it causes a continuous "machinery type" murmur. The murmur of ventricular septal defect does not change with position change. The murmur of PS would be expected to remain unchanged or perhaps increase with squatting. PS also causes a left precordial click, and often the murmur obscures the P_2 sound. Congestive heart failure causes dyspnea on exertion, orthopnea, or peripheral edema. Hypertrophic cardiomyopathy (hypertrophic obstructive cardiomyopathy is an unusual, but not rare, cause of sudden death during athletic exertion, accounting for half of nontraumatic athletic deaths. Therefore, diagnosis at the time of a preparticipation physical examination is crucial. The patient should be referred for echocardiogram or cardiac evaluation, and athletic activity should be forbidden until the condition is ruled out. Risk factors for this condition include family history of sudden cardiac death and history of syncope.

7. The answer is C. Right heart catheterization is needed to determine whether this candidate has pulmonary stenosis, the most common form being valvular stenosis. The criterion that determines whether this person should participate in competitive sports is the pulmonary artery (PA) pressure; it should be <75 mm Hg. Each of the other choices renders the diagnosis or results that are compatible with the diagnosis but will not quantify the pressure. Similarly aortic valvular stenosis with a gradient >40 mm Hg is a contraindication for physically competitive sports. Other cardiac contraindications are hypertrophic obstructive cardiomyopathy, congenital coronary artery anomalies, and cystic medial sclerosis of the aorta caused by Marfan syndrome.

8. The answer is D, to identify conditions that will place the athlete at risk of exacerbation of an existing illness or injury or at risk of incurring a new problem. This is the mission of the preparticipation examination itself. Furthermore, sports medicine implies that one will become a physician to athletes; thus, the second portion of the answer is important as well. All other objectives listed are worthy, including medicolegal mindfulness. However, they are overshadowed by the main theme of protection of the athlete from harm.

9. The answer is A. The testosterone-to-epitestosterone ratio is the current clinical test for anabolic steroid use or abuse. The forms of anabolic steroid that are used include androstendione and testosterone (trade name Dianabol). The follicle-stimulating hormone level is most directly involved in spermatogenesis rather than testosterone.

10. The answer is D. This injury is typical of the acromioclavicular separation and usually results in a visible and palpable nodule that is the lateral end of the clavicle, no longer tucked into the acromion in its normal position. Extremely painful for as long as it takes to heal soft tissue injuries (3 to 6 weeks, depending on the expected load of the tissues in normal function), this injury does not usually require surgical correction. A direct blow such as that occurred in the vignette could produce a traumatic rotator cuff tendonitis, though abduction of the shoulder would be more severely affected and that injury would produce no visible contour abnormality. Rotator cuff tears do not occur from the forces portrayed here and a complete tear would produce the phenomenon called "the arm drop," inability to maintain abduction to 90 degrees. The blow described could as easily result in a fractured clavicle, though would be unlikely, given the protection of the football pads, besides which the x-ray has ruled out a fracture. A herniated disc would produce referred pain to the shoulder and always neck pain.

MATCHING THE NUMBERED GRADE OF CONCUSSION WITH THE LETTERED CLINICAL PICTURE

11. Grade 1 concussion: **The answers are A and B,** Dazed without LOC, vertigo or amnesia for the event; confusion less than 15 minutes, no LOC nor amnesia.

12. Grade 2 concussion: **The answers are C, and D.** Confusion with amnesia and LOC less than 5 minutes, amnesia less than 24 hours; confusion longer than 15 minutes with pupil changes, LOC 3 minutes.

13. Grade 3 concussion: **The answer is E.** LOC, amnesia for the event more than 24 hours.

Discussion of Questions 11 through 13: The answers given are in line with a consensus among sports medicine experts. For first events, definitions and guidelines for continued participation are as follows: Grade I concussion is defined as head injury without loss of consciousness, dazed but no confusion or vertigo. Athlete may return to play within 15 minutes and may continue providing there are no symptoms for the following week and the mental status remains within normal limits. Grade II may be defined as loss of consciousness less than 5 minutes or amnesia for less than 30 minutes. Participation should be suspended for one week and the athlete must perform normally on an exertion test; Third degree concussions may be defined as associated with loss of consciousness for more than 5 minutes, vertigo or confusion for more than 15 minutes. Participation must be suspended for at least 2 weeks and computed tomography or magnetic resonance image of the head and brain must be normal. Restrictions become more stringent with recurrences and in view of recent viewpoints and research findings from NFL football, the foregoing are likely to be increasingly tighter.

References

Family Medicine Board Review (breakout session) 2009. Kansas City, Missouri; May 3–10, 2009.

Hellmann DB, Stone JH. Arthritis and musculoskeletal disorders. In: Tierney LM, McPhee SJ, Papadakis MA, eds. *Current Medical Diagnosis and Treatment*, 45th ed. New York: McGraw-Hill/Appleton & Lange; 2006:807–864.

Lombardo JA. Sports medicine. In: Rudy DR, Kurowski K, eds. *Family Medicine: House Officer Series.* Baltimore, MD: Williams & Wilkins; 1997:467–480.

Terrell TR, Leski JL. Sports medicine. In: Rakel RE, ed. *Textbook of Family Practice*, 6th ed. Philadelphia, PA: WB Saunders; 2002:845–890.

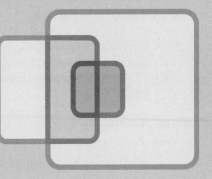

SECTION **X**

Infectious Diseases in Primary Care

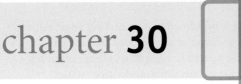

chapter **30**

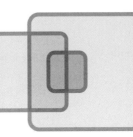

Acquired Infectious Diseases in Primary Care

Examination questions: *Unless instructed otherwise, choose the ONE lettered answer or completion that is BEST in each case.*

1 Which of the following ethnic groups has the lowest incidence of new acquired immunodeficiency syndrome (AIDS) cases in the United States?

(A) Asian and Pacific Islanders
(B) African-Americans
(C) Latinos
(D) Native Americans
(E) White Americans

2 Which of the following summarizes best in 2010, the application of antiretroviral therapy (ART) in treating AIDS?

(A) Treat opportunistic infections (OIs) only until the CD4 count falls to 50 cells/mcL or lower; then start ARTs.

(B) Treat as soon as the diagnosis is made by high dosage of one class of ARTs to avoid development of resistance to several ARTs.

(C) Treat with three nucleoside transcriptase inhibitors, ignoring OIs.

(D) Treat with three ARTs including at least two different classes, while treating OIs as needed.

(E) Initiate treatment with one of each of the six classes of ARTs followed by treatment of the OIs in detail.

3 A 25-year-old homosexual man comes to a family physician with a concern as to whether he may have AIDS. After taking a complete history, the physician orders a serologic test for the disease, the enzyme-linked immunosorbent assay (ELISA) screening test. Each of the following may be a criterion for making the diagnosis of AIDS, in conjunction with available laboratory testing except for which one?

(A) A positive human immunodeficiency virus (HIV) test consisting of Western blot antigen-antibody test after a positive ELISA

(B) A history of a CD4 T-cell lymphocyte count less than 200 cells/μL in an HIV-positive patient

(C) Dementia and weight loss to the point of wasting in a person with positive HIV serology

(D) Pneumocystis pneumonia, central nervous system lymphoma, and positive HIV serology

(E) CD4 lymphocyte count below 14% and positive HIV serology

4 Which of the following practices carries the highest risk of contracting AIDS?

(A) Insertive vaginal intercourse with a female who is HIV-positive

(B) Receptive vaginal intercourse with a male who is HIV-positive

(C) Accidental needle stick with HIV-infected blood

(D) Sharing of needles for illicit drug use with an HIV-infected person

(E) Receptive anal intercourse with an HIV-positive person participating in receptive anal intercourse

5 A 25-year-old male patient presents with fatigue and weight loss and is found to be positive for HIV, confirmed by the Western blot test. His CD4 count is 500 cells/mm³. Which of the following is the least likely cause of his weight loss?

(A) Mycobacterium avium complex (MAC)

(B) Tuberculosis

(C) Malabsorption

(D) Kaposi sarcoma

(E) Hairy leukoplakia

6 Each of the following infections is found virtually only when CD4 counts fall *to or below 50 cells/mcL* except which one of the following?

(A) Disseminated MAC

(B) Extrapulmonary histoplasmosis

(C) Cytomegalovirus (CMV) retinitis

(D) Primary lymphoma of the brain

(E) Cryptosporidiosis with diarrhea longer than 1 month

7 A 35-year-old homosexual man has been diagnosed recently with AIDS and manifests spotty bilateral sensory and motor symptoms as well as headaches and altered mental status. Blood pressure levels are within normal limits. A computed tomography (CT) scan of the brain shows scattered bilateral cerebral space-occupying lesions that are enhanced with contrast, which are distributed for the most part peripherally. Which of the following is the most likely diagnosis?

(A) Multiple sclerosis

(B) Non-Hodgkin lymphoma

(C) Multiple infarct dementia

(D) Toxoplasmosis

(E) Metastatic cancer to the brain

8 In evaluating an AIDS patient for visual disturbance, you notice perivascular hemorrhages and white fluffy exudates. Which of the following is the most likely cause?

(A) CMV

(B) Cotton wool exudates

(C) Cataracts

(D) Herpes virus

(E) Toxoplasmosis

9 A male homosexual patient who has tested positive for HIV infection complains of painful swallowing, and endoscopy shows white, adherent plaques that leave beefy red denuded areas when removed. The examination is negative except for white exudates in the oral cavity that leave a raw, slightly bleeding base. Which of the following is a clearly relevant statement regarding this patient's physical findings?

(A) He is presumed to have Ludwig angina due to beta-hemolytic streptococcal infection.

(B) The patient has esophageal herpes simplex related to his immunodeficient status.

(C) The patient has aphthous esophagitis related to his immunodeficient status.

(D) The patient has candidiasis of no more significance than coincidence as there is no oral thrush.

(E) The patient has esophageal candidiasis, of significance in an HIV-infected patient.

10 Which of the following is typical of the acute, initial infection with the HIV virus?

(A) Folliculitis

(B) Hairy leukoplakia

(C) Kaposi sarcoma

(D) Lymphadenopathy

(E) Vaginal candidiasis

11 Which of the following poses the least likely medium of contagion for HIV?

(A) Saliva

(B) Shared toothbrush

(C) Blood and blood products

(D) Semen

(E) Cerebrospinal fluid

12 A 28-year-old AIDS patient has begun to complain of intermittent difficulty writing clearly and of bouts of confusion interspersed with periods of lucidity. Neurological examination is otherwise unremarkable, as are a CT scan and magnetic resonance imaging of the brain. Which of the following is the diagnosis?

(A) Lymphoma of the brain

(B) Toxoplasmosis of the brain

(C) AIDS dementia complex

(D) Multiple infarctions of the brain

(E) Alzheimer disease

13 In the measurement of viral loads as they apply to diagnosis and follow-up of HIV infection, each of the following is correct and relevant, except for which statement?

(A) The test is a measure of active and proliferating HIV virus copies.

(B) The measurements correlate with disease progression.

(C) The measurements correlate inversely with response to antiretroviral drug treatment.

(D) The test may become positive before seroconversion of an exposed victim.

(E) A test of viral load before treatment that indicates any number of copies present is the equivalent of a positive HIV serological test confirmed by Western blot.

14 You are considering starting ART in a 30-year-old male patient who is positive for HIV. Which of the following would warrant initiating such treatment?

(A) Any patient with symptoms

(B) Seropositive patient with CD4 counts rapidly dropping

(C) Patients with viral load >100,000/mcL

(D) Seropositive asymptomatic patient with CD4 count 1000/mcL and convalescent hepatitis A

(E) Seropositive patients with risk factors for heart disease or cancer

15 A 25-year-old man who is a trash collector laborer in a run-down neighborhood grasps a plastic bag and is immediately stuck with 5 injection needles attached to syringes. The patient has no history of hepatitis B or other hepatitides nor is he a drug abuser nor has a history of HIV disease. Which of the following is the recommended course of treatment?

(A) Draw baseline serologic studies for hepatitides B and C and HIV.

(B) Draw baseline serologic studies for hepatitides B and C and HIV and repeat at 6 weeks, 12 weeks, and 6 months.

(C) Draw baseline serologic studies for hepatitides B and C and HIV; then institute a 4-week course of Combivir and repeat the serologic studies at 6 weeks, 12 weeks, and 6 months.

(D) Draw baseline serologic studies for hepatitides B and C and HIV; then institute a 4-week course of Combivir.

(E) Reassure that the risks of HIV disease and hepatitis are minimal.

Examination Answers

1. The answer is A. Asian and Pacific Islanders have the lowest incidence of new cases of AIDS, at 4.4/100,000. African-Americans have the highest incidence at 60.3/100,000 and AIDS is the leading cause of death in Africa-American women in the age group 25–34 years. Latino-Americans are next 20.8/100,00 followed by Native Americans 7.8/100,000 and then by White Americans 6.4/100,000.

2. The answer is D. Treat AIDS (as soon as diagnosed) with three ARTs including at least two different classes, while treating OIs as needed (see Question 14). In the recent past, it was felt that ART should be differed until opportunistic infects, such as MAC, were brought under control in 6 weeks on the assumption side effects of the ARTs or high-active antiretroviral therapeutic agents (HAART) would be worse if such infections were still in process. However, studies showed that if the ARTs and HAARTs were started immediately, while the OIs were dealt with simultaneously, AIDS progression was reduced by 50%. The principle at present is to start with at least three drugs with at least two from different classes. The six classes are (a) nucleoside reverse transcriptase inhibitors (e.g., zidovudine); (b) nucleo*tide* transcriptase inhibitors (tenofovir); (c) protease inhibitors (e.g., indinavir); (d) non-nucleoside reverse transcriptase inhibitors (e.g., nevirapine); (e) entry inhibitors (enfuvirtide); and (f) integrase inhibitors (raltegravir).

The most rapidly changing aspect of AIDS and HIV disease is the therapy, which has evolved as increasingly numerous, and varied drugs have become available and the disease has been converted into a chronic disease or clinically a carrier state. This presentation is based in great part on Chapter 31 in 2010 Current Medical Diagnosis and Treatment, with special attention to pages 23–34 and Table 31–6.

3. The answer is A. A positive HIV result consisting of Western blot antigen-antibody test after a positive ELISA is validly confirmed positive serological evidence of infection by the AIDS virus, and the person who exhibits this can pass the disease. However, positive HIV serology does not constitute the disease AIDS. Thus, the relative immune deficiency as evidenced by the low CD4 lymphocyte counts (by absolute number or percentage) and the various syndromes portrayed, each of them quite unusual in immunocompetent individuals, serve as criteria for the clinical diagnosis of AIDS. The latter obtains, of course, when the serology is positive as confirmed by the Western blot. Fortunately, early interventional therapy has made it likely that fewer patients will develop the aforementioned

criteria. Such therapy includes the antiretroviral agents, especially those regimens that include protease inhibitors and non-nucleoside reverse transcriptase inhibitors.

4. The answer is E. Receptive anal intercourse with an HIV-positive person participating in receptive anal intercourse carries the highest risk of those practices mentioned among the choices with a 1/30 to 1/100 risk. Sharing of needles for illicit drug use carries an approximately 1:150 risk. This presumably assumes repeated sharing but does not presume specific positivity for HIV in a given incident. Insertive vaginal intercourse carries a 1:10,000 risk (i.e., to the male), whereas receptive vaginal intercourse 1:1000 risk. Accidental needle stick with HIV-infected blood in a hospital setting carries a 1:300 risk of acquiring the virus.

5. The answer is A. MAC does not enter the picture in HIV disease until the CD4 count falls below 50 mm^3, whereas this patient has a CD4 count of 500. Each of the other conditions mentioned may occur as a result of HIV infection at lesser degrees of severity, wherein CD4 counts are less than the nominal 1,000 mm^3 (but more than 250). Other conditions that may be seen with the CD4 count at or below 200 include the following: toxoplasmosis, cryptococcosis, coccidioidomycosis, and cryptosporidiosis.

6. The answer is E. Cryptosporidiosis with diarrhea longer than 1 month may be found when CD4 T lymphocytes fall to the 250-µL range. The other conditions, all being OIs, although not unheard of in individuals without immune deficiency, are seen in significant prevalence only when the CD4 count drops below 50 µL.

7. The answer is D. Toxoplasmosis is the most common space-occupying lesion of the brain that appears as a complication of AIDS. Toxoplasmosis is a protozoan that may infect immunocompetent people in whom the clinical course usually resembles infectious mononucleosis with a limited and benign course. Often in AIDS patients and other immunocompromised individuals, the infection is not a primary but rather a reactivated disease in the face of the AIDS syndrome. Although multiple sclerosis is multicentric, the demyelinating lesions are not space occupying and visible on CT scan. Non-Hodgkin lymphoma is the second most common space-occupying lesion of the brain associated with AIDS. However, lymphoma is usually unifocal rather than multifocal. Multiple infarct dementia occurs in older people and is associated with long-standing hypertension. Metastatic cancer could be confused with the radiographic picture in some cases but would pose the dilemma of accounting for a clinical picture with more than one major diagnosis. In immuno-compromised patients, this infection must be treated for 4 to 6 weeks after cessation of symptoms. The first drug of choice is pyrimethamine given 25 to 100 mg daily plus sulfadiazine given 1 to 1.5 g 4 times daily. Folic acid is added to prevent marrow suppression.

8. The answer is A. CMV retinitis occurs in AIDS patients with CD4 counts under $50/\mu L$. It must be treated to prevent or retard the progression of the retinitis and to prevent retinal detachment. Treatment is by antiviral agents, such as ganciclovir, valganciclovir, and foscarnet. Cotton wool spots, different from the white fluffy exudates of CMV recognized by ophthalmologists, are benign and self-limiting.

9. The answer is E. Candidiasis is highly suggestive of immunoincompetence in adults, particularly in the esophagus, trachea, bronchi, or lungs. Of interest is that even oral candidiasis in an HIV-infected person strongly presages progression to AIDS, even correcting for CD4 count. Only 75% of patients with esophageal candidiasis have oral candidiasis so that oral candidiasis is not a reliable confirmatory indicator for esophageal candidiasis. Luwig angina is unusual and may well be suspicious for immunoincompetence but presents with a cellulitis apparent by external examination of the neck. The clinical picture does not include a description of herpetic or aphthous ulcers.

10. The answer is D. Lymphadenopathy. Fever, lymphadenopathy, sore throat, rash, and headache are typical symptoms of an acute infection with HIV. During the acute phase, none of the stigmatic conditions associated with HIV infection have yet appeared. The other presented entities are seen in later stages of HIV infection.

11. The answer is A. Saliva, a fluid functionally designed for secretion onto the exterior surface, is not an HIV risk unless there is a break in the mucosa that exudes blood into the saliva; thus, the shared toothbrush is a risk. Blood, semen, vaginal secretions, and synovial, pleural, peritoneal, and cerebrospinal fluids are all felt to contain significant amounts of the virus in an infected individual. Urine, saliva, perspiration, and even vaginal secretions normally (i.e., in the absence of contiguous breaks in skin or mucosa) pose little to no risk as media of transmission. Thus, fluids whose normal function is entirely within the body's envelope of skin and mucosae are not normally media of passage of the HIV virus.

12. The answer is C. AIDS dementia complex is a diagnosis of exclusion (see Question 5 and its discussion). Alzheimer disease may remit and exacerbate regarding cognitive changes but motor problems in Alzheimer disease follow a steady but slowly down hill course.

13. The answer is E. The statement is incorrect in that a count of *any* number of copies is not necessarily a confirmation of HIV. If the viral load is reported as a low level, say, <500 copies, it may be a false-positive result. All other statements regarding the use and applications of viral load measurements are true.

14. The answer is D. A seropositive asymptomatic patient with CD4 count 1000 mcL and convalescent hepatitis A is not an indication for initiation of ART, assuming no other indications exist. However, infection with hepatitis B C, risk factors for non-AIDS-associated cancers or for heart disease are each indication as HIV replication is thought to hasten progression of those conditions. Rapidly dropping CD4 counts or viral load at or above 100,000 mcL are firm indications as are symptoms that constitute grounds for a diagnosis with or without corroboratory laboratory evidence. Other indications are the clinical presence of the following OIs: candidiasis of esophagus or lower respiratory tract; extrapulmonary cryptococcosis; cryptosporidiosis with diarrhea lasting longer than 1 month; CMV in organs other than spleen or lymph nodes; mucocutaneous ulcer of herpes simplex virus (HSV) infection longer than 1 month or HSV bronchitis, pneumonitis, or esophagitis; Kaposi sarcoma in persons over 60 years of age; atypical mycobacteria of other than lungs, skin, or cervical or hilar nodes; pneumocystis jiroveci pneumonia; and progressive multifocal leukoencephalopathy and cerebral toxoplasmosis.

15. The answer is C. Draw baseline serologic studies for hepatitides B and C and HIV; then institute a 4-week course of Combivir and repeat the serologic studies at 6 weeks, 12 weeks, and 6 months. The situation would be very different if there had been a single known source, as occurs in a hospital setting, where both the source and the exposed patients could be tested or even retested. In that case, the exposed worker is simply tested in the manner outlined while the source patient is observed after baseline testing or retested if necessary and possible. Indeed, the risks, even in the vignette presented, are minimal, but the rare chances of disease, particularly HIV, are so immense that most clinicians would recommend the course of ART (which protects also against hepatitis B). Combivir is available as 150 mg lamivudine/300 mg zidovudine, taken twice daily for a recommended period of 4 weeks.

References

Katz ML, Zolopa AR, Hollander H. HIV infection. In: Tierney LM, McPhee SJ, Papadakis, MA, eds. *Medical Diagnosis and Treatment*. 45th ed. Lange; 2006.

McPhee SJ, Papadakis MA. *Current Medical Diagnosis and Treatment 2010*, 49th ed. New York/Chicago: McGraw-Hill/Lange; 2010.

Weinstock MB, Crane R. Adult acquired immune deficiency syndrome. In: Rudy DR, Kurowski K, eds. Baltimore: Williams & Wilkins; 1997:481–500.

chapter 31

Other Infectious Diseases in Primary Care

Examination questions: Unless instructed otherwise, choose the ONE lettered answer or completion that is BEST in each case.

1 A 38-year-old woman who has had an intrauterine device (IUD) for 15 years without changing it (had changed locations of residency several times) has noted a virtually painless 6 cm red area over the lower abdominal area for many weeks. This week the red area has broken down to exhibit purulent discharge. On pelvic examination, the adnexa are palpably fixed. The pap smear is negative for caner or precancerous findings. Which among the following is the most likely offending entity?

(A) Stage 3 carcinoma of the cervix
(B) *Streptococcus pyogenes*
(C) *Actinomyces israelii*
(D) *Staphylococcus aureus*
(E) Histoplasma capsulatum

2 A 25-year-old man returns from a trip to Lima Peru with diarrhea that had a sudden onset the day after arrival in the United States. The stools were grayish, turbid, without fecal odor, and voluminous in fluid volume. Cramping was minimal, and he was afebrile, but the patient was lightheaded when he stood up by the second day. Which of the following is clinically the most likely?

(A) Toxigenic *Escherichia coli* (bloody diarrhea)
(B) Cholera (rice water stools)
(C) Travelers diarrhea
(D) Shigellosis dysentery (bloody)
(E) Typhoid fever

3 A 12-hour-old female newborn has begun to exhibit apathy and poor feeding drive. The mother is 16 years old, gravida 1, para 1; she is single and has had no prenatal care. Her membranes had ruptured about 24 hours before her reporting to the emergency department of the hospital. On examination, the baby seems to be "floppy." A complete blood cell count reveals a leukopenia and absolute neutropenia of 100/mm³ mL, thrombocytopenia, and elevated C-reactive protein. Which of the following infections is most likely to be the cause of this clinical situation?

(A) *E. coli* sepsis
(B) Group B streptococcus (GBS)
(C) *Haemophilus influenzae*
(D) *Listeria monocytogenes*
(E) Coagulase-negative *S. aureus*

4 A 24-year-old male injection drug user complains of dry mouth, dysphagia, dysphonia, diplopia, nausea, and vomiting. In the past few hours, he has noted shortness of breath. He is alert and oriented. His temperature is normal. Breathing appears to be mildly labored and shallow, but the lung fields are "clear" to auscultation and percussion. Of the following that are present in the differential diagnosis of these symptoms, which one is the most likely?

(A) Tetanus
(B) Botulism
(C) Bowel obstruction
(D) Guillain–Barré syndrome
(E) Myasthenia gravis

5 A 50-year-old diabetic man complains of rapidly developing redness of the right (anatomical) leg over a period of 24 hours. You note a tense edematous area extending 10 to 12 cm along the mid right calf and some bulla formation. The man complains of pain that extends several centimeters beyond the area of visible inflammation while noting hypesthesia at the viable site. The area is warm to touch and the patient manifests systemic symptoms consisting of fever (temperature of 100.8°F), diaphoresis, and tachycardia. Which of the following is the most critical diagnostic test at this time?

(A) Culture and sensitivity of the bullae
(B) Blood culture
(C) Complete blood cell count
(D) Venogram
(E) Surgical exploration and biopsy

6 A 9-year-old boy is brought to you with complaints of 2 days of fever, headache, nausea, vomiting, and a macular rash of pink lesions that appears on the palms, soles, wrists, forearms, and ankles. The lesions blanch with pressure. He had been camping with his family in North Carolina from 2 weeks ago until about 5 days ago. Today, he has also begun to complain of headache, cough, and pleuritic chest pain. The boy has had no gastrointestinal complaints. Examination is unremarkable except for the rash. The neck is supple. Complete blood count shows thrombocytopenia, hyponatremia, and hyperbilirubinemia, with mostly indirect acting type. Which of the following is the most likely possibility to pursue?

(A) Rubeola
(B) Meningococcemia
(C) Rocky mountain spotted fever (RMSF)
(D) Varicella
(E) Typhoid fever

7 A 4-year-old Chinese American boy has had a fever for 5 days, with temperatures running between 100°F and 101°F. Upon examination, he manifests conjunctival injection, sore and fissured lips, palmar and solar erythema with desquamation of the tips of one index and one ring finger, transverse grooves in several fingernails, and enlarged cervical lymph nodes. Aside from the lips, the oral examination is unremarkable. Which of the following must be considered?

(A) Roseola
(B) Rubeola
(C) Scarlatina
(D) Erythema infectiosum
(E) Kawasaki disease

8 A 36-year-old man complains of diffuse macular rash, headache, and reddened eyes developing over 3 days. Today, his palms and soles show faintly and finely vesicular changes. He complains also of the recurrence over 4 days of soreness and focal redness on the left side of his nose, manifesting a flame-shaped region of erythema involving the left naris. He denies sore throat, and a rapid flocculation test for beta-hemolytic streptococcus is negative. In the past 24 hours, he has developed vomiting and diarrhea. Which of the following is the most likely diagnosis?

(A) Scarlatina
(B) Kawasaki syndrome
(C) Secondary syphilis
(D) Toxic shock syndrome
(E) Cirrhosis of the liver

9 A 25-year-old patient known to you is complaining of fever and malaise for 10 days. He complains also of arthralgia and painful violaceous lesions of the fingers and toes. Upon examination, you hear a heart murmur that was never mentioned in your notes, including two "complete physicals" over the past 4 years. His temperature is 101.3°F. He is alert but uncomfortable and manifests no neck stiffness. He says that he visited an urgent care center 2 weeks ago and was given a 7-day prescription for azithromycin and for 1 week felt better and was without fever. However, the fever recurred 5 days ago. You discover, with further investigation, that the young man has been using illicit intravenous recreational drugs. Which of the following is likely the cause of this illness?

(A) Acute hepatitis A
(B) Hepatitis B
(C) Hepatitis C
(D) Meningococcemia
(E) Bacterial endocarditis

10 Regarding the patient in Question 9, assume the febrile 25-year-old man had additional complaints of cough and pleuritic chest pain, and a chest x-ray shows infectious infiltrates in various places in both lungs. Which of the following sites would be most likely to be the seat of the infection?

(A) Deep veins of the thigh
(B) Aortic valve
(C) Tricuspid valve
(D) Mitral valve
(E) Pulmonic valve

11 Each of the following is a special risk factor for infectious bacterial endocarditis, except which one?

(A) Presence of prosthetic heart valves
(B) Previous bacterial endocarditis
(C) Complex cyanotic congenital heart disease
(D) Status 1 year post repair of ventricular septal defect
(E) Hypertrophic cardiomyopathy

12 A 35-year-old woman complains of a rash of variable lesions, fever, and headache. She had been camping in the New England states and had been in the wilderness for a week without an opportunity to bathe. She does not recall any prior skin lesions since the exposure in the field. Examination reveals a generalized rash of red lesions, some annular, some target like, some more intense centrally. Which of the following is the most likely cause of these symptoms?

(A) RMSF
(B) Tinea circinata
(C) Rubeola
(D) Secondary syphilis
(E) Lyme disease

13 Regarding the reemergence of pertussis, each of the following is true, except which one?

(A) The age group of victims is distributed from infancy throughout youth and into young adulthood.

(B) The organism can be cultured from the nasopharynx using a Dacron swab.

(C) Diagnosis can be made within 48 hours of the culture inoculation.

(D) Timely treatment with macrolide antibiotics reduces the severity and length of the period of symptoms.

(E) Pertussis should be considered in any patient whose cough lasts 2 weeks or more.

14 Each of the following is true regarding genital herpes simplex virus (HSV), except for which statement?

(A) Polymerase chain reaction testing is more sensitive than viral culture.

(B) Viral culture is useful in differentiating HSV-1 from HSV-2 infection.

(C) Early therapy with recently developed antiviral agents can cure the disease.

(D) Suppressant therapy can reduce the recurrence rate by 70% to 80%.

(E) Suppressive therapy reduces significantly the risk of heterosexual transmission in HSV-2 discordant couples.

15 A 57-year-old woman with diagnosed chronic obstructive pulmonary disease (COPD) who has smoked 2 packs per day for 40 years has developed fever, headache, purulent cough, and anorexia. She was recently discharged from a hospital, with likely diagnosis of Legionnaires disease in the patient. Which of the following would support the diagnosis of Legionnaires disease in this patient?

(A) A Gram stain of the sputum that reveals more bacteria than neutrophils

(B) Serum creatine kinase test

(C) Ear pain

(D) Constipation

(E) An incubation period of 2 to 4 weeks

Examination Answers

1. The answer is C *A. israelii.* The clinical presentation depicted is typical for actinomycosis with its slow and insidious course, characterized by granulomatous spread and fistula formation. It is best known as the cause of "lumpy jaw" but can involve the intestines, and in the present case, pelvic inflammatory disease, known, especially when an IUD has been left in too long. The pap smear virtually rules out cancer in a process so far advanced as that in the vignette. Clinically none of the bacterial infections match the case, nor does histoplasmosis follows the pathologic course shown here.

2. The answer is B Cholera. Cholera sets on suddenly, results in watery gray stools (rice water stools) and massive fluid loss. There is no fever, blood, nor severe cramps. The fluid loss in full-blown cases is massive, up to 15 L/day and sometimes 1 L/hour, and is the cause of death if fluid therapy is not aggressively pursued. Toxigenic *E. coli* and shigellosis are both forms of dysentery (bloody diarrhea). Typhoid fever causes acute systemic illness with high fevers. Travelers diarrhea generally causes severe cramps as well as diarrhea for a brief period but not the massive amounts of fluid loss. While stool cultures will reveal *Vibrio cholerae*, confirming the diagnosis, the disease is caused by the toxin adenylyl cyclase elaborated thereby. The disease is treated by aggressive fluid replacement (addressing physiological amounts of saline), and the course can be shortened by tetracycline, ampicillin, chloramphenicol, or azithromycin.

3. The answer is B. GBS is the most common infection of neonates. It occurs usually quite early after delivery in the form of pneumonia but may be expressed in more subtle clinical form as in this case, with hypotonia and poor feeding. Risk factors include prematurity, delayed delivery after membrane rupture, and GBS infection in the mother. However, infection may occur as late as at 2 weeks. In the latter case, GBS often presents as meningitis. Each of the other organisms, among the choices, may be found in the newborn as well.

4. The answer is B. Botulism is found in essentially three forms: the foodborne form, as in the ingestion of preformed toxin in canned, smoked, or vacuum-packed foods, which is potentially the most acute and deadly form; infant botulism, which occurs when the ingestion of botulinum spores (usually in honey) causes botulinum toxin to be produced in the gastrointestinal tract of infants, and wound borne botulism. The latter is found most often in injection drug users, probably most likely in those cases in which the addict has run out of functional surface veins

and resorted to what is known as skin popping. The symptoms are those of anticholinergic poisoning, and there is a curare-like effect on the skeletal muscles (i.e., flaccid paralysis in the advanced case). Dyspnea is due to paralysis of the diaphragm and intercostal muscles. Tetanus is not characterized by anticholinergic symptoms, and muscle tone is heightened, not reduced. Myasthenia gravis and Guillain–Barré syndrome should be considered, but not in the context of intravenous drug abuse.

5. The answer is E. Surgical exploration, probable debridement, and biopsy are crucial in the clinical picture shown. Narcotizing soft tissue infection, appreciated increasingly in the past 10 years, usually begins acutely, although on occasion over a more prolonged period. Originally thought to be caused by an evolved virulent strain of beta-hemolytic group A streptococcus, it has been found to be due to infections by several monomicrobial organisms, including *S. aureus* and *Clostridium perfringens* (69%). Often, there is polymicrobial infection that is most frequently due to *Staphylococcus epidermidis*, beta-hemolytic strep, Enterococcus organisms, *E. coli*, *Proteus mirabilis*, *Klebsiella pneumoniae*, *Pseudomonas aeruginosa*, and species of *Streptococcus*, *Bacteroides*, *Prevotella*, and *Clostridium*, as well as anaerobic cocci and fungi. Aerobic and anaerobic organisms may be found in combination. Each of the other studies mentioned are relevant, but none is diagnostic. The differential diagnosis includes uncomplicated cellulitis caused by group A beta-hemolytic strep and phlebitis. However, because necrotizing soft tissue infection, also called necrotizing fasciitis, is often so devastating in its course, suspicion must yield to surgical debridement. Biopsy permits the diagnosis of the etiologic organisms and of the pathophysiology. When the diagnosis is made, then the cornerstone of success in prevention of deaths and amputations is early debridement.

6. The answer is C. RMSF is a leading candidate for the cause of the symptoms and signs portrayed in the vignette, based on the rash, headache, and respiratory symptoms. The blanching macular rash evolves into a petechial eruption. The cause is *Rickettsia rickettsii*, passed through the bite of a tick with an incubation period of 7 to 14 days. The ticks that carry the rickettsia are by *Dermacentor andersoni* in the western states and by *Dermacentor variabilis* in the east (where the most cases are found). Contrary to the implications of its name, 56% of cases occur in one of five states, North Carolina, South Carolina, Tennessee, Oklahoma, and Arkansas. Up to 40% of patients do not recall the tick bite. There is a 3% to 5% case mortality, more likely in elderly and infirm. Typhoid and meningococcus must be ruled out.

About 10% occur without a rash. Diagnosis is made by serial serological studies, a process that may take 2 weeks, or by immunofluorescent antibody. The rash of Rubeola is morbilliform (i.e., like measles), not macular nor petechial. Meningococcemia, because of the seriousness, must be considered and ruled out. Varicella, chickenpox, presents with a centripetal vesicular rash, as opposed to the mostly centrifugal distribution of the rash of RMSF, albeit spreading centripetally. Typhoid fever is characterized by a rash, but nearly always manifests gastrointestinal symptoms, usually evolving into "soupy diarrhea." Diagnosis of meningococcal meningitis is made by spinal tap for identification of *Neisseria meningitidis*, presumptively by smear and definitively by culture. Doxycycline or tetracycline is the treatment of choice for RMSF, even in children, continued until 3 days after defervescence. Chloramphenicol is effective but is reserved for pregnant women to avoid tetracycline side effects in the fetus. The other agents mentioned are not effective.

7. The answer is E. Kawasaki disease is the only entity among the choices that fits the clinical picture presented. The disease is an inflammatory response to an unknown agent, perhaps one of several that may engender the vasculitis that is the essence of the disease. Asians are more susceptible. Timely diagnosis is important to prevent vasculitides, especially coronary vasculitis that can lead to myocardial infarction. Roseola affects younger children and is characterized by very high fever for several days that breaks precisely as a morbilliform rash appears. Rubeola features high fever, malaise, and the generalized morbilliform rash that appears along with the first symptoms and persists throughout, as do the Koplik spots that are most often seen opposite the second molars or in the vaginal mucosa. Rubella is also called the "three day measles," and the adenopathy occurs in the retroauricular and suboccipital regions. Scarlatina is "scarlet fever," a Group A beta-hemolytic streptococcal infection that releases the erythrotoxin. With the cervical adenopathy and the desquamation of the fingertips, scalatina must be considered as well, but can easily be diagnosed as streptococcus disease with the 10-minute flocculation "Rapid Strep" screen from the pharynx. *Erythema infectiosum* is "fifth disease," occurs in infants younger than 2 years, and is known for the slapped cheek appearance, caused by a diffuse flush as opposed to the other rashes described in this vignette. Therapy of Kawasaki syndrome is based on anti-inflammatory modalities, for example, aspirin and, in the opinions of some, glucosteroids. Diagnosis is based on fever lasting at least 5 days and satisfaction of clinical criteria as in other inflammatory conditions. Four of the following clinical criteria must be met:

1. Bilateral non-exudative conjunctivitis
2. Mucous membrane changes of at least one of the following types: injected pharynx, erythema, swelling or fissure of the lips, strawberry tongue
3. Peripheral extremity changes, palmar or solar erythema, desquamation, induration or Beau's lines (transverse grooves in the fingernails)
4. Polymorphous rash
5. Cervical lymphadenopathy

8. The answer is D. Toxic shock syndrome now occurs as frequently in non-female menstrual situations as in the originally described association with the retained tampon. The vesicular changes of the palms and soles lead to the well-known desquamation seen in the late stages. Toxic shock, which may carry a case mortality as high as 15% as a result of hypotension and heart failure, is due to the toxin elaborated. Thus, early cultures may be unhelpful. Scarlatina may be considered long enough to rule out quickly because the rash of scarlatina is quite different, described as pampiniform (pinpoint red spots). Kawasaki syndrome occurs nearly always in children 5 years old or younger, albeit characterized by desquamation of the palms and the soles. Although secondary syphilis manifests palmar and solar changes, they are nonvesicular and consist of macules, papules, and pustules. Cirrhosis of the liver is mentioned because of palmar erythema seen in the face of patients with advanced compromise of liver function. Again, however, vesicle formation and desquamation is not characteristic of such a situation.

9. The answer is E. Febrile disease associated with a new heart murmur or a changing heart murmur must be considered to have bacterial endocarditis until proven otherwise, by serial blood culture. The disease is also called infectious endocarditis to distinguish it from autoimmune endocarditis. The major risk factors are previous valvular heart disease and intravenous drug abuse. However, neither of the foregoing may be present for there to be bacterial endocarditis. The painful lesions of the fingers and toes fit the description of Osler's nodes. Other stigmata of endocarditis of bacterial endocarditis include Janeway nodes (painless erythematous lesions of the palms or soles), splinter hemorrhages of the nails, and Roth spots (retinal exudates). Although the patient is at risk for hepatitides B and C because of his drug abuse history, and thus they should be ruled out in any febrile illness, they do not present with heart murmurs nor are well known for skin lesions. Meningococcemia is unlikely in the absence of meningismus. *S. aureus* causes 60% of endocarditis cases in intravenous drug users. This has effected a change in the overall concepts of bacterial endocarditis over the past 30 years. Staph disease in endocarditis follows a more acute course than *Streptococcus viridans* disease; thus, in the past, the synonym for endocarditis was *subacute bacterial endocarditis*, or SBE.

10. The answer C. The tricuspid valve is the one most often involved in intravenous drug abuse and, as a right-sided lesion, is subject to septic emboli. Deep venous thromboembolic disease may result in pulmonary emboli as well, but the patient is not febrile and the emboli are not; hence, they show up as radiographic densities after a period of delay, rather than seen as infectious infiltrates.

11. The answer is D. Although the presence of a ventricular septal defect (VSD) (as well as atrial septal defect) is a risk factor for bacterial endocarditis, the risk has disappeared 6 months after clinically satisfactory repair. Each of the other conditions is a risk factor. Mitral valve prolapse associated with a murmur is a risk, but not so MVP with a click if unassociated with a murmur.

12. The answer is E. Lyme disease. Classically, Lyme disease consists of three stages. Stage 1 features flulike symptoms (arthralgia, headache, malaise, and weakness) and the typical single skin lesion of erythema migrans at the site of the tick bite. Stage 2, after a latent period, features a rash similar to the one described here and systemic symptoms similar to those of stage 1. Stage 3, after a greatly varying prolonged asymptomatic period, ranging from months to years, features synovitis, arthritis, central nervous system impairment, dermatitis, keratitis, and neurologic and myocardial abnormalities. Stage 3 greatly resembles an autoimmune mechanism. An important point is that a great percentage of cases do not follow this neatly described sequence. Moreover, a significant proportion of afflicted patients give no history of a tick bite. Stage 2 disease may be seen quite early; erythema migrans may not occur or go unrecognized.

13. The answer is C. Diagnosis of pertussis *cannot* be made within 48 hours of the culture inoculation, although culture is taken from the nasopharynx. Direct fluorescent antibody testing is not available for rapid diagnosis as of this writing. The culture requires at least 7 days for reporting out. All other statements given are true. Although approximately 29% of cases occur in the classic age group, infancy, the remainder are spread throughout all age groups, and 20% are found in people over the age of 20 years. Timely treatment with macrolide antibiotics reduces the severity and length of the period of symptoms. In the milieu of 2007, pertussis should be considered in any patient whose cough lasts 2 weeks or more.

14. The answer is C. Early therapy with recently developed antiviral agents cannot cure the disease. Herpes simplex remains an incurable disease. Genital or (classically) type 2 disease is more liable for recurrence over time but decreasingly over time, whereas type 1 recurs at a rapidly decreasing rate. The vast majority of cases is treated according to clinical diagnosis, but culture of vesicular fluid is the standard; type-specific serological testing is available. Polymerase chain reaction testing is 95% sensitive but not in general use mostly due to the costs incurred. Viral culture is only 70% sensitive but when positive differentiates HSV-1 from HSV-2 infection. Suppressant therapy is employed with any of a number of antiviral agents, for example, acyclovir and related famciclovir, valacyclovir, and the newer trifluridine, vidarabine, foscarnet, and cidofovir. These can reduce the recurrence rate by 70% to 80% and can also significantly reduce the risk of heterosexual transmission in HSV-2 discordant couples.

15. The answer is B. A recent review of the literature indicates that, of all the common laboratory studies usually performed, only an elevated creatine kinase level separates the other pneumonitides from Legionnaire. This is a typical presentation of Legionnaire disease. A cough may be nonexistent or mild compared to the remaining clinical picture, including chest x-ray. The incubation period for Legionnaire disease is only 2 to 10 days. Diarrhea, not constipation, is an associated finding. Ear pain from an associated otitis media can be seen with mycoplasma pneumonia and even with some streptococcal infections but is not typical of Legionnaire disease. Many more neutrophils than bacteria are usually seen in Gram stains from patients with Legionnaire disease. Anorexia, myalgia, and hyponatremia are also frequently seen. Treatment is accomplished with the macrolides and rifampin.

References

Bauman JG. Genital herpes: A review. *Am Fam Physician.* 2005; 72(8):1527–1534, 1541–1542.

Bratton RL, Corey GR. Tick-borne disease. *Am Fam Physician.* 2005; 71:2323–2330, 2331–2332.

Campos-Altcalt D. Practice alert – pertussis: A disease re-emerges. *J Fam Practice.* 2005; 54:699–702.

Chambers HF. Infectious diseases: Bacterial and chlamydial. In: Tierney LM, McPhee SJ, Papadakis MA, eds. *Medical Diagnosis and Treatment.* 45th ed. New York/Chicago: Lange; 2006.

Haddy RI. Less common infectious diseases in primary care. In: Rudy DR, Kurowski K, eds. *Family Medicine: House Officer Series.* Baltimore: Williams & Wilkins; 1997:501–512.

Hay WW, Levin MJ, Sondheimer JM, Deterding RR, eds. *Current Diagnosis & Treatment Pediatrics.* New York/Chicago: McGraw-Hill/Lange; 2009.

Headley AJ. Narcotizing soft tissue infections: a primary care review. *Am Fam Physician.* 2003; 68:323–328.

Moran A, Shandera WX. Infectious diseases: Viral and ricketsial. In: Tierney LM, McPhee SJ, Papadakis MA, eds. *Current Medical Diagnosis and Treatment.* 45th ed. New York: McGraw-Hill/Appleton & Lange; 2006:1349–1399.

Rakel RE, Bope ET, eds. *Conn's Current Therapy 2009.* Philadelphia: Saunders/Elsevier; 2009.

Endocrinology in Primary Care

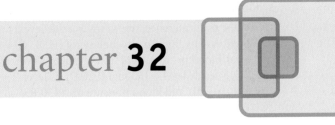

chapter **32**

Diabetes Mellitus

Examination questions: *Unless instructed otherwise, choose the ONE lettered answer or completion that is BEST in each case.*

1 Which of the following ethnic groups should be screened for diabetes mellitus (type 2) at the lowest body mass index (BMI) and age to meet statistical criteria to justify screening?

(A) Caucasian
(B) Asian
(C) Latino-Americans
(D) African-Americans
(E) Aboriginal Americans

2 Each of the following is a correct statement regarding the incretin-like new antidiabetic drug, exenatide, except for which one?

(A) It is delivered by subcutaneous injection twice daily.
(B) It reduces insulin resistance in type 2 diabetes.
(C) It promotes a significantly higher insulin response than an equivalent dose of glucose.
(D) It carries a lower risk of hypoglycemic reaction than sulfonylureas.
(E) It suppresses hyperglucagonemia stimulated by insulin surging.

3 Which of the following insulins is characterized by the longest effective activity?

(A) Glargine
(B) Lispro
(C) Aspart
(D) Regular (Lilly)
(E) Glulisine

4 A 55-year-old obese male patient, known to have diabetes type 2, is found to be stuporous after complaining of lethargy for 2 days during a bout of gastroenteritis in which he passed between six and eight loose stools per day. A hemoglobin A1C level taken 2 weeks before was 7.5%. His blood sugar is 600 mg/dL; serum acetoacetate and beta-hydroxybutyrate are normal and serum osmolality is 310. The blood urea nitrogen (BUN) level is 110 mg/dL. Which of the following is the best description of the patient's condition?

(A) Diabetic ketoacidosis (DKA) precipitated by viral infection
(B) Hyperosmolar state precipitated by high-solute-containing foods
(C) Hyperosmolar hyperglycemic state (HHS) precipitated by dehydration
(D) Hyperosmolar state precipitated by acute renal failure

(E) Hyperosmolar state precipitated by inadequate blood sugar control

5 Which of the following statements about the HHS is true?

(A) It carries a mortality rate considerably lower than that of DKA.

(B) It is known for a significant anion gap.

(C) The major precipitants are medication noncompliance, ethanol, and cocaine use.

(D) The presence of gastroparesis effectively rules out hyperosmolar state in favor of ketoacidosis and diabetes type 1.

(E) The most rapidly effective therapy is insulin.

6 Which of the following families of oral agents applicable to diabetes type 2 can facilitate weight loss?

(A) Sulfonylurea agents, such as glyburide

(B) Biguanides, metformin

(C) Non-sulfonylurea secretagogues such as repaglinide

(D) Thiazolidinediones ("glitazones"), for example, pioglitazone

(E) Alpha-glucosidase inhibitors, such as acarbose

7 A 47-year-old 257-lb (116.4-kg) man whose height is 5 ft, 7 in. (1.7 m) has been followed for type 2 diabetes for the past 2 years. His treatment has consisted of escalating institutions and additions of, first, 10 to 20 mg of glyburide; 500 to 2 g of metformin daily; and 4 mg of pioglitazone daily. During that time, his weight has increased from an initial level of 215 lb (97.4 kg) 2 years ago to the present weight given here. His latest hemoglobin A1C level was 8.5%. He now complains of burning pains in his legs and feet and asks why that would be so and what should be done about it. For you to address the base cause, which of the following is the most clearly relevant information?

(A) The pains are caused by noncompliance by the patient.

(B) The pains are caused by ischemic peripheral vascular disease.

(C) The pains are a side effect of the metformin.

(D) The pains are caused by long-standing hyperglycemia.

(E) The pains are caused by lumbar radiculopathy.

8 In performing a routine periodic history and physical examination on a 56-year-old Mexican woman who weighs 175 lb (79.3 kg), you included a glycohemoglobin (HbA1C) study to supplement a complete blood cell count, comprehensive metabolic panel, and fasting lipids. Her fasting glucose level was 115 mg/dL, and a 2-hour postprandial (PP) blood sugar level was 160 mg/dL. BUN and creatinine levels are normal.

The complete blood cell count shows a hemoglobin level of 8 g/L and a hematocrit measure of 31. The HbA1C level was 5.9% (normal is ≤6%). Which of the following factors *could not* explain a lower than expected HbA1C?

(A) Thallassemia

(B) Recent blood loss

(C) Patient's diabetes is not severe enough to create a sustained level of hyperglycemia.

(D) A hemoglobin variant that co-elutes with hemoglobin A

(E) Hereditary spherocytosis

9 Which of the following list of factors is included by both the World Health Organization and the Adult Treatment Panel III in defining metabolic syndrome X?

(A) Waist circumference, serum triglyceride level, high-density lipoprotein cholesterol (HDL-C) level, blood pressure, and fasting glucose level

(B) Triglyceride level >150 mg/dL, HDL-C level <40 mg/dL, and blood pressure of >130/85

(C) Triglyceride level >150 mg/dL, HDL-C level <35 mg/dL, waist-to-hip ratio >0.9, and blood pressure >140/90

(D) Central obesity, type 2 diabetes mellitus, and hypertension

(E) Dyslipidemia and diabetes mellitus

10 A 45-year-old type 2 diabetic male patient weighing 240 lb (109 kg) at a height of 5 ft, 10 in. (1.77 m) has not lost weight as mandated by his physician. Recently a coworker underwent leg amputation as a result of uncontrolled diabetes. Now the patient is newly motivated to lose weight and wishes to review the correct diet for control of his diabetes. Which of the following is the correct diet for control of his diabetes, assuming he has stable weight?

(A) An intake of 3,000 cal as 412 g of carbohydrate (CHO), 113 g of protein, and 113 g of fat

(B) An intake of 2,000 cal as 250 g of CHO, 75 g of protein, and 75 g of fat

(C) An intake of 1,700 cal as 233 g of CHO, 64 g of protein, and 64 g of fat

(D) An intake of 1,200 cal as 164 g of CHO, 45 g of protein, and 45 g of fat

(E) An intake of 800 cal as 100 g of CHO, 40 g of protein, and 30 g of fat

11 A 16-year-old girl, who weighs normally 140 lb at a height of 5 ft, 8 in., is brought to you with complaints of weight loss, increasing fatigue, thirst, and polyuria accelerating over the past 3 weeks. Her blood sugar is 450 mg/dL and serum bicarbonate level is 19 mmol. You hospitalize her and start fluid therapy (1 L of normal saline for the first 90 minutes), after a 20-unit bolus of regular human insulin, and slow infusion of regular insulin at 10 units/hour until the blood sugar has fallen to 250 mg/dL. After slowing the progress of remission, adding 5% dextrose in half-normal saline (0.45% NaCl) intravenously, you find that she emerges from acidosis and is ready for discharge home after 36 hours. Her premorbid weight was 120 lb (54.4 kg) at a height of 5 ft, 4 in. (1.63 m). Which of the following insulin daily dosages would be the most reasonable for an initial regimen?

(A) 120 units daily
(B) 60 to 120 units daily
(C) 27 to 54 units daily
(D) 25 units daily
(E) 15 units daily

12 In evaluating a patient regarding his renal status, you now estimate the progress of disease by noting the results of the 24-hour urine collection just received. Which of the following findings in the 24-hour urine specimen should command the most attention in evaluating this patient's renal status?

(A) 10 mg albumin/dL
(B) ≥20 mcg/minute in an overnight specimen
(C) 500 mg protein/dL
(D) Positive urine culture
(E) 3.5 g of protein/24-hour urine output

13 A 35-year-old woman, gravida 3, para 2, is in her 25th week of pregnancy. Although her weight is normal for her period of gestation, her mother has type 2 diabetes, as does an older sister who is overweight. She undergoes the 1 hour, 50-g glucose tolerance test and the blood sugar at 1 hour is 155 mg/dL (8.6 mmol/L). You decide to place her on a limited CHO diet to prevent the complications in diabetic progeny such as macrosomia and neonatal hypoglycemia. Which of the following ranges is considered the minimum necessary to prevent such complications?

(A) ≤105 mg/dL
(B) ≤190 mg/dL (10.5 mmol/L)
(C) ≤165 mg/dL (9.2 mmol/L)
(D) ≤145 mg/dL (8 mmol/L)
(E) ≤73 mg/dL (4 mmol/L)

14 A pregnant patient is treated with diet therapy alone for 3 weeks. You now check her home blood sugar recordings to assess the degree of success on this regimen, prepared to start insulin if control of the diabetes is not satisfactory. At which of the following fasting and 2-hour PP limits would you pose as the minimum requirement to start insulin therapy?

(A) ≤75 mg/dL fasting, 95 mg/dL at 2 hours
(B) ≤105 mg/dL fasting, 120 mg/dL at 2 hours
(C) ≤120 mg/dL fasting, 150 mg/dL at 2 hours
(D) ≤150 mg/dL fasting, 160 mg/dL at 2 hours
(E) ≤100 mg/dL fasting, 105 mg/dL at 2 hours

15 Diabetologists consider three stages of glucose tolerance or intolerance. Which of the following fasting blood sugar (FBS) levels fits the definition of impaired glucose regulation (vs. normal or diabetes mellitus)?

(A) >90 mg/dL FBS
(B) ≥100 mg/dL 2 hours PP
(C) 100 to 125 mg/dL fasting
(D) ≥150 to 200 mg/dL 2 hours PP
(E) ≥200 mg/dL PP

16 A 16-year-old girl who is known to be a type 1 diabetic has gone through a period of rebellious denial and stopped taking her insulin 7 days ago. Now she is feeling very thirsty and frightened. She wishes to resume her diabetes management. She is alert. Which of the following laboratory findings would indicate that it is safe to manage her case outside the hospital?

(A) Serum bicarbonate level of 10 to 15 mEq/L
(B) Arterial pH of 7.25 to 7.30
(C) High level of beta-hydroxybutyrate; alert patient
(D) Blood sugar of ≤250 mg/dL
(E) Urine ketones positive; alert patient

17 A 36-year-old male insulin-dependent diabetic of 15 years complains of blurred vision in his left eye. You discover that he did not keep his ophthalmologist's appointments over the past 3 years. The eye chart shows his near visual acuity to be 20/50 OS and 20/20 OD; his far visual acuity is 20/40 OS and 20/25 OD. One year ago, his visual acuity was 20/25 OU far and 20/20 OU near. Random blood sugar was 130 by finger-stick performed by the office nurse as the patient entered today. A hemoglobin A1C level drawn last week was 8.5%. Which of the following pathophysiologic mechanisms is the cause of this condition?

(A) Retinal surface proliferative changes impede light transmission to the retina.
(B) Microaneurysms interfere with retinal function.
(C) Dot hemorrhages interfere with retinal function.
(D) Cotton-wool exudates interfere with retinal function.
(E) Changes in average blood sugar affect refraction density of the aqueous fluid.

18 You order a serum creatinine and 24-hour urine for creatinine and for *total and complete protein* for an 40-year-old Caucasian diabetic type 1 male. His height is 6 ft 1 in. and he weighs 180 lb. From these data, you calculate a creatinine clearance of 50 mL/hour. Each of the following statements is relevant regarding this finding except for (which) statement?

(A) Closer blood sugar control is indicated.
(B) Among cases of this condition, more are caused by type 2 diabetes than by type 1.
(C) Blood pressure control is important.
(D) Pharmacological means to raise the glomerular filtration rate is indicated.
(E) Dietary protein control is indicated.

Examination Answers

1. The answer is B. Asian. This group develops type 2 diabetes at lower BMIs and lower ages than other groups. Furthermore, they appear to be most subject to renal disease due to diabetes. This may be surprising because Latinos and blacks are known to be developing diabetes at increasingly lower ages but that is clearly because of the appearance of increasingly lower ages of obesity. The same may be said for Latino-Americans and some aboriginal tribes. As for blacks in America, insulin resistance is greater for given levels of BMI (but without a commensurate increase in atherosclerotic risk, as compared to Caucasians).

2. The answer is B. The incorrect statement is that exenatide reduces insulin resistance in type 2 diabetes. Each of the other statements about the much-lauded exenatide (Byetta) is true. Suppression of glucagon appears to be somewhat clinically significant in that blood sugar control is improved and HgbA1c adequately controlled. Perhaps more important is that a side effect is weight loss. Exenatide must be delivered by subcutaneous injection twice daily, promotes a higher insulin response than an equivalent dose of glucose, and carries a lower risk of hypoglycemic reaction than sulfonylureas.

3. The answer is A. Glargine (Lantus by Sanofi-Aventis), the longest acting of the insulins presented. Its onset occurs at about 1.5 hours after injection and lasts for 24 hours. As to lispro (Humalog by Lilly), glulisine (Apidra by Sanofi Aventis), and Aspart insulin (Novolog by Novo Nordisk), all have onsets of action within 5 to 15 minutes peaking at 1 to 1.5 hours and lasting 3 to 4 hours. Regular insulin sets on in 30 to 60 minutes, peaks in 2 hours and lasts 6 to 7 hours.

4. The answer is C. HHS precipitated by dehydration is the best description of the pathophysiology of this patient's condition. Required for this development is type 2 diabetes, a measure of at least temporary poor control, and a clinical stimulus for dehydration. As serum osmolality exceeds 310 mosm/kg, the patient develops lethargy and confusion with coma supervening at 320 to 330. DKA, found virtually only in type 2 diabetes, is ruled out by the lack of ketosis. The hyperosmolar state is certainly somewhat related to diabetes control, but the latter is not the proximate cause. In the present case, dehydration would have been caused by the gastroenteritis. Even egregiously noncompliant or poorly controlled patients seldom develop the hyperosmolar state. The BUN of 110 mg/dL is common in the hyperosmolar state and does not denote renal failure. The azotemia will respond to aggressive fluid and electrolyte repletion therapy.

5. The answer is C. The major precipitants of HHS, although the final common pathway is dehydration, are medication noncompliance and ethanol and cocaine use. Although it has been written that "causes" include myocardial infarction, stroke, hyperthermia and hypothermia, pulmonary embolus, and many other diseases, no one develops HHS who does not have a type 2 diabetic diathesis. According to the article by Stoner cited in the references, the case mortality of this syndrome is greater than that of DKA. A significant anion gap is more characteristic of DKA, and infarct is not a particular characteristic of HHS. Although gastroparesis is generally thought of as a complication of type 2 diabetes, it may be found in HHS during the acute phase when dehydration is marked. Because the basic pathophysiology of HHS is dehydration, that is, neither hyperglycemia per se nor acidosis, the quickest response is fluid therapy while using modest means to reduce the blood sugar level, which will fall even without insulin as fluid and sodium repletion proceeds.

6. The answer is B. Only the biguanides, of which the only presently approved example is metformin, facilitate weight loss while reducing blood sugar without stimulating insulin production. It accomplishes the latter by decreasing hepatic glucose production, mainly through reduction of gluconeogenesis. Because of its ability to reduce blood sugar without stimulating insulin production, it functionally reduces insulin resistance. Sulfonylurea agents decrease blood sugar levels by stimulating production of insulin (i.e., they are secretagogues for insulin), hence contributing to higher insulin levels and ultimate exhaustion of the beta-cells of the pancreas. Non-sulfonylurea secretagogues work similarly to sulfonylurea secretagogues but more rapidly. Thiazolidinediones enhance insulin sensitivity by activating a nuclear transcription factor and modulating many genes that regulate CHO metabolism. The net effect is to increase insulin sensitivity. Alpha-glucosidase inhibitors work by delaying intestinal absorption of CHOs and thus reducing PP glucose levels. Their effectiveness is not impressive, and the side effect of flatulence has made the agent acarbose less popular with time.

7. The answer is D. The pains are caused by long-standing hyperglycemia. The patient has diabetic neuropathy (i.e., neuropathy did not cause the pains; the pains were evidence, part and parcel, of diabetic neuropathy). The United Kingdom Prospective Diabetes Study Group results published in four separate journal articles (two in *Lancet* and two in the *British Medical Journal*, all in 1998) showed for type 2 diabetes the same as the DCCT Group showed for diabetes type I (*Diabetes Care*, 1996); that is, virtually all the complications of diabetes, particularly neuropathic complications, are preventable by strict control of blood sugar. Thus, control of diabetes is the route to prevention of complication. Although noncompliance contributes to poor diabetes control, it is neither the direct nor the proximate cause.

8. The answer is D. A hemoglobin variant that co-elutes with hemoglobin A apparently constitutes an additional substance with an affinity for glucose as the red cell is formed, thus causing a *falsely elevated* HbA1C level. HbA1C elevation is 91% specific and 85% sensitive. False low levels can be caused by conditions associated with shortened red blood cell life, such as hemolytic anemias (e.g., thalassemia and spherocytosis), or in which red cells are disproportionately recently extruded from the marrow, as in recovery from recent blood loss. Finally, of course, hyperglycemia must be persistent enough to affect a significant proportion of the red cells as they are newly created; that is, the diabetes must be of adequate severity to result in elevation of the HbA1C level. Hemoglobin A1C is but one of three A1 hemoglobins. The other two, hemoglobins A1a and A1b, involve phosphorylated glucose and fructose, respectively. They are not measured in clinical medicine.

9. The answer is A. The point of the question is to show that, although there may be differing opinions and details in varying definitions as to what constitutes the metabolic syndrome, qualitatively, there is wide agreement; waist circumference (related to hip circumference), serum triglyceride level, HDL-C level (HDLC), blood pressure, and fasting glucose are listed in the definitions of metabolic syndrome X by both the World Health Organization and the Adult Treatment Panel III. These items constitute risk factors that tend to occur together in the same individuals and families, such as dyslipidemia, hypertension, and diabetes. Obviously, the definition is thus arbitrary. However, all agree that insulin resistance exists and that it is characterized by increased central obesity, elevated triglyceride levels, decreased HDL-C levels, tendency to or existing hypertension, and some degree of compromised glucose tolerance. Of greatest clinical significance is that the syndrome in full expression presents an array of vascular risk factors. Diagnosis neither requires all the elements to be present nor needs to be official for the syndrome to be treated by diet and medications as appropriate to management of the separate disease manifestations. Each of the other choices as answers to the question is relevant to the syndrome, but few choices are present in all cases.

10. The answer is C. The correct maintenance diet for diabetes (or for anyone) is based on the following: At 70 in. of height, his ideal weight is 106 lb + 6 lb for each inch over 5 ft (100 lb + 5 lb for each inch over 5 ft for females) = 166 lb for the patient in this vignette. Total maintenance caloric requirement is ideal weight in pounds × 10 = (rounded) 1,700 calories for this patient. Fifty five percent (45% to 65%) of these calories should be in CHOs = 935 cal. Grams of CHO = 935/4 cal/gm = 233 gm. Fifteen percent of calories should be in protein. 1,700 × .15 = 255 cal. As protein, 255 cal/4 cal/gm = 64 gm. This leaves 30% of calories to be consumed as fat, or 510 cal (of which no more than 7% should be in saturated fats) 510 cal/8 cal/gm = 64 gm fat.

11. The answer is C. Giving 27 to 54 units daily fits the guideline of 0.5 to 1 unit of insulin/kg (120 lb/2.2 = 54 kg).

12. The answer is B. In the recent past, the definition of microalbuminuria was defined as at least 295 mg/24-hour specimen. Although this remains a valid definition, it was been facilitated by the more convenient and hence more reliable procedure of the timed overnight specimens overnight collections where normal is ≤15 mcg/minute. Microalbuminuria is then defined as ≥20 mcg/minute. One hundred and fifty to three hundred milligrams of albumin/24 hours is the earliest diabetic clinical sign of diabetic nephropathy, signaling the initiation of Kimmelstiel–Wilson basement membrane lesions in the glomeruli. Note the distinction between protein and albumin in this definition: that is, *microproteinuria* is defined in mg/24 hours of albumin, a *component* of urinary protein. This amount on a single voided specimen is as little as 20 mg/dL on urinalysis.

13. The answer is A. ≤105 mg/dL (5.8 mmol/L) is the accepted FBS in a 50-g, 1-hour glucose tolerance test; the goal being to keep the FBS 60 to 90 mg/dL. These should be measured at the latest during 24 to 28 weeks of pregnancy and should call for aggressive diet therapy for diabetes.

14. The answer is B. Blood sugar exceeding 90 mg/dL fasting or 120 mg/dL at 2 hours surpasses ideal blood sugar control in pregnancy; hence, if consistently in those ranges, consideration for starting insulin is signaled.

15. The answer is C. 110 mg/dL to 125 mg/dL blood sugar; 140 mg/dL to 199 mg/dL defines this state at the 2-hour point in a 100-g glucose tolerance test. This may appear to be an academic exercise because any patient with prediabetes, diabetes, or simply to harbor risk factors for diabetes deserves qualitatively similar therapeutic approach. However, research has been devoted to prevention of delay of the onset of diabetes type 2 and has shown that the stage of impaired regulation yields success through lifestyle change that rivals that of metformin.

16. The answer is B. An arterial pH level of 7.25 to 7.30 is only mildly depressed and is compatible with an alert person in early DKA. At this level of acidosis, the patient may be managed as an outpatient. A moderately acidotic pH level is defined as 7 to 7.224 and severe is defined as <7. Urine ketones would be positive in all three degrees of severity. Similarly, hydroxybutyrate might be elevated to high levels in all three categories of severity, and blood sugar levels above 120 mg/dL are to be found in all three categories. Bicarbonate levels of 10 to 15 mEq/L are in the moderately acidotic category and <10 is considered severe. Mild DKA is reflected by a bicarbonate level of 15 to 28 mEq/L.

17. The answer is A. Retinal surface proliferative changes are directly related to visual loss (and distinctly so compared to the other factors mentioned). The fact that the visual loss is unilateral (OS = left eye) and that random blood sugar determination is nearly normal rules out a change in refraction brought about temporarily by hyperglycemia. The elevated glycolated hemoglobin allows the inference that long-term control, however, has been less than optimal. Thus, the patient likely suffers from retinopathy. Such retinopathy occurs in approximately one-half of all diabetics after 10 years of living with type 1 disease and after a variable duration in type 2. This retinal lesion is the reason that diabetes is the leading cause of blindness in the United States. For this reason, the standard of care is for routine ophthalmologic examination scheduled annually after 5 years of disease or after a proliferative lesion has been seen. The other changes, microaneurysms, dot hemorrhages, and cotton-wool exudates as well as hard exudates, are commonly seen in diabetes, microaneurysms being virtually pathognomonic of the disease, *but no authors have stated that they are causes of blindness.*

18. The answer is D. This man's creatinine clearance is significantly less than would be expected for a man of his age and size. If this problem is not acted upon, he is likely to be headed ultimately for end-stage renal disease. One-third is the approximate proportion of cases of end-stage renal disease that are caused by diabetes. The following table puts diabetes, hypertension, and renal disease into a perspective of their clinical interaction.

Diseases	Percentage
Diabetes mellitus	31
Hypertension	27
Glomerulonephritis	14
Obstructive uropathy	5.7
Polycystic renal disease	3.6
Others	5.7
Unknown	13

Used with permission from Rudy and Kurowski (1997). The diseases listed in the left column are responsible for the corresponding percentages of end-stage renal disease.

References

Family Medicine Board Review 2009 M 3–10, 2009. Kansas City, Missouri Kimmel B and Inzucchi SE: Oral Agents for Type 2 Diabetes. *Clinical Diabetes* 2005; 23(2):65–75.

Masharani U. Diabetes mellitus and hypoglycemia. In: Tierney LM, McPhee SJ, Papadakis MA, eds. *Current Medical Diagnosis and Treatment*. 45th ed. New York/Chicago: Lange; 2006.

McPhee SJ, Papadakis MA. *Current Medical Diagnosis and Treatment 2010*, 49th ed. New York/Chicago: McGraw-Hill/Lange; 2010.

Rudy DR. Hypertension. In: Rudy DR, Kurowski K, eds. *Family Medicine: House Officer Series*. Baltimore: Williams & Wilkins; 1997.

Stoner GD. Hyperosmolar hyperglycemic state. *Am Fam Physician.* 2005; 71:1723–1730.

Turok DK, Ratcliffe SD, Baxley EG. Management of gestational diabetes. *Am Fam Physician.* 2003;68:1967–1972, 1075–1076.

Tzagournis M, Rudy DR. Diabetes mellitus. In: Rudy DR, Kurowski K, eds. *Family Medicine: House Officer Series*. Baltimore: Williams & Wilkins; 1997:513–542.

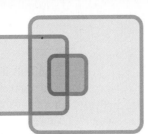

chapter 33

Thyroid Diseases

Examination questions: *Unless otherwise instructed, choose the ONE lettered answer or completion that is BEST in each case.*

1 Each of the following statements is true regarding management of myxedema crisis except for which one?

(A) Hypothermic patients may be treated by warm intravenous (IV) fluids.
(B) Levothyroxine 400 µg given IV is often indicated.
(C) IV glucocorticoid may be indicated.
(D) Maintenance dosage of levothyroxine IV may be as low as 50 µg.
(E) Infections coexisting must be treated more aggressively than in euthyroid patients.

2 Which of the following starting dosages of levothyroxine is most appropriate for hypothyroid pregnant women?

(A) 25 to 50 µg daily
(B) 50 to 100 µg daily
(C) 75 to 100 µg daily
(D) 100 to 150 µg daily
(E) 200 to 250 µg daily

3 A 35-year-old woman has developed digital clubbing, digital swelling, and a periosteal reaction in bones of the extremities, along with sinus tachycardia as well as ophthalmopathy. Which of the following is this condition?

(A) Chronic obstructive pulmonary disease
(B) A variant of hepatic cirrhosis
(C) Toxic multinodular goiter
(D) Paget disease
(E) Thyroid acropachy

4 A 55-year-old Caucasian woman has been on maintenance amiodarone to prevent recurrent atrial fibrillation for 2 years, and bipolar disorder has also been on a lithium preparation. She begins developing upper lid retraction (Dalrymple sign), lid lag with downward gaze (Graefe sign), and a stare (Kocher

sign). Each of the following processes may be the mechanism of thyrotoxicosis except for which one?

(A) Toxic nodular goiter
(B) Side effect of lithium
(C) Graves disease
(D) Factitious hyperthyroidism
(E) Amiodarone side effect

5 In screening for primary thyroid disease (hypothyroidism or hyperthyroidism), which of the following serum tests is the most sensitive?

(A) Free tetraiodothyronine (FT_4)
(B) Triiodothyronine (T_3) resin uptake
(C) Total tetraiodothyronine (T_4)
(D) Thyroid-stimulating hormone (thyrotropin, or TSH)
(E) Antithyroglobulin antibodies

6 A 25-year-old woman complains of fatigue and cold intolerance increasing over the past 3 months. On examination, she manifests a somewhat dry skin, which she says is a change from her usual. She admits to being puzzled and saddened over the situation. Her apical heart rate is 68 in a regular rhythm. Blood pressure is 110/68. The TSH level is 0.3 µIU/mL (0.4 to 4.8). She gives a further history of being on bromocriptine for a microprolactinoma. Which of the following is the likely cause of her condition?

(A) Hashimoto thyroiditis
(B) Panhypopituitarism
(C) Secondary hypothyroidism
(D) Primary hypothyroidism
(E) Primary hyperthyroidism

7 A 45-year-old white woman is undergoing a routine annual preventive health examination. After reviewing the routine mammogram and before performing the routine breast and pelvic examination, you proceed to a head-to-toe brief physical examination. You discover a palpable thyroid nodule that seems to be about 2.5 cm in diameter. Which of the following blood tests would be the most logical, in addition to certain routine medical profiles?

(A) Serum lipids
(B) Free T_4 and TSH
(C) Protein-bound iodine
(D) T_3 resin uptake and total T_4
(E) Timed Achilles heel reflex

8 The results of routine testing of the patient in Question 7 are FT_4 3 ng/dL (0.2 to 2.1) and TSH 0.2 μIU/mL (0.4 to 4.8). Which of the following would be the next most logical action?

(A) Order serum antithyroid peroxidase antibodies
(B) Order exploratory surgery of the thyroid
(C) Order a bone scan for metastatic lesions
(D) Order sodium iodide I^{123} thyroid uptake
(E) Perform a fine-needle aspiration

9 Regarding the patient in Question 7, if the thyroid function studies had indicated a euthyroid state, what would be the best next action?

(A) Order serum antithyroid peroxidase antibody test
(B) Order exploratory surgery of the thyroid
(C) Order a bone scan for metastatic lesions
(D) Order I^{123} thyroid uptake
(E) Perform FNA biopsy

10 A 25-year-old woman manifests a single palpable nodule, and it has tested out to be euthyroid by FT_4 and TSH and did not take up I^{123} on scan. An FNA biopsy is planned. Her mother inquires as to which of the results would be most favorable if the finding were to be cancer. Which of the following is the least aggressive thyroid cancer?

(A) Papillary thyroid carcinoma
(B) Follicular thyroid carcinoma
(C) Medullary thyroid carcinoma
(D) Anaplastic carcinoma
(E) Metastatic melanoma

11 Each of the following clinical or laboratory findings may be found as statistically more likely in hypothyroidism, except which one?

(A) Hyponatremia
(B) Amenorrhea
(C) Menorrhagia
(D) Delayed recovery of deep tendon reflexes
(E) Onset of obesity

12 You have been following a 45-year-old man for hypothyroidism for the past 2 years without significant complaints. He was prescribed 100 μg of levothyroxine 1 year ago, when the diagnosis was made, and his TSH fell to normal levels at the 3-month and 6-month visits. He returns for a routine annual recheck and manifests a normal blood pressure and apical heart rate of 80, regular. As he has a family history of adenomatous colon polyps, you arrange for colorectal cancer screening annually this decade. Then you draw routine fasting lipids because he has gained 5 lb (2.26 kg) during the past year and also draw in the same specimen serum TSH. The test results return normal except for TSH, whose level is 6.2 μIU/mL (normal is 0.4 to 4.8). Each of the following may constitute explanations for this finding, except which factor?

(A) Failure of patient to comply with the prescribed dosage of levothyroxine.
(B) Inadequate dosage of levothyroxine prescribed.
(C) The prescribed levothyroxine is malabsorbed.
(D) The patient has secondary hypothyroidism.
(E) There may be a comorbid autoimmune condition.

13 A 45-year-old white woman complains of an 8-lb (3.6-kg) weight loss, despite eating normally, if not more than her usual amount, over the past 3 months. She admits to being more irritable than is her custom. Upon examination, she exhibits a stare and lid lag. The thyroid gland is diffusely palpable. Her skin is moist and velvety, and her peripheral and apical pulses are identical: 104 and regular. Blood pressure is 140/60. Her deep tendon reflexes are uniformly hyperactive, including the presence of the Hoffman reflex bilaterally. Which of the following combinations of test results distinguishes this as thyroiditis as opposed to primary hyperthyroidism?

(A) Suppressed TSH, elevated FT_4, abnormally low I^{123} uptake
(B) Suppressed TSH, elevated FT_4, elevated I^{123} uptake
(C) Elevated TSH, elevated FT_4
(D) Suppressed TSH, normal FT_4, normal T_3
(E) Suppressed TSH, elevated FT_4

14 A 55-year-old white woman has noted for the past month an increasing tightness in her neck when wearing certain high-buttoned clothing. The thyroid gland is diffusely palpable, somewhat enlarged, and finely nodular. She denies changes in heat or cold tolerance; her vital signs are unremarkable and there are no other physical findings. TSH and FT_4 levels are within normal limits. Which of the following is the most logical next step among those mentioned?

(A) FNA biopsy
(B) Temperature graph recorded at home, to be returned in a week
(C) Serum T_3 determination
(D) Open biopsy
(E) Serum antithyroid peroxidase

15 A previously healthy 35-year-old man complains of painful neck for the past 2 weeks, along with malaise and night sweats. In addition, he notes increased nervousness and irritability. He manifests a sinus tachycardia at 108 beats per minute. He denies treatment for cancer and human immunodeficiency virus (HIV) disease and risk factors for HIV. The thyroid is diffusely palpable and mildly tender. The eyes exhibit a mild stare, but exophthalmos is not present. The TSH level is 0.2 μIU/mL (0.4 to 4.8) and the FT_4 level is 3 ng/dL (0.9 to 2.1). A radioactive iodine (RAI) uptake and scan shows a very low uptake. Which of the following is the diagnosis?

(A) Graves disease
(B) Riedel struma
(C) Hashimoto thyroiditis
(D) Ludwig angina
(E) Subacute thyroiditis

16 Which of the following is the most reasonable therapeutic approach for the patient in Question 15, at the present time?

(A) Institute methimazole treatment as 30 mg daily by mouth
(B) Start propylthiouracil 300 mg daily
(C) Start propranolol 20 mg daily
(D) Treat with I^{131}
(E) Consult and arrange for subtotal thyroidectomy

17 A 45-year-old female has completed treatment for subacute thyroiditis for 3 months. Now, however, she complains of decreasing energy and increased sleep requirements. Her skin is dry and the eyes mildly "puffy" compared with her former appearance, even before the acute phase of the recent illness. Each of the following statements regarding this development is true except for which one?

(A) The patient's case has evolved into hypothyroidism.
(B) Treatment of this condition will remain in place for life.
(C) This complication occurs in nearly one-half of patients.
(D) The patient may, at a later date, develop hyperthyroidism.
(E) A significant proportion of patients with this condition will have persistent elevations of antithyroid peroxidase antibodies

18 A 35-year-old woman enters your office complaining of a 20-lb (9-kg) involuntary weight loss over a period of 4 months. At 5 ft, 4 in. (1.63 m), she weighs 110 lb (50 kg), down from her usually stable weight of 130 lb (59 kg). Her skin is moist and velvety in texture. Her sclerae are visible above her corneae and she shows an asymmetrical ocular proptosis. Her thyroid gland is diffusely palpable and non-nodular. She is at risk for each of the following diseases, except which one?

(A) Alopecia areata
(B) Diabetes mellitus type 1
(C) Vitiligo
(D) Coronary atherosclerosis
(E) Adrenal insufficiency

19 For a 37-year-old woman with Graves disease, which of the following is the *least* favored choice of treatment for this woman, assuming she wants no more children and is not pregnant?

(A) Methimazole
(B) Propylthiouracil
(C) I^{131} therapy
(D) Thyroidectomy
(E) Short-term propranolol

20 A 45-year-old white man complains of weight loss for several weeks and his wife complains that he often sets the heating system down, a change from his prior comfort zone in which the two had always had agreement. He has lost weight from his usual 185 lb (84 kg) at 5 ft, 10 in. (1.78 m) to 165 lb (74.7 kg) over the past 3 months. His wife reminds him that while they were living in another city several years ago, he was diagnosed as having a goiter, which was treated with thyroid hormone, but his prescription lapsed after they had moved and he had not sought further treatment. His thyroid gland is enlarged and palpably nodular in both lobes. Examination of his eyes externally is normal. This entity is preceded by which of the following conditions?

(A) Single "cold" thyroid nodule
(B) Single "hot" thyroid nodule
(C) Autoimmune thyroiditis
(D) Nontoxic multinodular goiter
(E) Factitious hyperthyroidism

21 Regarding the patient in Question 20, which of the following is the most likely treatment of choice?

(A) Respective surgery
(B) I^{131} therapy
(C) Propylthiouracil
(D) Methimazole
(E) Propranolol

Examination Answers

1. The answer is A. The incorrect statement is that critically myxedematous hypothermic patients may be treated by warm IV fluids. In fact, such aggressive address of hypothermia may precipitate cardiovascular collapse. Warming should be accomplished with blankets. Levothyroxine 400 µg loading dose given IV is indicated and may result in improvement within hours. IV glucocorticoid may be indicated because adrenal insufficiency may coexist with myxedema itself. Myxedema interferes with gastrointestinal absorption of oral thyroid preparations. Thus, medications may have to be given IV. Relatively low maintenance IV dosage (e.g., 50 µg) is selected initially in patients with known coronary artery disease. Coexisting infections must be treated more aggressively.

2. The answer is D. 100 to 150 µg daily, a relatively high levothyroxine starting dosage, is appropriate for pregnant women. This addresses the facts that (a) fetuses are not thyroid sufficient until term; (b) high estrogen levels, as obtained during pregnancy, require increased dosing to achieve euthyroidism. Maternal hypothyroidism is a risk for fetal central nervous system development in the second trimester, adding to the need for emphasizing adequate dosing in pregnancy. Dosages range downward in nonpregnant people; for example, a starting dosage for cardiac patients is perhaps 25 µg, advancing in increments. They may range upward to 250 to 300 µg daily.

3. The answer is E. Thyroid acropachy, an extreme and unusual manifestation of Graves disease, that is, an autoimmune disease that includes periosteal reaction. Ophthalmopathy is the tip that Graves disease is in the picture. Multinodular goiter, while likely featuring a stare or lid lag, is not characterized by ophthalmopathy (inflammatory exophthalmos). Paget disease manifests typical bone changes easily seen on x-ray but not clubbing. Chronic obstructive pulmonary disease and hepatic cirrhosis are known to be associated with digital clubbing but without ophthalmopathy.

4. The answer is B. Side effect of lithium does *not* have a side effect of thyrotoxicosis as hypothyroidism is an effect of lithium therapy. Amiodarone has the effect of causing thyrotoxicosis as a proximate effect of its heavy content of iodine, which becomes free iodine in metabolism. This effect is likely and more marked in a patient with iodine deficiency (and of course in geographic areas where that exists).

5. The answer is D. TSH, sensitive assay, is the most sensitive screening test for overactive and underactive thyroid disease. Although not a direct measurement of metabolism, as total and free T_4 (tetraiodothyronine) and T_3

(triiodothyronine), the TSH responds in suppression before T_3 and T_4 begin to rise in hyperthyroidism and by elevation before T_3 and T_4 begin to fall. Obviously, in both the foregoing instances, the patient would be asymptomatic.

6. The answer is C. Secondary hypothyroidism. Abnormally low or suppressed TSH occurs most often in Graves disease or other forms of primary hyperthyroidism, as a result of suppression by the feedback on excessive circulating thyroid hormones. However, this patient manifests symptoms and signs of hypothyroidism rather than thyrotoxicosis. Abnormally low TSH occurs, of course, in hypopituitarism as well, causing secondary hypothyroidism. In this case, rather than panhypopituitarism, the patient most likely has secondary hypothyroidism that is due to suppressed TSH as a side effect of bromocriptine. Hashimoto thyroiditis presents in several phases but generally results in primary hypothyroidism in the long term, with TSH elevation.

7. The answer is B. Free T_4 and TSH are generally thought of as constituting the best combination of initial tests of thyroid physiology. TSH is the most sensitive screen for both hyperthyroidism and hypothyroidism. Free T_4 is the metabolically active form of tetraiodothyronine, which in turn accounts ultimately for the overwhelming proportion of hormone output by the gland, with triiodothyronine accounting for the remainder. I^{123} thyroid uptake is unnecessarily involved for an initial investigation of the activity status of the thyroid gland, if the TSH is suppressed and the FT_4 is elevated. Protein-bound iodine is an outmoded test for thyroid hormone activity, being directly related to the T_4 content. It is no longer in use because not only is it not a direct measurement of hormone but it also is subject to too many inaccuracies. Similarly, the Achilles tendon reflex exhibits time of recovery inversely related to the state of metabolism regulated by the thyroid. It too has inadequate sensitivity and specificity. T_3 resin uptake is an indirect measurement that has also fallen out of use, in favor of the free T_4 and TSH.

8. The answer is D. I^{123} thyroid uptake is indicated in a solitary palpable thyroid nodule with hyperthyroid functional status. The radioactive radioiodine (RAI) uptake can distinguish a hot nodule from an incidental or cold nodule in a hyperthyroid gland.

9. The answer is E. FNA biopsy is indicated for most solitary nodules, the exception being a hot nodule, as judged by the I^{123} thyroid uptake and scan. This is the only way to rule out carcinoma, short of open exploration.

10. The answer is A. Papillary thyroid carcinoma is the least aggressive and happily the most common, comprising 76% of all thyroid cancers. Follicular thyroid carcinoma is the most well differentiated of the thyroid cancers; the second most well differentiated is papillary carcinoma. Medullary carcinoma of the thyroid occurs equally frequently in male and female individuals, whereas anaplastic carcinoma occurs 56% of the time in female individuals. Follicular carcinoma constitutes 16% of all thyroid carcinomas. Because of good differentiation, follicular carcinoma is also amenable to I^{131} therapy after total thyroidectomy. To a lesser degree, this applies to papillary carcinoma as well. Patients with medullary carcinoma have a 6% chance of dying of the disease; those with follicular carcinoma have a 24% chance of dying of the disease. Although papillary carcinoma is the least aggressive, it tends to be multifocal and presents frequently with lymph node metastases. These, however, tend to respond to I^{131} therapy.

11. The answer is E. Contrary to popular lore, hypothyroidism, although rendering it more difficult to lose weight because of reduced basal requirements, does not cause true obesity. Along with reduced basal energy requirements, the appetite appears to be reduced proportionately. Each of the other choices is well known to be powerfully associated with hypothyroidism except for amenorrhea. Conventional wisdom as taught to medical students is that thyrotoxicosis is associated with oligomenorrhea or amenorrhea, whereas hypothyroidism is associated with menorrhagia. Actually, either amenorrhea or menorrhagia may be found in hypothyroidism. Thus, any form of menstrual irregularities warrants routine thyroid function studies.

12. The answer is D. "The patient has secondary hypothyroidism" is an incorrect statement. Secondary hypothyroidism occurs as a result of failure of the pituitary gland, specifically, inadequate TSH production, and hence it manifests lower than normal TSH levels, not elevated levels. Each of the other choices results in elevated TSH in primary hypothyroidism. Malabsorption of thyroid medication can occur because of concurrent administration of binding substance, sprue or diarrhea of any kind, or bile acid-binding agents like cholestyramine. In some autoimmune conditions, false elevations of TSH may occur through interference with the laboratory assay.

13. The answer is A. Suppressed TSH, elevated FT_4, and an abnormally low I^{123} uptake are typical of acute thyroiditis. However, for confirmation, thyroglobulin should be checked and found to be elevated. Otherwise, the diagnosis may be hypermetabolism caused by exogenous thyroid hormone. Acute thyroiditis causes a release of thyroid hormone resulting in a suppression of TSH, all of which occurs in the absence of active production of hormone by the parenchyma; thus, there is no increase and may be a decrease in I^{123} uptake. Choice B, suppressed TSH, elevated FT_4, and increased I^{123} uptake, is typical of primary hyperthyroidism. If the increased uptake is diffuse, the picture is that of classical Graves disease. A nodular I^{123} uptake scan result may be multiple in toxic multinodular goiter or single in the case of a toxic adenoma. Choice C, elevated FT_4 and elevated TSH, assuming no spurious cause of TSH elevation, can occur only in secondary hyperthyroidism (i.e., increased production of pituitary TSH). Choice D, suppressed TSH, normal FT_4, and normal T_3, is evidence of subclinical hyperthyroidism, treated hyperthyroidism (perhaps dosed slightly above therapeutic), pregnancy, or rarely nonthyroid illness. Choice E, suppressed TSH, elevated FT_4, indicates exogenous thyroid hormone, as may occur in Choice D.

14. The answer is E. Serum antithyroglobulin, taken on a blood sample, if elevated, makes the diagnosis of Hashimoto thyroiditis in 90% of Hashimoto and to lesser sensitivity in other thyroiditides 40% of Hashimoto manifest antithyroglobulin titers. Hashimoto thyroiditis is the most common thyroid disorder in the United States. RAI uptake with I^{123}, in the subacute phase, as with all thyroiditides, will be very low as opposed to Graves disease or normal. However, as the disease becomes chronic, in euthyroid or hypothyroid patients, the RAI uptake tends to be normal or elevated with an uneven distribution. FNA biopsy would be indicated if there was a single prominent nodule. In the absence of thyrotoxicosis, T_3 determination is not indicated and then only if TSH is suppressed and FT_4 is normal. Hashimoto thyroiditis (also called lymphocytic thyroiditis or, archaically, struma lymphomatosa) uncommonly causes a thyrotoxic phase but often leads to hypothroidism, remitting then in 5% of cases.

15. The answer is E. Subacute thyroiditis, accounting for about 5% of clinical thyroid disease, is usually painful but may be silent, the latter understandably causing confusion with Hashimoto thyroiditis. It is often associated with systemic symptoms of viral-like illness during the early phase. It has also been called de Quervain thyroiditis. Graves disease causes exophthalmos in addition to other signs of hyperthyroidism and manifests an increased RAI uptake. Riedel struma does not cause thyrotoxicosis. Hashimoto thyroiditis does not present with a tender gland and only rarely manifests hyperthyroidism. Ludwig angina is a streptococcal infection of the floor of the mouth and descending inferiorly. Though anterior neck pain would be characteristic, hyperthyroidism would not.

16. The answer is C. Start propranolol at 20 mg daily. In subacute thyroiditis, the thyrotoxic phase usually is mild and lasts about 2 months. Therefore, thiourea drugs (e.g., methimazole and propylthiouracil) are not necessary and would not be effective because their action depends on active hormone production by the gland. The same statements are true for I^{131}. From the foregoing, it is clear that thyroidectomy is not warranted.

17. The answer is B. Typical of subacute or de Quervain thyroiditis is not only a brief thyrotoxic phase but also 6 to 9 months of hypothyroidism that follows virtually on the heels of the toxic phase. Thus, treatment of this condition will rarely remain in place for life. The complication occurs in nearly one-half of patients, although the vast majority revert to a euthyroid state without elevated antithyroid antibodies. Approximately 5% of patients will not remit from the hypothyroid phase; a few will have recurrent subacute phases, and uncommonly some will undergo change to Graves disease. About one-third of subacute thyroiditis patients will have persistent elevations of antithyroid peroxidase antibodies and a persistent goiter.

18. The answer is D. Coronary atherosclerosis is not a particularly strong risk in Graves disease, the most common cause of hyperthyroid disease, illustrated in the vignette presented. As an autoimmune disease, Graves is associated statistically with all the other diseases mentioned among the choices and as well with coeliac disease, myasthenia gravis, cardiomyopathy, and hypokalemic periodic paralysis. The female-to-male ratio among those afflicted with Graves disease is approximately 8:1. Lifetime incidence (sometime prevalence of this disease) is thus 2.2% for female individuals and about 0.3% for male individuals. Indeed, the vast majority of all thyroid problems occur more in female than in male individuals.

19. The answer is D. Thyroidectomy is the least likely choice, with the patient having the final vote, assuming she is well informed of all side effects and contraindications. In the short term, when the patient is uncomfortable or seriously in jeopardy because of the severity of the thyrotoxicosis, nonselective beta-adrenergic blocking drugs such as propranolol are used while the definitive therapy takes effect. I^{131} therapy is well tolerated but is usually followed ultimately by hypothyroidism and the need for replacement therapy. The thiourea drugs have the advantage of often succeeding after finite periods of 1 to 2 years. Between the two most often utilized, propyl-

thiouracil is safe even in pregnancy, if kept below 200 mg/day to avoid fetal hypothyroidism. Thyroidectomy is less and less frequently elected because of its obvious invasiveness and the fact that it too must generally be followed by permanent hypothyroidism and the need for replacement therapy.

20. The answer is D. This patient has toxic nodular goiter, preceded as happens in a certain proportion of cases, by nontoxic nodular goiter. This disorder is not characterized by exophthalmos, unlike Graves disease, although the eyes may manifest the stare and the lid lag of thyrotoxicosis. It occurs most frequently in older individuals (i.e., ≥55 years) and begins as a grouping of nodules, apparently under the influence of an elevated TSH caused by incipient hypothyroidism. In a certain proportion of cases, the nodules become autonomous and hyperfunctional. This form of thyrotoxicosis is a less severe form of hyperthyroidism, whether measured in terms of clinical symptoms and signs or laboratory measurement of FT_4, T_3, or I^{123} uptake.

21. The answer is B. Therapy with I^{131} is ideal in this disease because it occurs most frequently in older people (but would be the best choice in any adult with toxic multinodular goiter, as will be clear from subsequent commentary). Surgery is eschewed for the same reasons as discussed elsewhere, unless there is reason to expect a cancerous nodule or nodules. Thiourea agents are not effective over the long term, as they are followed by a 95% chance of recurrent multinodular disease. Beta-blocking agents are not needed during the early treatment phase in most cases because in the vast majority the degree of thyrotoxicosis is mild.

References

Fitzpatrick PA. Endocrinology. In: Tierney LM, McPhee SJ, Papadakis MA, eds. *Medical Diagnosis and Treatment.* 45th ed. New York/Chicago: Lange; 2006.

Larsen PR, Davies TF, Hay ID. The thyroid gland. In: Wilson JD, Foster DW, Kronenberg HM, Larsen PR, eds. *William's Textbook of Endocrinology.* 9th ed. Philadelphia: WB Saunders; 1998:389–515.

Reid JR, Wheeler SF. Hyperthyroidism: Diagnosis and treatment. *Am Fam Physician.* 2005;72:623–630, 635–636.

Rudy DR, Tzagournis M. Thyroid problems in primary care. In: Rudy DR, Kurowski K, eds. *Family Medicine: House Officer Series.* Baltimore: Williams & Wilkins; 1997:543–566.

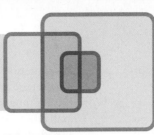

chapter 34

The Adrenal and Parathyroid Glands

Examination questions: *Unless instructed otherwise, choose the ONE lettered answer or completion that is BEST in each case.*

1 Which of the following findings is most specific for primary hyperparathyroidism?

(A) Increased sleep requirement
(B) Polyuria and polydipsia in the face of total calcium level of 12 mg/dL (8.5 to 10.5 mg/dL; 2.2 to 2.8 mmols/L) and parathormone level (PTH) unobtainable
(C) Prolonged P-R interval on resting electrocardiogram (ECG) with total calcium level of 12 mg/dL (8.5 to 10.5 mg/dL; 2.2 to 3 mmols/L) and PTH of 40 ng/L (0 to 60 ng/L)
(D) Calcium-containing kidney stones
(E) Diminished deep tendon reflexes with calcium level of 14 mg/dL (8.5 to 10.5 mg/dL, 2.2 to 3 mmols/L)

2 The NIH consensus, Question 1 notwithstanding, for diagnosis of hyperparathyroidism in 2009 requires all of the following factors except for which one?

(A) Serum calcium more than 1 mg/dL above normal
(B) Urinary calcium greater than 400 mg/dL
(C) Abnormally low bone density
(D) Carpopedal spasm
(E) Age less than 60 years

3 Each of the following conditions can be confused with Cushing disease or syndrome either chemically or clinically. Which one is NOT characterized by elevated serum cortisol?

(A) Factitious hypercortisolism
(B) Ingestion of gamma-hydroxybutyrate
(C) Familial cortisol resistance
(D) Anorexia nervosa
(E) Depression

4 A 34-year-old type 1 diabetic man had been controlled on 36 units daily of human insulin, both short (R) and intermediate (N) acting, in the form of 16 units of human N and 8 units of human R in the mornings and 8 units of human N and 4 units of human R after the evening meal. Three days ago, the man was involved in an auto accident in which he incurred abdominal blunt trauma and was hypotensive several hours before undergoing transfusion and splenectomy for rupture. There had been no apparent head injury. Yesterday, in the hospital, he began running a fever, with a temperature of 39°C (102.2°F). There are no apparent sites of infection. Blood cultures were drawn and are incubating. This morning, 3 hours after his morning insulin, he experienced a severe episode of hypoglycemia with a blood sugar measurement of 45 mg/dL. The fasting blood sugar before the morning insulin doses was 85 mg/dL. The patient complains of nausea, vomiting, and diarrhea. Initial laboratory results show a mild eosinophilia and hyperkalemia at 5.3 mEq/L. Which of the following is the most likely explanation of these developments?

(A) Sepsis secondary to surgical wound infection
(B) Sepsis secondary to primary wound infection at the sites of abdominal trauma
(C) Viral gastroenteritis
(D) Acute adrenal insufficiency
(E) Neurologic complication of the trauma involving temperature control

5 Adrenal insufficiency may be primary or secondary (i.e., secondary to pituitary failure). In addition to abnormally low levels of corticotropin (adrenocorticotropic hormone, or ACTH), which of the following findings would favor secondary adrenal insufficiency?

(A) Abnormally low level of serum cortisol
(B) Hypovolemia, hyponatremia, and hyperkalemia
(C) Physical findings of hyperpigmentation in the skin creases, skin over extensor surfaces (e.g., knuckles, elbows), and posterior neck
(D) Abnormally low level of serum cortisol, moderate neutropenia, lymphocytosis, and neutrophilia

(E) Hypovolemia, normal sodium concentration, normal serum potassium, and normal skin color

6 Your 33-year-old female patient has been diagnosed with primary adrenal insufficiency. She had manifested, among other things, hyperkalemia. Which of the following would be the most likely acceptable regimen for replacement therapy?

(A) Dexamethasone 0.75 mg daily, given in divided doses as 0.5 mg in the morning and 0.25 mg in the afternoon
(B) Prednisone 5 mg daily
(C) Hydrocortisone 24 mg daily, given as 16 mg in the morning and 8 mg in the afternoon, plus fludrocortisone 0.3 mg daily in the morning
(D) Prednisone 10 mg daily and fludrocortisone 0.3 mg daily
(E) Prednisone 15 mg daily, given as 10 mg in the morning and 5 mg in the afternoon

7 Which of the following is the basis of standard treatment for the most common form of adrenal hyperplasia, the androgenizing condition, 21-hydroxylase deficiency (also called P-450$_{c21}$ deficiency)?

(A) Conjugated estrogens
(B) Orchidectomy
(C) Hydrocortisone in replacement dosages
(D) Fludrocortisone
(E) Syntropin

8 A 35-year-old woman complains of weakness, fatigability, polyuria, and polydipsia. She had become hypertensive during the past few months and has been treated with a combination of hydrochlorothiazide/triamterene with fair results. Her most recent blood pressure readings have averaged 120/88. A spot blood sugar test 3 hours after her latest meal showed a level of 95 mg/dL. She complains also of muscular weakness, on occasion exhibiting paralysis for brief periods. Which of the following routine chemistries is likely to be the most critical in making a diagnosis that encompasses the hypertension and the weakness?

(A) Blood urea nitrogen
(B) Serum potassium
(C) Serum creatinine
(D) Serum sodium
(E) Serum bicarbonate

9 A 45-year-old woman has been followed for four visits for hypertension (blood pressure of 150 to 160/90 to 100) discovered during a routine examination, at which time, she was also found to have type 2 diabetes. Initially, an angiotensin-converting enzyme inhibitor failed to effect a fall in blood pressure from her baseline measurements. On the third visit, the

blood pressure had responded to hydrochlorothiazide/triamterene and her blood sugar had fallen to 120 to 130 at 2 hours postprandially as prescribed glipizide took effect. You notice that she is not only obese but also that her obesity is centripetal with proximal muscle wasting, associated with a plethoric face and purple striae about the trunk and that she complains of menstrual irregularity. She manifests also supraclavicular fat pads. Which of the following is the most likely comprehensive clinical diagnosis?

(A) Metabolic syndrome
(B) Essential hypertension
(C) Type 2 diabetes
(D) Cushing syndrome
(E) Morbid obesity

10 Regarding the patient in Question 8, which of the following tests will differentiate Cushing disease (Cushing syndrome caused by pituitary overproduction of ACTH) from Cushing syndrome caused by an ectopic source, primary adrenal disease, or extrinsic origin?

(A) Serum cortisol test
(B) 24-hour urine catecholamine test
(C) Dexamethasone suppression test
(D) Serum prolactin test
(E) Melanocyte-stimulating hormone test

11 A 56-year-old ambulatory white woman undergoes routine periodic physical examination and evaluation that includes mammogram, Pap smear, review of systems and medications, and routine laboratory hemogram and chemistries. All results are normal except that the serum calcium level is confirmed to be elevated. Which of the following is the most likely cause of the hypercalcemia, assuming no other information is available?

(A) Carcinoma of the breast
(B) Hypervitaminosis D
(C) Hypervitaminosis A
(D) Sarcoidosis
(E) Primary hyperparathyroidism

12 Regarding the patient in Question 11, a parathyroid hormone (PTH) level and urinary calcium-to-creatinine clearance ratio (Ca/CC) were ordered. At that time, you found the patient had been taking vitamin D supplements. Which of the following results would you expect if the cause of hypercalcemia were vitamin D intoxication?

(A) Elevated PTH and Ca/CC >0.02
(B) Normal PTH and Ca/CC >0.02
(C) Low PTH and Ca/CC >0.02
(D) Low PTH and Ca/CC <0.01
(E) Normal PTH and Ca/CC <0.01

13 After diagnosing primary hyperparathyroidism, you find that the condition has occurred in other family members. You wish to seek further the possibility of coexistence of each of the following diseases except for (which) one?

(A) Colonic adenomatous polyps
(B) Pheochromocytoma
(C) Parathyroid adenoma
(D) Facial angiofibromas
(E) Medullary carcinomas

14 Primary adrenal insufficiency, as distinct from secondary disease, is characterized clinically by hyperpigmentation, among other stigmata. Which of the following other endocrinopathies is also associated with hyperpigmentation and also with hyperkalemia?

(A) Thyrotoxicosis
(B) Parathyroid adenoma
(C) Adrenocortical adenoma
(D) Nonpituitary adenoma
(E) Pancreatic adenoma

15 A 35-year-old man has been having bouts of palpitations, pounding heart, and headaches, lasting several minutes. Last evening, he had such an attack during intercourse. He denies flushing during the attacks. During one attack, his wife, a medical assistant, measured his peripheral pulse at 130 beats per minute, but the pulse was easily counted and regular. Looking back, the man feels he has had at least one attack daily for the past 2 weeks. Vital signs are normal, with blood pressure being 115/75 and pulse 78 and regular. Temperature was 97.8°F at 9 AM. The doctor considers first that the patient has had panic attacks as a part of panic disorder. However, feeling that panic disorder should be considered only after ruling out organic causes of the attacks, which of the following would be the most reasonable diagnosis for the doctor to investigate and pursue?

(A) Thyrotoxicosis
(B) Carcinoid syndrome
(C) Pheochromocytoma
(D) Supraventricular tachycardia
(E) Sepsis

Examination Answers

1. The answer is C. Prolonged P-R interval on resting ECG with total calcium level of 12 mg and PTH of 40 ng is virtually certain to be caused by hyperparathyroidism, which is not the same as saying all cases of hyperparathyroidism exhibit this combination of factors and others that follow in this discussion; that is, high specificity does not translate to high sensitivity. The main message here is that any measurable level of PTH in the presence of hypercalcemia signifies that PTH is the driver. Each of the other symptoms listed as well as calcium-containing renal stones and decreased deep tendon reflexes are found in hyperparathyroidism but are not specific. Other findings and symptoms include prolonged Q-T interval and decreased P-R intervals on ECG, pruritus, intellectual fatigue, and depression. It has been said that hyperparathyroidism causes problems with "bones, stones and abdominal groans, psychic moans."

2. The answer is D. Carpopedal spasm. That is, it is *not* a required characteristic by NIH consensus for diagnosis of hyperparathyroidism. Actually, carpopedal spasm is a sequela of hypocalcemia. Hyperparathyroidism causes hypercalcemia. Each of the other characteristics must be present by those criteria: serum calcium >1 mg/dL above normal; urinary Ca >400 mg/dL; abnormally low bone density; age less than 60 years.

3. The answer is D. Anorexia nervosa is characterized by increased urinary cortisol but not elevated serum cortisol. Ingestion of gamma-hydroxybutyrate occurs in its use as a party drug and results in ACTH-dependent reversible Cushing syndrome. In familial cortisol resistance, serum cortisol is elevated, but by definition, relatively ineffective and the resultant errors of metabolism lead to hypergonadism and hypertension. Factitious hypercortisolism is by definition caused by planned deception. In this case, when elevated cortisol level is encountered, it is most likely due to factitious self-treatment with ACTH and can be very difficult to prove.

4. The answer is D. Acute adrenal insufficiency may be precipitated by hypotension, trauma, or hemorrhage. The fact that this is an acutely ill patient, who is a type I diabetic yet manifests hypoglycemia, as opposed to markedly increased insulin requirements, rules against, if not eliminates, sepsis or other infectious causes. Neurologic sequelae from trauma would be unexpected in a person who suffered neither loss of consciousness nor symptoms of concussion.

5. The answer is E. Hypovolemia, normal sodium concentration, normal serum potassium, and normal skin color, in association with abnormally low levels of cortisol, are all signs of adrenal insufficiency that is due to pituitary failure as opposed to primary adrenal insufficiency. In primary disease, ACTH is elevated, and increased skin pigmentation is an indirect result of this. Also, in primary adrenal insufficiency, most often as a result of destructive processes in the physical site of the adrenal glands, the zona glomerulosa is destroyed as well so that hyperkalemia, resulting from absence of aldosterone, occurs; this is not so in secondary adrenal insufficiency. Peripheral blood cell changes, neutropenia, relative eosinophilia, and lymphocytosis occur in primary or secondary adrenal insufficiency.

6. The answer is C. Hyrocortisone 24 mg daily, given as 16 mg in the morning and 8 mg in the afternoon, plus fludrocortisone 0.3 mg daily. Important points to remember are (a) that the glucocorticoid should be given as two-thirds of the replacement dosage in the morning with the remainder in the afternoon and (b) that many patients with primary adrenal insufficiency require replacement of the mineralocorticoid as well. In this example, fludrocortisone replaces aldosterone. The dexamethasone replacement dosage is 0.75 mg daily in divided doses, with two-thirds in the morning and one-third in the afternoon. However, as the most pure synthetic product among those presented, it has the least mineralocorticoid activity. Thus, nearly always there must be mineralocorticoid replacement, if dexamethasone is used to treat primary adrenal insufficiency. If prednisone is used for glucocorticoid replacement, then the dosage is 5 mg, but also in divided doses (two-thirds and one-third). From the foregoing, it is easily inferred that prednisone is five times as potent, milligram for milligram, as hydrocortisone and that dexamethasone has 33 times the potency of hydrocortisone.

7. The answer is C. Hydrocortisone in replacement dosages not only repletes the serum cortisol that tends to be insufficient but, through negative feedback, suppresses ACTH, removing the stimulus driving the aberrant pathway. About 50% of cases lack also minealocorticoid (salt wasting) and bear treatment with fludrocortisone. Little is known about that polyuria and polydipsia may accompany this disease. Three other types, all rare, manifest elevated 17-hydroxypregnenolone (3-beta-hydroxy) and decreased 17-alpha-hydroxy steroid (17-hydroxylase deficiency).

8. The answer is B. A low serum potassium may explain the combination of hypertension and weakness as being caused by primary aldosteronism. Certainly, serum potassium level is mandatory before inaugurating therapy for hypertension. If one suspects primary hyperaldosteronism in a patient on antihypertensive medication, the drugs must be withheld for 2 weeks before serum potassium measurement can be reliable.

9. The answer is D. Cushing syndrome is associated with and precipitates, if not causes, both hypertension and diabetes type 2. The purple striae are not specific for Cushing syndrome, as they are associated with recent and rapid development of obesity. However, Cushing syndrome brings with it not only recent and rapid obesity but also the protein catabolic aspects of the syndrome, and attendant weakening of protein structures allows a significantly lower threshold for development of the striae. The same may be said for the facial plethora but to a lesser degree. The metabolic syndrome is also associated with hypertension and diabetes type 2, but the purple striae and rubor are a virtual stigma of Cushing syndrome when seen with hypertension and diabetes. On occasion, in a primary care setting, a physician may encounter seemingly mysterious supraclavicular fat pads in a patient seen for unrelated reasons. In such cases, one needs to be mindful of the possibility of Cushing syndrome. Morbid obesity, weight equal to or exceeding 100 lb (45.3 kg) in excess of the ideal, would not explain proximal muscle wasting.

10. The answer is C. There are several levels of precision and sensitivity in the dexamethasone suppression tests. In Cushing disease, cortisol precursors and their metabolic by-products are responding to excessive production of ACTH by the anterior pituitary. In the overnight dexamethasone suppression test, the baseline plasma cortisol level is measured before administration of 1 mg of dexamethasone and should be suppressed to less than 50% of that value on the next morning. In addition, baseline ACTH is measured and expected to be similarly suppressed, and the same with 24-hour urine 17-hydroxycorticosteroids. Another version of the overnight dexamethasone suppression test employs administration of 1 mg of dexamethasone orally at 11 AM and the collection of serum cortisol on the following morning at 8 AM. A morning cortisol level of <5 μg/dL by fluorometric assay or of <2 μg/dL by high-performance liquid chromatography is 98% specific to rule out Cushing syndrome. Thus, cortisol was suppressible. This would not apply to Cushing disease caused by exogenous hydrocortisone (medication). Thus, Choice A, serum cortisol, is part (but only part) of the test. None of the other choices is relevant to this case.

11. The answer is E. Primary hyperparathyroidism is the most common cause of hypercalcemia in ambulatory patients. However, there are numerous causes of elevated serum calcium, and they include not only the other choices given here but also several more. Sarcoidosis would be more likely in a person of black African descent. Carcinoma of the breast is associated with extreme hypercalcemia in late, virtually always metastatic, disease, and can be life-threatening. Malignancy is the most frequent cause of hypercalcemia in hospitalized patients. Both hypervitaminoses D and A are causes of hypercalcemia. In addition to the foregoing, other causes and concurrent conditions include prolonged immobility (especially in a patient with Paget disease of the bone), thiazide diuretics, severe thyrotoxicosis, aluminum toxicity (usually with renal dialysis), and, for reasons not understood, Addison disease.

12. The answer is D. Low PTH and Ca/CC <0.01 would be found in vitamin D intoxication. Elevated PTH and Ca/CC >0.02 are what one would find in primary hyperparathyroidism. Even with a normal PTH level, a Ca/CC of >0.02 constitutes strong evidence for primary hyperparathyroidism. Low PTH levels are generally secondary, through the feedback mechanism, to other causes of hypercalcemia. Normal PTH and Ca/CC <0.01 is the normal state.

13. The answer is A. Colonic adenomatous polyps are not associated with hyperparathyroidism. Each of the others is among the conditions associated with hyperparathyroidism in the multiple endocrine neoplasia (MEN) syndromes, types I and II (MEN I and MEN II, respectively). Besides hyperparathyroidism, MEN I has the strongest associations with facial angiofibromas and collagenomas, pancreatic and pituitary adenomas, and, to a lesser extent, adrenocortical adenomas and subcutaneous lipomas. In MEN II, medullary carcinoma is associated with hyperparathyroidism and pheochromocytoma in 20% to 50% of the cases and 20% to 35% of the cases, respectively. Hyperparathyroidism is not a part of MEN III, which is a cluster, more or less, of mucosal and gastrointestinal ganglioneuromas, medullary carcinomas, and pheochromocytomas.

14. The answer is D. Nonpituitary ACTH-producing adenomas, the most prominent example of which is from a small-cell lung carcinoma, may produce ACTH at quantities that dwarf the average pituitary adenoma. In those situations, melanocyte-stimulating hormone may be activated and hyperpigmentation ensues.

15. The answer is C. Pheochromocytoma, although uncommon, best fits the clinical picture presented. Although all other diagnoses listed may be considered to some degree and would in reality be ruled out, their likelihoods would be small. Carcinoid syndrome is the second in consideration because it causes cataclysmic bouts, not unlike pheochromocytoma, and is generally tested for at the same time as pheochromocytoma. This patient did not exhibit hypertension in the office, if pheochromocytoma were caused by epinephrine production, he could have normal blood pressures between attacks. Carcinoid is famous for causing flushing during attacks but not hypertension. Thyrotoxicosis rarely occurs without sinus tachycardia or atrial fibrillation, as the former is steady, not paroxysmal; the latter perhaps occurs in bouts. For that matter, any type of supraventricular tachycardia is unlikely, given the regular rhythm found at home by the spouse. Sepsis would be unlikely, given the basically well state in which the patient presented to office the morning after an attack.

References

Family Medicine Review. Kansas City, Missouri; May 3–10; 2009.

Fitzpatrick PA. Endocrinology. In: Tierney LM, McPhee SJ, Papadaki MA, eds. *Medical Diagnosis and Treatment*. 45th ed. Lange; 2006.

McPhee SJ, Papadakis MA. *Current Medical Diagnosis and Treatment 2010*, 49th ed. New York/Chicago: McGraw-Hill/Lange; 2010.

Orth DN, Kovacs WJ. The adrenal cortex. In: Wilson, Foster, Kronenberg, et al., eds. *Williams Textbook of Endocrinology*. 9th ed. Philadelphia: WB Saunders; 1998:598–607.

Sandarum V, Falko JM. Triage of problems of the adrenal gland. In: Rudy DR, Kurowski K, eds. *Family Medicine: House Officer Series*. Baltimore: Williams & Wilkins; 1997: 567–576.

chapter 35

Growth and Development

1 A 15-year-old boy is 5 ft 5 1/2 in. in height and complains of short stature. His father's height is 5 ft 9 in. and his mother 5 ft 2 in. The boy's sexual maturity is appropriate in its chronology and appropriate for his age; his upper to lower segment ratio is normal (0.9). Which of the following is the most likely cause?

(A) Constitutional growth delay
(B) Prader–Willi syndrome
(C) Achondroplasia
(D) Hypopituitarism
(E) Familial short stature

2 Each of the following traits is characteristic of Turner syndrome except for which one?

(A) XO genotype
(B) Frequent occurrence of web neck
(C) Lower than normal IQ
(D) Risk of bicuspid aortic valve
(E) Wide set nipples

3 You are approached by the parents of a 15-year-old boy who is concerned that he is not as sexually developed as his class peers. Upon inspection, you see that pubic hair is only lightly pigmented and elongating but not curly. The penis is only slightly enlarged as compared with that expected in the preadolescent state. Which of the following should be your next disposition?

(A) Order serum follicle-stimulating hormone (FSH) level test
(B) Order serum luteinizing hormone (LH) level test
(C) Order x-rays for bone age
(D) Reassure the parents that the boy's level of sexual maturation is within normal limits
(E) Start the boy on testosterone at a dosage of 50 mg daily

4 You are treating a 5-year-old girl introduced for growth hormone deficiency with growth hormone injections 6 times a week. She has no other complaints and feels well. Her physical examination remains normal except for her small size. When reassessing her 1 year later, you find that her growth remains poor. Besides checking for compliance and rechecking her bone age, which of the following would you recommend?

(A) Stop growth hormone treatment, as this must be constitutional growth delay
(B) Check the serum cortisol level
(C) Perform the dexamethasone suppression test
(D) Repeat the karyotype testing
(E) Check TSH, T_3, and FT_4

5 Given that the pubertal maturation scale before puberty is defined as stage I, on the Tanner scale, in which stage is a female who manifests breast bud development, as opposed to enlargement of the breasts?

(A) Tanner I
(B) Tanner II
(C) Tanner III
(D) Tanner IV
(E) Tanner V

6 At which Tanner stage is a male who has penile enlargement and pubic hair limited to the area immediately surrounding the base of the penis?

(A) Tanner I
(B) Tanner II
(C) Tanner III
(D) Tanner IV
(E) Tanner V

7 You are examining an obese 16-year-old girl who has never had a period and is at Tanner I on examination. She has no complaints. She is 2 standard deviation (SD) below mean height for her age. A TSH test is normal. A urine pregnancy test is negative. Her bone age is appropriate for her short stature. Her dehydroepiandrosterone sulfate level is appropriate for her age. Her FSH and LH levels are elevated. Among the options presented, which of the following accounts for her condition?

(A) Prader–Willi syndrome
(B) Prolactinoma
(C) Gonadal failure
(D) Constitutional delay
(E) Dramatic recent weight loss (≥20% of body weight)

8 Regarding the patient featured in Question 7, there are other possible causes not mentioned among the choices given. Each of the following is an additional possible etiology for the disorder of the patient described in Question 6, except for which one?

(A) Polycystic ovary syndrome (PCOS)
(B) Over 3,000 rads of radiation to the ovaries
(C) Autoimmune gonadal failure
(D) Alkylating agent chemotherapy
(E) Turner syndrome

9 During your examination of a 19-month-old female infant, you note unilateral breast bud development in the right breast. The child has otherwise been well and is on no medications. The vaginal mucosa appears as expected at 19 months. She remains at about the 50th percentile for both height and weight. Which of the following do you recommend?

(A) Reassure the parents
(B) Order a right breast ultrasound
(C) Order a bilateral mammogram
(D) Suggest a breast surgeon consultation for surgical excision of lesion
(E) Check estradiol, FSH, and LH levels

10 You are evaluating a 14-year-old girl who is manifesting virilization. She otherwise has no complaints and has not been ill. She used to take an albuterol inhaler but has not needed that in the past 2 years. She has clitoral enlargement and facial hair, but motor and sensory examination, including deep tendon reflexes, are normal. Visual fields are intact to gross confrontation. You appreciate no masses on abdominal examination. Which of the following would be part of your *initial* work-up?

(A) Serum testosterone level
(B) Serum progesterone level
(C) Karyotype testing
(D) Serum estrogen (total) level
(E) A magnetic resonance imaging of the pituitary gland

11 A 25-year-old man and his 23-year-old wife express their concern regarding failure to achieve pregnancy after 2 years of marriage and monthly attempts at conception. An initial screening sperm count shows significant azospermia. The husband possesses an elongated lower body segment but otherwise is of normal weight for height. His education level was high school. His testicles measure 3 cm and 3.5 cm, respectively. Otherwise, secondary sex characteristics are normal except for a suggestion of gynecomastia. His past development was normal in regard to secondary sex characteristics and the timing of their onset. LH and FSH levels are within normal limits. Which of the following is the most likely diagnosis?

(A) Kallmann syndrome
(B) Prader–Willi syndrome
(C) Klinefelter syndrome
(D) Laurence–Moon syndrome
(E) Bardet–Biedl syndrome

12 A phenotypical male newborn shows no testicles in the scrotum. Which of the following should be the most timely action to be taken in the newborn period in regard to this finding?

(A) Consult a surgeon for possible orchiopexy
(B) Consult a surgeon for orchiectomy
(C) Observation for likely descent of the testicles within the first 3 months
(D) Ascertain the presence of testes in the abdomen
(E) Early institution of hormonal therapy to bring about descent of testes

13 Which of the following statements is correct regarding the prognosis of undescended testicles if they had been brought into the scrotum within the first year?

(A) Fertility can be expected to revert to normal when the child comes of age if correction is made by time the child reaches the age of 1 year.
(B) Potential for malignancy in an undescended testicle reverts to normal after medical or surgical correction if accomplished by the time the child reaches the age of 1 year.
(C) Neither fertility nor potential for malignancy can be expected to be comparable with those in males without the affliction, even if the condition is corrected by the time the child reaches the age of 1 year.
(D) Both fertility and potential for malignancy will revert to normal after correction if it is made by the time the child reaches the age of 1 year.
(E) Surgical or medical correction of cryptorchidism serves only a cosmetic function, as it has no effect on the long-term course of the individual who suffered from the condition.

14 The parents of a 7-year-old boy bring him to you for evaluation. They have noted bilateral breast development. There is no history of exogenous estrogen use. His vital signs are normal, including a regular heart rhythm at a rate of 88. He has otherwise been well and is on no mediations. There is no history of ambiguous genitalia at birth. On examination, the testes are approximately 1 cm each bilaterally. The penis is small. Breast tissue is palpable bilaterally with discernible areola development. There are no abdominal masses. The boy is 40th percentile for height and weight. Which of the following do you recommend?

(A) Reassure parents that it is just benign gynecomastia and is probably transient
(B) Begin treatment with testosterone enanthate 50 mg IU each month
(C) Begin search for estrogen-secreting tumor
(D) Obtain surgical consultation for excisional biopsy of breast masses
(E) Review the family history for similar occurrences

15 An 8 1/2-year-old boy has deepening voice and early growth of facial hair. His testicles measure 2.8 cm bilaterally. Bone age is advanced for his height and chronological age. FSH and LH are in the pubertal range that is, above the low prepubertal levels. True sexual precocity is diagnosed. Which of the following medications would be appropriate for treatment of this condition

(A) Gonadotropin-releasing hormone (GnRH) agonist
(B) Human chorionic gonadotropin
(C) Cyproterone acetate
(D) Medroxyprogesterone acetate
(E) Spironolactone

Examination Answers

1. The answer is E. Familial short stature is most likely cause of the boy's height unsatisfactory as it may be to him. The issue is whether his height falls within about 1 SD from the midparental height (MPH) or about at 25% of the distance from the 3rd percentile on the standard pediatric height chart to the MPH [from tables such as 32–2 from *Current Medical Diagnosis and Treatment Pediatrics*, 19th edition, 2009]. The MPH is calculated by adding 13 cm (5 in.) to the mother's height for boys (subtracting 5 in. from the father for girls) and averaging the result with the father's height – in this case, the MPH is 5 ft 8 in. and 1 SD below the MPH would be 3.3 in. below the MPH, encompassing the boy's height. Constitutional growth delay does not fit the case because sexual maturation had been on schedule. By the same token, Prader–Willi syndrome is characterized by hypogonadism as is hypopituitarism. The normal U:L segment ratio rules out achondroplasia.

2. The answer is C. Lower than normal IQ is not a characteristic of Turner syndrome. However, there may be learning difficulties with Turner syndrome patients. Turner syndrome, of course, is defined as the presence of a single sex chromosome, an X, so that patients are phenotypically females and lack of development of secondary sex characteristics. The web neck is common; bicuspid aortic valve occurs at greater than normal frequency, and wide-set nipples are common. Other anomalies include aortic dissection and coarctation of the aorta.

3. The answer is D. Reassure the parents and the boy that the boy's level of sexual maturation is within normal limits. Delayed puberty is defined as the onset of puberty at an age later than the age onset of puberty for the sex type. For boys that is 13.5 ± 4 years. For girls, the mean age ± SD is 13 years ± 7. Thus, although the 15-year-old boy is in an age above average for the time of clear progress in development of puberty, he does not warrant expensive and anxious measures of diagnosis at this time.

4. The answer is E. Thyroid function studies. That hypothyroidism was ruled out before embarkation on growth hormone therapy notwithstanding, growth hormone sometimes induces hypothyroidism, and this is a significant possible etiology of poor growth of patients *on therapy*. Even patients who are growing normally should have thyroid function testing every year. Stopping growth hormone treatment would be self-defeating because the girl's growth rate remains an issue. Cortisol levels would be relevant only if she exhibited signs or symptoms of adrenal insufficiency or excess, as would the dexamethasone suppression test. The karyotype (XO karyotype) was already tested and found to be normal.

5. The answer is B. Tanner II. Sparse pubic hair can also be noticed just on the labia during this stage. Tanner III is best defined as breast enlargement without separation of the contours of the areola and the papilla, in formation of a single mound. Stage IV features contour development, with the nipple being the only projection of the breast but without the full adult pattern (i.e., triangular form). Stage V thus is defined by full pubic hair development.

6. The answer is B. Tanner II. In keeping with the theme that Tanner I is prepubertal, Tanner II is the first identifiable stage of pubertal development. Stages III and IV in the case of males are definable only by degree of testicular, penile, and pubic hair growth (i.e., without clear-cut boundaries). Tanner V in males, as in females, is defined by the full adult pattern of public hair (i.e., for males, spread of the hair onto the thighs). Arbitrary as the Tanner stage definitions may be, they provide the language necessary for communication among physicians when questions of sexual development must be discussed.

7. The answer is C. The increased LH and FSH levels indicate primary ovarian failure; in other words, the fact that gonadotropins were in the stimulatory range, yet the gonads failed to respond, shows that gonadal failure was the basis for the abnormality. Turner syndrome is one likely cause of primary ovarian failure. Weight loss, prolactinoma, and Prader–Willi syndrome can all cause a delay in puberty, but through insufficient hypothalamic release of LH and FSH (and thus low levels are detected). Constitutional growth delay also results in *low* FSH and LH levels (i.e., the cause of delays being a hypothalamic–pituitary cause as opposed to ovarian failure).

8. The answer is A. PCOS is a potential etiology of infertility, but not of ovarian failure. FSH and LH have not failed. Other aspects of PCOS include amenorrhea, androgenization, and insulin resistance, leading to type 2 diabetes. Weight loss is the single best therapy for PCOS. Radiation to the ovaries, autoimmune gonadal failure, alkylating chemotherapy, and Turner syndrome can each account for ovarian failure. Viral infections (such as mumps or coxsackie B virus) also can produce acute gonadal failure.

9. The answer is A. Reassure the parents that this can sometimes be seen at this age and have them contact you if any other secondary sex characteristics develop. This case demonstrates premature thelarche, which is most commonly seen at ages younger than 2 years or older than 6 years. Reassurance alone is required unless there is evidence of pubertal development in other tissues or if growth or bone age is affected. Breast ultrasound mammogram, surgical consultation, and serum estradiol, FSH, or LH level testing are not called for, given the foregoing facts.

10. The answer is A. Serum testosterone. Virilization is likely to be secondary to an androgen-secreting tumor, congenital adrenal hyperplasia, hyperprolactinemia, hypothyroidism, or drugs. It is not produced by an estrogen or progesterone deficiency, and therefore, checking these levels is not appropriate. Checking testosterone, testosterone-binding globulin, and prolactin levels is appropriate. A magnetic resonance imaging would be indicated only if laboratory studies showed hyperprolactinemia or a suspected gonadotropin-dependent disorder. A general rule in endocrinology is to first define the hormonal abnormality before ordering imaging studies.

11. The answer is C. Klinefelter syndrome is the most common cause of male infertility. As a matter of economics, the evaluation of couple infertility should begin with a sperm count on the male partner. Normal secondary sex characteristics and pubertal timing are typical of Klinefelter syndrome. Unlike Turner syndrome, testosterone levels and growth are normal in Klinefelter syndrome patients until about age 14. Klinefelter syndrome is a congenital disorder, classically with an XXY karyotype. Each of the other choices is a form of hypogonadotropic hypogonadism. Kallmann syndrome features delayed puberty, anosmia, and small genitalia. Prader–Willi syndrome is characterized by childhood obesity. Laurence–Moon syndrome manifests hypogonadotropic hypogonadism and spastic paraplegia with developmental delay in virtually all cases. Bardet–Biedl syndrome shows hypogonadotropic hypogonadism, polydactyly, and obesity.

12. The answer is D. Ascertaining the presence of testes in the abdomen is crucial to ruling out the possibility of the newborn being a fully virilized female with potentially fatal salt-losing congenital adrenal hypoplasia as opposed to a case of undescended testicles. This can be effected by measurement of plasma testosterone level after human chorionic gonadotropin stimulation. After that has been accomplished, watchful waiting is justified for as long as 1 year before the commitment to surgery must be made. Fifty percent of cryptorchid testes will descend by the time the child reaches the age of 3 months; 80% will descend by the time the child reaches the age of 1 year.

13. The answer is C. Neither fertility nor potential for malignancy can be expected to be comparable with those in males without the affliction, even if the affliction is corrected by the time the child reaches the age of 1 year. Thus, the abnormalities attendant to cryptorchidism are part of

the cause of the condition; the nondescent is not the cause in itself. In fact, when one side descends within the medically satisfactory time interval of 1 year, even the opposite testicle, normally descended, will exhibit malignant potential, greater than normal, accounting for 25% of malignancies of the testicles in cases of cryptorchidism. Nevertheless, the recommendation is for medical or surgical correction to occur in time for at least partial amelioration of infertility and malignant potential, improved opportunity for close observation over time, and for cosmetic effect.

14. The answer is C. Begin search for an estrogen-secreting tumor. In contrast to boys in puberty, in which over 30% have at least a transient gynecomastia, breast development in males before puberty causes concern about estrogen exposure, from either an estrogen-secreting tumor (adrenal, testicular, or bronchogenic) or exogenous estrogen exposure. Interesting is that fact that hyperthyroidism is sometimes associated with excess estrogen, but not hypothyroidism. Besides the obvious difference in setting between benign transient gynecomastia and an endocrinologically significant condition (pubertal vs. prepubertal), there may be the question of gynecomastia versus enlarged breast in an obese male. In case of obesity, there is neither palpable breast bud nor particular areola development. Thus, reassurance is inappropriate; treatment with testosterone is premature, as is surgical consultation for excisional biopsy. This condition is associated with no identifiable familiality. Thyroid function is not feasibly an issue in this case.

15. The answer is A. Leuprolide, a GnRH agonist, when administered in a steady (as opposed to pulsing) dosage, suppresses the GnRH pulsating release, which is necessary for the physiologic stimulation of FSH and LH. Use of human chorionic gonadotropin has no application in precocious puberty. Cyproterone is a testosterone antagonist, which is appropriate for peripheral precocity (pseudoprecocity). Medroxyprogesterone acetate is the most widely prescribed progestogen, which is not relevant in this case. Spironolactone is, of course, the sole clinically applied aldosterone; it is used in primary and some secondary forms of aldosteronism.

References

Hay WW, Levin MJ, Sondheimer JM, et al., Deterding eds. *Current Diagnosis & Treatment Pediatrics.* New York/Chicago: McGraw-Hill/Lange; 2009.

Schuster DP, Falko JM. Problems of growth and development. In: Rudy DR, Kurowski K, eds. *Family Medicine: House Officer Series.* Baltimore: Williams & Wilkins; 1997:577–590.

Zeitler PS, Travers SH, Barker J, et al. Endocrine disorders. In: Hay WW Jr, Levin MJ, Sondheimer JM, et al. eds. *Current Pediatric Diagnosis and Treatment.* 17th ed. New York: McGraw-Hill; 2003:961–1005.

Allergies

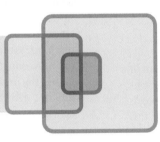

chapter **36**

Atopic, Food, and Contact Allergies

Examination questions: *Unless instructed otherwise, choose the ONE lettered answer or completion that is BEST in each case.*

1 Which of the following is a correct statement regarding montelukast (Singulair)?

(A) The drug is applicable to acute attacks of asthma.

(B) It may be used as monotherapy for the treatment of exercise-induced asthma.

(C) Rescue medication is contraindicated when a patient is on montelukast maintenance.

(D) It is indicated for prevention and maintenance therapy in asthma.

(E) It is indicated in status asthmaticus.

2 Each of the following defines Type I (Immunoglobulin E (IgE)-mediated) allergic response except for which one?

(A) Immune hemolytic anemia

(B) Allergic asthma

(C) Atopic dermatitis

(D) Allergic gastroenteropathy

(E) Anaphylaxis

3 A 30-year-old woman develops wheezing, throat tightness, and urticaria 2 minutes after being stung by a yellowjacket. Her pulse is 104. Her respiratory rate is 30 and her blood pressure is 110/70. She appears to be in significant distress. There is diffuse expiratory wheezing. Which of the following best describes the pathophysiology of her situation?

(A) Circulating antigens reacting with tissue-based antigen, producing inflammatory injury

(B) Deposition of circulating immune complexes into the tissues, where they produce inflammatory injury

(C) IgG response to injected antigen

(D) Mast cell granule release in response to membrane-bound IgE that is cross-linking with a specific allergen

(E) A so-called late-phase reaction produced through inflammation

4 Regarding the patient in Question 3, which of the following therapeutic measures is the best clinical response?

(A) Epinephrine, 1:100, injected subcutaneously

(B) Epinephrine, 1:100, injected intravenously

(C) Diphenhydramine, 50 mg, injected intramuscularly

(D) Epinephrine, 1:1,000, injected intramuscularly

(E) Cromolyn/nedocromil by nasal inhalation

5 Which of the following might be a cause for accidentally increasing the dosage of epinephrine in an emergency situation?

(A) Increased body mass index of the patient
(B) Blood pressure rising to 170/110
(C) Current medications being taken by the patient include propranolol.
(D) Patient has a history of frequent attacks of allergic symptoms.
(E) The patient is Celtic ethnicity

6 Twelve hours after successful epinephrine treatment of anaphylaxis, a 35-year-old woman manifests angioneurotic edema and urticaria. Which of the following is the most reasonable approach for treatment of this development?

(A) Diphenhydramine 25 to 50 mg given orally every 6 hours
(B) Repeated injections of epinephrine
(C) Increase the volume of fluid therapy per unit time by 50%
(D) Theophylline, 0.5 mg/kg/hour, after a loading dose
(E) Beta-adrenergic medication given orally

7 A 35-year-old female patient has begun experiencing hives at various times, usually within 30 minutes after a meal. If you were to actuate a trial of food eliminations, adding back one eliminated food every 5 days until the occurrence of allergic symptoms, which of the following groups of four foods would you choose first, to obtain the earliest conclusion as to cause?

(A) Beef, rice, apples, bananas
(B) Tomatoes, peaches, wheat, potatoes
(C) Peanuts, tree nuts, vertebrate fish, shellfish
(D) Chicken, green beans, peas, corn
(E) Kidney beans, lima beans, lettuce, radishes

8 A white 18-year-old young woman who lives in the Midwest (Ohio Valley; northwest of the Appalachian mountains, east of the Mississippi River) complains of rhinorrhea and sneezing that begins during the months of May and June, peaks at about July 4, and then tapers off in September and October. Which of the following is true regarding this condition?

(A) The condition is precipitated by exposure to *Cladosporium* (previously known as *Hormodendrum*) and *Alternaria* mold spores.

(B) The symptoms are caused by exposure to ragweed pollen.
(C) The peak age for symptoms is between 10 and 15 years.
(D) Females are twice as likely to be affected as males.
(E) Symptoms will respond to antibiotics.

9 A 35-year-old man has been your patient since moving into the area from his lifelong home in California. He comes to you in the first week of September complaining of coryza and occasional wheezing that seems not to evolve through the various stages of a cold. It occurred about this time last year, but it is now more severe; it has lasted more than 2 weeks since its onset in the last half of August. The nasal discharge is thin and watery, without yellowish mucus or mucosanguinous characteristics. He has tried taking the antihistamine loratidine (Claritin), which did not give him significant relief; you prescribed cetirizine (Zyrtec), which also failed to relieve the symptoms. You then suggested over-the-counter diphenhydramine (Benadryl) and chlorpheniramine. These two antihistamines relieved the symptoms but caused intolerable drowsiness. Which of the following is the most practical approach for his acute symptoms, assuming he has no other significant medical problems?

(A) Skin testing to confirm the offending allergen, followed by allergen immunotherapy (desensitization)
(B) Prescription of clarithromycin, 500 mg, XL tablets, twice daily for 7 days
(C) Prescription of prednisone, given orally at a starting dosage of 40 mg daily, reduced every 2 days to taper off over a 2-week period
(D) An increase in the dosage of Benadryl
(E) Counseling the patient to remain indoors in an air-conditioned environment for the duration of the allergy season

10 A patient with medically refractory allergic rhinitis was found to be reactive to ragweed and you plan on initiating desensitization in the coming year. Meanwhile, which of the following foods, if any, would you advise him to avoid while attempting other means to give relief of symptoms?

(A) Peanuts
(B) Shellfish
(C) Vertebrate fish
(D) Chocolate
(E) Bananas

11 From the physiological point of view, which of the following is the goal of immunotherapy in the treatment of atopic allergies, for example, rhinitis and conjunctivitis, in regard to allergen-specific antibodies?

(A) Increase IgE antibodies specific to the allergen
(B) Decrease IgG antibodies specific to the allergen
(C) Increase in IgE, decrease in IgG
(D) Increase in IgG, decrease in IgE
(E) Decrease in both IgG and IgE

12 A 34-year-old man has noticed increasing incidents of being stung by bees and increasingly severe reactions from the stings. Instead of normal erythema and swelling, when he was stung 2 weeks ago on the ankle, the whole leg became swollen with an angry redness. At that time, he went to another doctor, who diagnosed cellulitis and treated with antibiotics. Then, today he was stung on the arm with rapid development of the same type of response as last week, and this time, he is experiencing hives and having some shortness of breath. The sting occurred an hour ago. He appears to be in mild distress with the dyspnea and discomfort at the sting site. Auscultation of the lungs reveals bilateral wheezes with adequate respiratory excursion. You opt for an intramuscular injection of 1:1,000 epinephrine, and the patient's dyspnea responds rapidly. Which of the following is the best long-term management plan for this patient?

(A) Prescribe 5 years of specific venom immunotherapy
(B) Prescribe epinephrine unit-dose syringes (EpiPen Auto-Injector) for use immediately after he is stung
(C) Prescribe prednisone in 2-week tapering dosages for initiation whenever he is stung
(D) Prescribe 8 mg chlorpheniramine given orally whenever he is stung
(E) Prescribe cromolyn for inhalation at the time of a bee sting
(F) Prescribe diphenhydramine, 50 mg, for oral use immediately upon being stung

13 A 12-year-old boy has been followed for asthma for the past 2 years. Until recently, he has been satisfied with self-treatment with albuterol inhalations once or twice per week, and they are needed once or twice per month at night. However, in the past 2 weeks, he has required albuterol 3 or 4 times per week. His forced expiratory volume in 1 second (FEV_1) is measured at 85% of normal. Which of the following would be an accepted therapeutic adjustment to this development?

(A) Increase albuterol inhalations to every 6 hours as needed
(B) Start oral albuterol at a dosage of 8 mg every 12 hours
(C) Start inhaled glucocorticoids
(D) Start both inhaled cromolyn and inhaled glucocorticoids
(E) Start long-acting beta-2 agonist, inhaled glucosteroids, and oral glucosteroids

14 A teenaged boy with asthma has begun to require albuterol daily and once or twice weekly in the night. His FEV_1 and PEF have fallen to 65% of predicted levels. In addition, the variability of the PEF ranges from 20% to 30% of predictability. What should be the next therapeutic regimen?

(A) Perform skin testing and prepare for immunotherapy
(B) Start oral albuterol at a dosage of 8 mg every 12 hours
(C) Start inhaled glucocorticoids
(D) Start both inhaled glucocorticoids and a long-acting beta-2 agonist
(E) Start a long-acting beta-2 agonist, inhaled glucosteroids, and oral glucosteroids

15 Considering infectious precipitants, which of the following organisms is thought to be most often implicated in the initiation of an asthmatic diathesis?

(A) Adenoviruses
(B) Herpes viruses
(C) Arboviruses
(D) Respiratory syncytial virus
(E) *Streptococcus pneumoniae*

16 A 17-year-old with a long-standing history of asthma (since age 5) has been on short-acting beta-agonist inhalers or cromolyn inhalers (step 2) with fair daytime symptom control, but he is now awakening almost every night with attacks of wheezing and dyspnea. The PEF is 75% of the predicted level. In keeping with recategorizing the stage of asthma, hence the care step, which of the following inhalers has the longest duration of action and thus specifically would be the best choice to control his nocturnal symptoms?

(A) Albuterol
(B) Terbutaline
(C) Pirbuterol
(D) Ipratropium
(E) Salmeterol

Examination Answers

1. The answer is D. Montelukast is indicated for prevention and maintenance therapy in asthma. The drug is *not* applicable to acute attacks of asthma; it should *not* be used as monotherapy for the treatment of exercise-induced asthma because it should not be used in acute attacks (although it is quite conceivable that a person could be subject to exercise-induced asthma while on Montelukast and should be treated accordingly); not only is rescue medication not contraindicated when a patient is on montelukast but should be used if an attack occurs while the patient is on montelukast. The drug is not indicated in status asthmaticus – again because status is acute and montelukast is a maintenance medication.

2. The answer is A. Immune hemolytic anemia is *not* mediated by IgE antibodies. It is a Type II or cytotoxic hypersensitivity reaction mediated through IgG antibody. Each of the other conditions is IgE mediated: allergic asthma, atopic dermatitis (and other atopic manifestations such as rhinitis and food allergies), allergic gastroenteropathy, and anaphylaxis. The last includes manifestations such as hypotension, bronchospasm, gastrointestinal and uterine muscle spasm, urticaria, and angioedema. IgE antibodies are formed immediately after the exposure of a sensitive person to the allergen. Each of these allergic reactions is treatable at the most conservative level by H-1 antihistamines and most aggressively by epinephrine. Type III reactions entail immune complex–mediated reactions including serum sickness. Type IV reactions are T-cell mediated and are delayed, such as contact allergies (e.g., rhus), and the autoimmune diseases lupus erythematosus and glomerulonephritis result in chronic inflammation but not anaphylaxis.

3. The answer is D. Mast cell granule release in response to membrane-bound IgE cross-linking with a specific allergen. This is a classic immediate hypersensitivity (Type I) response. This individual must have had prior exposure to the antigens (but may not recall the first uneventful sting), which previously led to the production of these IgE antibodies on the mast cell surface. The early phase response is characterized by capillary permeability and fluid leakage. It is invoked in allergy skin testing as another example of its applicability. Late-phase responses (not to be confused with delayed hypersensitivity, Type IV) include local invasion by basophiles, eosinophils, monocytes, and lymphocytes. Analogous clinical situations include the rapid onset and recovery (15 to 30 minutes) of bronchospasm in asthmatic exposure to inhaled allergenic antigens. The late response in asthma occurs 3 to 8 hours later and can last up to 24 hours. There are mucosal and conjunctival counterparts to these reactions. The late phase resembles the actual clinical picture in asthma, for example, resulting in air trapping.

4. The answer is D. Epinephrine, 1:1,000, injected intramuscularly, or on occasion intravenously, is the treatment for anaphylaxis. The greatest single error made in the management of acute anaphylaxis is timidity; failure to act in a timely and aggressive manner. Epinephrine, 1:100, injected would be a dangerous overdose and has occurred by accident with fatal consequences. Diphenhydramine, 50 mg, injected intravenously would be too mild a response, given the rapidly developing systemic involvement of the anaphylaxis. Cromolyn–nedocromil by nasal inhalation is a preventive treatment for allergic rhinitis and has no application in anaphylaxis. To combat hypotension, besides the epinephrine, fluid therapy and other vasopressors may be employed, for example, dopamine, norepinephrine and phenylephrine. Specific therapy for persistent bronchospasm should be treated with beta-agonists such as albuterol by inhalation.

5. The answer is C. If the patient with anaphylaxis has been taking the nonselective beta-adrenergic blocking agent, propranolol, the effective dosage of epinephrine for reversing the pathophysiology may well be increased. This occurs, of course, because of the blocking effect on the beta-adrenergic portion of the action of epinephrine. None of the other choices has any bearing on the treatment of anaphylaxis.

6. The answer is A. Late occurrence of anaphylactoid symptoms and signs is frequent after anaphylaxis, due to the late-phase reaction discussed in Question 3, manifestations of which are possible for up to 24 hours and form the basis for the continued monitoring of anaphylaxis patients for that period. If these include angioneurotic edema and urticaria, oral diphenhydramine (Benadryl) is appropriate. If late manifestations involve bronchospasm, a frequent part of the acute syndrome, rescue medication such as albuterol is appropriate. Fluid therapy applies only in the case of hypotension, a development not to be expected during the late-phase reaction.

7. The answer is C. Peanuts, tree nuts, vertebrate fish, and shellfish account for 90% of all food allergies. An elimination diet is a practical technique available in primary care. Additional foods that are often involved in food allergy situations include beer, chocolate, tomatoes, and egg (albumen). In practice, it may be helpful to include all eight of the foregoing groups in an elimination diet. Foods are added back individually with 2 days between each addition. When the urticaria or angioneurotic edema reappears, the most recently added food item is assumed to be at least one of the causes of the symptoms. That food can then be avoided. Food allergies in many cases appear for a certain epoch of a patient's life, followed by remission. The period of the most intense symptoms, in some cases, may seem to coincide with life stressors, such as crises in a marriage or child rearing.

8. The answer is A. The condition is precipitated by exposure to mold spores, that is, *Cladosporium* and *Alternaria* organisms, in a person sensitive specifically to the antigens. These are the second and third most intense and prevalent pollen allergens in the United States, generally confined to the eastern half of the country. Ragweed, the most prevalent and severe offending allergen, has a season that begins on approximately August 15 at the 40th parallel, occurring earlier as one moves north (the allergy season is timed with the drying ripened flower). The peak age group for allergic rhinitis is between 15 and 25 years. There is no particular difference in the prevalence of allergic rhinitis between the sexes.

9. The answer is C. Prednisone, given orally at 40 mg daily, with the dosage reduced every 2 days to taper off over a 2-week period, is a regimen justified in cases such as the one presented, which is typical for allergic rhinitis that is due to a ragweed allergy in the eastern half of the United States. Skin testing and desensitization will not be able to address and relieve symptoms in the year in which the program is initiated. However, the need to employ glucocorticoids in a given season for the relief of severe, otherwise nonresponsive symptoms should be the trigger to initiate skin testing, as systemic glucocorticoids should not be prescribed lightly. The patient had no symptoms of sinusitis or of any other bacterial infection; thus, clarithromycin is not indicated and any other antibiotic would not be justified. Benadryl was already shown to cause drowsiness at a therapeutic dosage, and increasing the dosage would only be expected to worsen the drowsiness. Avoidance may be effective in cases of animal dander allergy but is not practical for the management of pollen allergy.

10. The answer is E. Bananas and also melons cross-react with ragweed and therefore should be avoided during the season of allergic symptoms (mid-August until the temperature drops below 40°F). Other cross-reacting foods include apples and carrots with birch pollen. These foods may increase the symptoms of rhinitis. The other foods presented as choices are prominent classic food allergens. Symptoms of classic food allergies are more likely to be angioneurotic edema or urticaria, rather than coryza.

11. The answer is D. An increase in IgG and decrease in IgE antibodies specific to ragweed, in this case. The immediately reacting IgE is the offending antibody. Successful immunotherapy (desensitization) leads to a transient slight rise in IgE followed by a fall to much lower levels than beforehand and a rise in the blocking antibody IgG. (Remember: the "G" in IgG is "good," applying to immunity to both allergens and infections in virtually all disease states to which it is relevant.)

12. The answer is A. Five years of specific venom immunotherapy. This program is 98% effective in preventing systemic reactions to specific stinging insects, such as honey bees, wasps, hornets, yellow jackets, and immigrant fire ants. Epinephrine unit-dose syringe injections are necessary for the acute reaction after the sting but should not comprise the long-term management. Prednisone (or other oral glucocorticoids) is not suited to acute-phase (IgE) reactions and is not suited to long-term prevention. Both antihistamines chlorpheniramine and diphenhydramine are inadequate for acute treatment and have no place in prevention. Cromolyn by inhalation is a preventative, specific for reactive airway disease, which must be taken thrice daily for effect but, unlike immunotherapy, does not have preventive effects for longer than the term of administration.

13. The answer is C. Start inhaled glucocorticoids (or inhaled cromolyn). The patient has progressed from the mild, intermittent stage (symptoms requiring use of a beta-2 agonist inhaler no more than twice weekly and no more than twice in the night monthly), which could be called stage 1. When he began having symptoms more than twice weekly (but not as frequently as daily), he entered the stage called mild persistent, or stage 2. In the first two stages described, the FEV_1 and the PEF should be greater than 80% of those predicted for age. The foregoing and the complete spectrum of the staging of asthma are based on guidelines published by the National Asthma Education and Prevention Program (NAEPP).

14. The answer is D. Start both inhaled glucocorticoids and a long-acting beta-2 agonist (e.g., salmeterol or formoterol). The inhaled glucocorticoids, dosed mildly in the second step of therapy, are prescribed as a medium-dosed product at step 3 and a high-dosed product at step 4. The patient has entered the third stage of asthma, which is moderate persistent asthma. It is defined as symptoms that occur daily and more than once per week at night. Either the FEV_1 or the PEF is between 60% and 80% of the predicted values. Stage 4 is defined as continuous symptoms and limited physical activity caused by asthma. Because long-acting beta-2 agonists and inhaled steroids are not rapidly acting, they must still be supplemented with rapid-acting medications such as albuterol. As stated previously, albuterol alone is not adequate in persistent asthma. Immunotherapy would have no application for treating symptoms in the present or near future. Albuterol alone is not appropriate as a stable plan, as was pointed out in the definition of stage 2 asthma. Long-acting beta-2 agonists, inhaled high-dose glucosteroids, and oral glu- costeroids, all three, would be appropriate in stage 4 dis- ease (i.e., as step 4 therapy). Below is a table outlining the stages of asthma, modified slightly from the scheme of NAEPP, Expert Panel Number 2, in the NIH Publication No. 97–4951.

TABLE 36–1   Stages of Asthma Modified from NAEPP Expert Panel No. 2 NIH Publication 97-4951

Stage	Symptoms	Night Symptoms	Lung Function
1. Mild	≤2×/wk	≤2×/mo	FEV_1 or PEF intermittent none; normal PEF ≥80%; PEF between bouts var <20%
2. Mild	>2×/wk <1 daily	>2×/mo	FEV_1 or PEF persistent ≥80 PEF var 20%–30%
3. Moderate persistent	Daily short beta-2 Ag Activity affected Attacks ≥2×/wk May last for days	>1×/wk	FEV_1 or PEF >60%, <80% PEF var >30%
4. Severe persistent	Contin symptoms Limited physical activity	Frequent	FEV_1 or PEF <60% PEF var >30%

Source: The table is modified slightly from the scheme shown by the National Asthma Education and Prevention Program (1997).
var, variability; *beta-2 Ag,* beta-2 agonist.

15. The answer is D. Respiratory syncytial virus. Up to 50% of children with bronchiolitis caused by respiratory syncytial virus will have recurrent wheezing until they reach the age of 3 years, although most children with this combination of circumstances have atopic constitutions and family histories of similar problems. Bacteria are less likely than viruses to provoke asthma. In the case of *S. pneumoniae,* the organism is the most likely bacterium to complicate symptomatic lower respiratory tract infec- tions, especially those that are community acquired, and sometimes asthma, but it is not an initiator of reactive air- way disease. However, the 50% rate of such sequelae to respiratory syncytial virus is far above the expected rate in the population.

16. The answer is E. Salmeterol, a long-acting beta-2 agonist. The patient has moved to the moderate persistent stage or, one could say, stage 3. The effects of salmeterol may last up to 30 hours and salmeterol is many times stronger than albuterol as a beta-2 agonist. Terbutaline and pirbuterol are beta-2 agonists that are intermediate in their duration of activity. Anticholinergic medications (e.g., ipratropium) are rather short in length of activity (4 to 6 hours). The following is a table outlining step care that corresponds to the four stages of asthma.

TABLE 36–2   Therapeutic Modalities for Steps Analogous to the Stages of Asthma

Step	Long-Term Control	Quick Relief
1	None	Short beta-2 Ag
2	Daily inh Ster LD	≤2×/wk ≥beta-2 Ag/day signifies or cromolyn or nedocromil move to step 3
3	Daily MD inh Ster, long beta-2 Ag or both	See step 2
4	Same as step 3 + PO Ster	See step 2

beta-2 Ag, beta-2 agonist; *inh,* inhaled; *Ster,* (gluco) steroid; *LD* and *MD,* low and medium dose (steroids); *PO,* oral.

References

Boguniewicz M. Allergic disorders. *Chapter in Current Pediatric Diagnosis and Treatment,* 17th ed. McGraw-Hill; 2003.

Family Medicine Review. Kansas City, Missouri; May 3–10; 2009.

McPhee SJ, Papadakis MA. *Current Medical Diagnosis and Treatment 2010,* 49th ed. New York/Chicago: Lange; McGraw-Hill; 2000.

Mengel MB, Schwiebert LP, eds. *Family Medicine Ambulatory Care & Prevention;* 5th ed. New York: Lange; McGraw-Hill; 2009.

Schwer WA. Atopic, food, and contact allergies. In: Rudy DR, Kurowski K, eds. *Family Medicine: House Officer Series.* Baltimore: Williams & Wilkins; 1997:591–604.

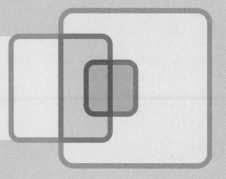

Preventive Health Care

chapter **37**

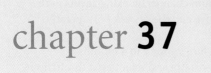

Preoperative Clearance

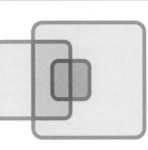

Examination questions: Unless instructed otherwise, choose the ONE lettered answer or completion that is BEST in each case.

1 A 65-year-old male has scheduled elective knee replacement surgery. Fifteen days before the appointed date, he was diagnosed as having stable angina and underwent anterior descending coronary stent placement 1 week before the replacement was to have been performed. There was no evidence of myocardial infarction (MI). The patient is a nonsmoker and his blood pressure is 128/78. When would it be safe to carry on with the knee replacement?

(A) Immediately upon being pronounced as stable post-stent procedure
(B) One week after stent placement
(C) Two weeks after stent placement
(D) Six weeks after stent placement
(E) Three months after stent placement

2 Each of the following operations except for which one confers *at least* a 5% risk of perioperative coronary events?

(A) Surgery involving valvular heart disease
(B) Emergency abdominal exploration for suspected ruptured viscus

(C) Peripheral vascular surgery
(D) Aortic surgery

3 A 45-year-old female patient with a history of smoking is to undergo a thoracotomy to biopsy a coin lesion. The patient denies wheezing and shortness of breath. Which of the following is the bare minimum requirement for preoperative pulmonary evaluation in this patient who will be operated upon under general anesthesia?

(A) Arterial blood gases
(B) Digital oxygen saturation
(C) Standard spirometry
(D) Examination to rule out decreased breath sounds, prolonged expiratory phase, and adventitious sounds
(E) Chest posteroanterior and left lateral x-ray

4 A 58-year-old Caucasian man had an interrupted MI (thrombolysis) 5 years ago and must undergo colon resection for a malignant polyp at stage B by biopsy during colonoscopy. His medications are atenolol, amlodipine, lisinopril, hydrochlorothiazide/triamterene (Hctz/tmp, Dyazide), and clonidine. Which of the following should be held on the day of surgery?

(A) Atenolol
(B) Amlodipine
(C) Clonidine
(D) Lisinopril
(E) Hctz/tmp

5 A 45-year-old male patient is scheduled for elective cholecystectomy and common duct exploration. He has neither history nor finding of hypertension, diabetes, heart disease, or bleeding diathesis, nor any other significant system review. Specifically, he denies and manifests on examination no excessive bruising. He underwent general anesthesia for emergency appendectomy in the past. He is athletic and runs routinely without symptoms of chest pain or undue dyspnea. Which of the following would be the minimally acceptable set of ancillary studies to order for preoperative clearance?

(A) Complete blood cell (CBC) count, prothrombin time (PT), partial thromboplastin time (PTT), electrocardiogram (ECG), routine liver and kidney function blood studies, and chest x-ray
(B) CBC count, PT, PTT, and routine liver and kidney function blood studies (no chest x-ray)
(C) CBC count, PT, PTT, and kidney function studies (neither liver function studies nor chest x-ray)
(D) CBC count, PT, and PTT
(E) No ancillary testing

6 A 55-year-old white man is scheduled for abdominal surgery to resect a segment of colon from which an adenomatous polyp was snared, which revealed at least stage B carcinoma (tumor in muscularis or serosa). All but which one of the following situations significantly increases the risk of a MI or other coronary event during or after surgery?

(A) Angina symptoms limited to strenuous physical activity such as shoveling dirt at a rapid pace
(B) Angina when walking one or two blocks on level ground
(C) History of congestive heart failure (CHF)
(D) Anginal pains with any significant physical activity
(E) Insulin treatment for diabetes

7 A 58-year-old man with a history of angina treated successfully with percutaneous transluminal angioplasty 3 months ago is now asymptomatic. He must undergo a femoropopliteal graft for peripheral vascular disease. For a low-risk patient with known coronary artery disease, the perioperative cardiac mortality risk is 4%. Each of the following preoperative measures can reduce that risk, except for which one?

(A) Alpha$_2$ agonist agents (e.g., clonidine)
(B) Beta-blocking agents (e.g., metoprolol)

(C) Albuterol
(D) Statins (e.g., atorvastatin)
(E) Smoking cessation

8 A 60-year-old woman has been diagnosed with cholelithiasis without evidence of common duct involvement. Although she has had several moderately severe attacks of abdominal pain after meals, currently she is asymptomatic. Elective surgery is indicated, but she has a history of an uncomplicated MI 2 months ago. Which of the following is the best preoperative strategy for maximizing her cardiovascular safety through the period of surgery and the 2-week postoperative period?

(A) Institute preoperative beta-adrenergic blocking agents for 2 weeks before and 30 days after surgery
(B) Start calcium channel blocking agents in the preoperative and the 4-week postoperative periods
(C) Postpone surgery for 2 to 4 months
(D) Start atorvastatin and maintain it throughout the postoperative period
(E) Institute an alpha-adrenergic agonist before surgery and throughout the postoperative period

9 A 56-year-old male patient with cholelithiasis has had two attacks of abdominal pain caused by gallbladder disease. Currently, he has been abdominal symptom free for 2 weeks, but upon system review, he is shown to have a history of anginal pains precipitated by climbing a single flight of stairs and by walking one block. His course had been stable, and he has apparently been in denial of his chest pains until the history was extracted as a part of preoperative clearance for his gallbladder problem. In fact, the anginal pains appear to be precipitated with increasingly less activity. Which of the following is the best strategy for minimizing his perioperative cardiovascular risk?

(A) Institute preoperative beta-adrenergic blocking agents for 2 weeks before and 30 days after
(B) Proceed with evaluation for coronary revascularization
(C) Postpone surgery for 2 months
(D) Start atorvastatin and maintain it throughout the postoperative period
(E) Prescribe nitroglycerin sublingually and a long-acting nitrate for 2 weeks before proceeding with surgery

10 A 67-year-old black female patient has been treated for 3 months for CHF caused by uncontrolled hypertension; her blood pressure readings have been running

180 to 220/100 to 140. She had been in pulmonary edema that responded to after-load reducing agents and loop diuretics. Her blood pressure readings are now under control at 120 to 125/75 to 80 through the use of a combination of angiotensin-converting enzyme inhibitors and a potassium-sparing combination of a thiazide diuretic and triamterene. Now she is to undergo a semi-urgent uterine suspension for stress incontinence. For the past 8 weeks, she has not been dyspneic, and she exhibits no peripheral edema, hepatomegaly, or neck vein distention. Which of the following is true or correct regarding the upcoming surgery?

(A) The patient should undergo her surgery after an aggressive program of loop diuresis.

(B) The patient will be at increased risk for MI.

(C) The patient will be at increased risk of the onset of angina.

(D) The patient will be at increased risk of pulmonary edema.

(E) Because the patient is well compensated, she will be subject to no excess risk.

11 A 55-year-old man must undergo laparotomy to resect a descending colon segment at the site of a malignant polyp discovered at routine colonoscopy. He had a MI 6 months ago, which was diagnosed too late for successful thrombolytic therapy. However, his course has not been complicated by symptoms of CHF, and he has had no chest pains since then during an orderly cardiac rehabilitation program. Because of this history, the patient's preoperative clearance included measurement of the cardiac ejection fraction, whose result was 45%. Which of the following is true or correct regarding the patient's upcoming surgery and postoperative period?

(A) He should be anticoagulated before surgery.

(B) The patient will be at increased risk for MI.

(C) The patient will be at increased risk for the onset of angina.

(D) The patient will be at increased risk of CHF.

(E) Because the patient is well compensated, he will be subject to no excess risk.

12 A 45-year-old man with hypertension must undergo abdominal exploration for an asymptomatic mass that was suggestive of lymphoma. His blood pressure readings, on hydrochlorothiazide/triamterene and lisinopril, have averaged 145 to 150/95 to 98 over the past 7 days. CBC and serum electrolyte levels are within normal limits. Which of the following decisions regarding his preoperative and intraoperative management is correct in light of current thinking?

(A) Continue the current medications, including the dose(s) that is due on the day of surgery, and proceed with the surgery

(B) Delay surgery and add a calcium channel blocking drug; proceed with surgery when the blood pressure is consistently below 140/90

(C) Add a ganglionic blocking drug for 2 days and proceed with surgery

(D) Order an ECG and proceed with surgery if there is no evidence of left ventricular hypertrophy

(E) Consult a cardiologist for preoperative clearance and advice on management of postoperative hypertension

13 If the patient in Question 12 had had a blood pressure of 190/115 without symptoms, which of the following would have been the most acceptable therapeutic approach?

(A) Continue the current medications, including the dose(s) that is due on the day of surgery, and proceed with the surgery

(B) Delay surgery and step up the care of the hypertension, such as adding a calcium channel blocking drug; proceed with surgery when the blood pressure is consistently below 140/90

(C) Order a thallium stress test

14 A 45-year-old man presents with a left upper lobe mass on a chest x-ray, ordered because of bloody mucus production from his previously long-standing cough. The patient has resumed smoking after a period of cessation lasting 3 weeks. Spirometry is repeated because of the passage of a year since this ongoing smoker was cleared for surgery and operated upon. It now shows a forced expiratory volume in one second (FEV_1) of 2.2 L; a Maximal voluntary ventilation (MVV) of 45% of predicted value; and a diffusing capacity in the lungs for carbon monoxide of 45% of predicted value. Because of these findings, a ventilation–perfusion (V/Q) scan is ordered. Which of the following is a criterion that must be met for this patient to qualify for a pulmonary resection without leading to the probability of ventilator dependency?

(A) The contribution of the lobe being considered for resection must not exceed 1,400 mL.

(B) A V/Q mismatch must not be found.

(C) A diagnosis of pneumonia constitutes a permanent contraindication for lobectomy.

(D) The V/Q criterion for resectability depends on the tissue diagnosis of the mass.

(E) V/Q results may be interpreted only in the context of the spirometric findings.

15 A 43-year-old male alcoholic is scheduled for biliary surgery after discovery of an impacted common bile duct stone. Which of the following preoperative parameters is the most significant prognostic indication of his postoperative hepatic status in regard to ascites, encephalopathy, and gastrointestinal bleeding?

(A) Direct-acting bilirubin
(B) Presence or absence of ascites
(C) Level of serum albumin
(D) Preoperative Child–Turcotte–Pugh classification of cirrhosis score

16 A 34-year-old woman is being prepared for hysterectomy, indicated by menometrorrhagia in a woman who is gravida 4, para 4, and desires no more pregnancies. In preparing for surgery, you are aware that her hemoglobin (Hgb) may be decreased as a result of an iron deficiency, which at various periods over the past 3 years has required iron therapy. She has been inconsistent in her compliance with the prescriptions. Which of the following is felt to be the point below which the risk of perioperative complications in otherwise healthy individuals is significantly increased?

(A) 12 g/dL
(B) 10 g/dL
(C) 8 g/dL
(D) 6 g/dL
(E) 4 g/dL

17 A 65-year-old man has been diagnosed with a symptomatic ventricular septal defect (VSD), but surgical correction is indicated because of the emergence of concentric cardiomegaly (diastolic dysfunction). The blood pressure is 140/65. The patient is also diagnosed, in the course of his overall evaluation and the discovery of a bruit over the right carotid artery, as having a 75% right carotid artery stenosis caused by atherosclerosis. While awaiting repair of the septal defect, the patient experiences a 2-minute bout of a visual scotoma involving the right lower quadrant of both fields homonymously. Which of the following is the most logical sequence of actions?

(A) Perform repair of the VSD followed by carotid endarterectomy.
(B) Perform coronary bypass grafting procedure followed by repair of the VSD.
(C) Perform carotid endarterectomy followed by repair of the VSD.
(D) Carotid artery angiography followed by reevaluation before making further decision.
(E) Treat the cardiac hypertrophy aggressively medically followed by carotid endarterectomy when the cardiac status is stable and satisfactory.

18 Which of the following ranks as the most specific and earnest preoperative preparation for an elective abdominal operation on a 55-year-old man who is in chronic renal failure on dialysis?

(A) Preoperative ECG within 24 hours of the operation
(B) Blood urea nitrogen and creatinine levels within 24 hours of the surgery
(C) CBC within 1 week of surgery
(D) Dialysis within 24 hours and electrolytes studies just before surgery

19 A 35-year-old female patient with chronic diarrhea has been diagnosed as having Crohn disease and is being considered for exploratory laparotomy. Considering the recent severe diarrhea, the patient's state of nutrition is a factor in preparing for surgery and planning postoperative care. Below what level of serum albumin, may she be considered to be severely malnourished?

(A) ≤4 g/dL
(B) ≤3.5 g/dL
(C) <2 g/dL
(D) <1.5 g/dL

20 A 63-year-old woman is being scheduled for an operation to relieve partial bowel obstruction that is due to a descending colon carcinoma. Her symptoms consist of alternating constipation (cessation of movements, normally daily) for periods of 2 to 3 days, followed by diarrhea for 1 to 2 days. She says her appetite has waned during the period of these symptoms, approximately 6 weeks. Her weight is 120 lb (54.4 kg) at a height of 5 ft, 6 in. (1.68 m). In evaluating her for the possible need of supplemental feeding, at least orally, before surgery to take place in 1 week, what dietary intake should she be able to ingest (caloric and percentage of protein oral intake), which would be adequate to obviate the need for an oral supplement (e.g., Ensure)?

(A) 35 kcal/kg, of which 20% should be protein
(B) 30 kcal/kg, with 30% protein
(C) 40 kcal/kg, with 80 g of protein
(D) Adequate oral intake as confirmed subjectively by the patient will suffice to ensure that the patient is taking in an adequate amount to carry her through major surgery.
(E) This calculation is not needed as long as the patient's serum albumin and transferrin levels are within normal limits.

21 Prophylactic antibiotics after surgery have become a much more accepted practice over the past 20 years. However, there are guidelines and a theme for this practice. Which of the following *does not* merit prophylactic antibiotic therapy after surgery?

(A) Lymph node biopsy in the neck area
(B) Thoracotomy
(C) Hysterectomy
(D) Biliary surgery
(E) Urinary cystotomy

22 For which of the following preexisting conditions is preoperative antibiotic prophylaxis against bacterial endocarditis recommended?

(A) Patients who have undergone coronary bypass surgery
(B) Patients with cardiac pacemakers
(C) Patients with hypertrophic cardiomyopathy
(D) Patients with previous Kawasaki disease
(E) Patients with implanted defibrillators

Examination Answers

1. The answer is D. Six weeks after stent placement is the conservative safe period for elective surgery after placement of a stent in the absence of evidence of acute MI beforehand. There is approximately a 5% chance of a coronary event occurring within 6 weeks; the first 6 weeks, much higher with 2 weeks (one study found a 32% mortality rate within 2 weeks). Three months is the minimum recommended period of delay after a proven MI.

2. The answer is E. Breast surgery in general is categorized as low risk. The remaining choices convey risks of 5% or greater for coronary events in the perioperative period. Operations of highest risk are any emergency surgery, especially in patients over 75 years of age; aortic, cardiac valve surgery, and other vascular procedures. Operations conveying intermediate risk (1% to 5%) are carotid endarterectomy, head and neck surgery, intraperitoneal and intrathoracic procedures, and orthopedic procedures. Other operations listed as being of low risk (less than 1% chance of coronary events) are endoscopic procedures, superficial procedures, and cataract surgery. The following is an adaptation of Lee's Revised Cardiac Risk index, with permission from The American Family Physician. It consists of two tables, combining patient-centered risk and procedure-centered risks, using a point system:

Clinical Variable	Points
High-risk surgery	1
(Patient with) coronary artery disease	1
Congestive heart failure	1
History of cerebrovascular disease	1
Insulin treatment for diabetes	1
Preoperative serum creatinine >2.0 mg/dL (180 μ/L)	1

Interpretation of Risk Factors

Risk Class	Points	Risk of Complications (%)
I Very low	0	0.4
II Low	1	0.9
III Moderate	2	6.6
IV High	3+	11.0

3. The answer is D. Examination to rule out decreased breath sounds, prolonged expiratory phase, and adventitious sounds (rales, rhonchi, wheezes) in the absence of symptoms is as good as spirometry or the other functional studies mentioned for discovering factors that might indicate increased risk in surgery. Statistically, 1,000 chest x-rays would be preformed for any one case in which it influences operative preparation or outcome.

4. The answer is E. Hydrochlorothiazide/triamterene (or hydrochlorothiazide by itself) should be held on the day of surgery, likely due to potential electrolyte changes during anesthesia. Beta-blockers (e.g., atenolol) and alpha$_2$ agonists (clonidine) are in certain cases protective against cardiac events in the perioperative phase and should be given on the morning of surgery. Calcium channel blockers (amlodipine) and Ace inhibitors (e.g., lisinopril) also should be given on the day of surgery, based on the fact that they do not interfere with safe anesthesia and surgery and, assuming they were well indicated, need not be foregone.

5. The answer is E. No ancillary testing is recommended for healthy patients under the age of 50, given the complete historical and physical findings given in the vignette. In the first edition of this work, the cutoff age was given as 40 years. To be sure, this presupposes a careful history for cardiovascular health and exercise tolerance and care in exposing liability for hemorrhagic diathesis. Regarding the latter group, a checklist of historical and physical information should include whether there have been unprovoked bruising on the trunk >5 cm in diameter; frequent epistaxis or gingival bleeding; menorrhagia with iron deficiency; hemarthrosis with mild trauma; history of excessive surgical bleeding; family history of abnormal bleeding; or presence of severe kidney or liver disease.

6. The answer is A. Angina symptoms limited to strenuous physical activity, such as shoveling dirt at a *normal* pace, are not considered to be severe and are classified in the Canadian Cardiovascular Society system as level II. Level I is angina that appears with *rapid strenuous* but not with ordinary walking or climbing stairs. Levels I and II pose low risk of intraoperative and postoperative cardiac complications. Levels III and IV pose significant risks and call for noninvasive preoperative testing. Angina when a person is walking one or two blocks on level ground is classified as level III; level IV is characterized as angina with any significant physical activity. CHF uncompensated within 1 year of elective surgery increases the risk of cardiovascular complication significantly, as does the presence of insulin-dependent diabetes.

7. The answer is C. Albuterol. This is, course, a beta$_2$ agonist and could aggravate cardiac stress during anesthesia. On the contrary, beta-adrenergic blocking drugs, for example, atenolol and metoprolol, and clonidine, an alpha$_2$ agonist, have been shown significantly to reduce such perioperative risk. In addition, 45 days of a statin, such as atorvastatin, beginning 2 weeks before surgery has also an effect, a markedly reduced perioperative coronary disease risk status. Smoking cessation not only reduces morbidity and mortality in dozens of ways but also reduces respiratory complications in anesthesia in a relatively short time before surgery.

8. The answer is C. Postpone surgery for 2 months. An MI within 3 to 6 months poses a significant risk of perioperative cardiovascular mortality and morbidity. If the planned surgery is elective, delaying the operation is the correct strategy, rather than instituting risk-reducing agents, effective although they may be.

9. The answer is B. One should proceed with evaluation for coronary revascularization. This is another example of a high-cardiovascular-risk situation in that the patient has class III angina, according to the Canadian Cardiovascular Society system (see discussion of Question 2), that is now accelerating. Although there have been some recently published data that might shed doubt on correcting stable coronary artery disease before elective noncardiac surgery, all agree that patients with clear-cut indications for a revascularization procedure without regard for contemplated surgery must have such a procedure before proceeding with elective surgery. Nitroglycerin and long-acting nitrates have their place in maintaining the patient's stability.

10. The answer is D. The patient will be at increased risk for pulmonary edema but not for other cardiac events. This applies specifically to patients who have a history of CHF but are well.

11. The answer is D. The patient will be at increased risk of CHF on the basis of the preoperative ejection fraction of <50%. Such patients have 4 times the chance of CHF (12% vs. 3%) compared with those patients with ejection fractions >50%.

12. The answer is A. Continue the current medications, including the dose(s) that is due on the day of surgery, and proceed with the surgery. Current thinking and inferences from certain studies suggest that mild to moderate hypertension does not pose a significant cardiac risk in the perioperative period. By the same token, however, it is felt that antihypertensive medications should be continued up to the day of surgery and postoperatively as required for control of the blood pressure.

13. The answer is B. Delay surgery and take more aggressive steps to control the blood pressure, such as adding a calcium channel blocking drug; proceed with surgery when the blood pressure is consistently below 140/90. One should put this or another effective method of lowering the blood pressure into play before allowing the operation to proceed. This is the thinking of experts for repeated blood pressure readings >180/110.

14. The answer is A. The contribution of the lobe being considered for resection must not exceed 1,400 mL. This is based on the fact that the postoperative FEV$_1$ must be at least 800 mL. Thus, as the preoperative FEV$_1$ was 2.2 L, the contribution of the tissues to be resected being greater than 1,400 mL would leave less than 800 mL after the surgery. (One may encounter a more liberal opinion, i.e., that the FEV$_1$ may be as low as 500 mL after surgery.) MI or death is 8% to 30%; after 6 months, such risk falls to 3.5% to 5%.

15. The answer is D. Preoperative Child–Turcotte–Pugh classification score is an indicator for postoperative hepatic status in a patient with lever disease. This score is a combination of graduated scores regarding several manifestations of cirrhosis. Five conditions are listed (below), each of the five with a score from 1 point to 3 points (1 is normal, 2 is moderately abnormal, and 3 is severely abnormal). Thus, normal risk is defined as no more than 1 point in each of the 5 categories (ascites, encephalopathy, bilirubin elevation, serum albumen insufficiency, and elevation of prothrombin international normalized ratio [INR] time), and maximum risk denoted by overscore in the 5 categories of 15. The risk of postoperative hepatic complications is reasonably directly related to the Child–Turcotte–Pugh score. The following table is a representation of the Child–Turcotte–Pugh scoring.

Parameter	Numerical Score		
	1	2	3
Ascites	None	Slight	Moderate to severe
Encephalopathy	None	Slight to moderate	Moderate to severe
Bilirubin (mg/dL)	<2	2–3	>3
Albumin (g/dL)	>3.5	2.8–3.5	<2.8
PT (seconds increased)	1–3	4–6	>6

The table is modified from Friedman (2006); used with permission.

16. The answer is C. Measure of 8 g/dL is the accepted level below which the Hgb should be corrected before elective surgery in those patients with no major risk factors for coronary artery disease or factors of age, nutrition, or alcohol. However, for those with baseline risk factors, risk of coronary disease perioperatively is significantly increased if the Hgb falls below 10 g/dL. In addition, Hgb <10 g/dL is associated with an increased risk of postoperative delirium.

17. The answer is C. Perform carotid endarterectomy followed by VSD repair. The main point to be made is that the carotid stenosis is not only severe enough to indicate a repair but also that the repair became more urgent when the carotid stenosis became symptomatic (ipsilateral quadrantanopia, a variant of amaurosis fugax). Although there is less than a 1% chance of stroke fatality after noncardiac surgery, it occurs in up to 6% of cases after cardiac surgery. Such perioperative stroke carries up to a 22% mortality rate. If both cardiac surgery and carotid endarterectomy are indicated, the first to be performed is a matter of judgment. In the vignette, the carotid procedure became more urgent with the advent of the symptom. The cardiac condition, with concentric hypertrophy, must be repaired as well, but it does not represent decompensation such as would be manifested by systolic dysfunction.

18. The answer is D. Dialysis within 24 hours and electrolytes studies just before surgery. Patients on renal dialysis exhibit a 20% to 30% risk of postoperative hyperkalemia requiring emergency dialysis. Another complication particularly likely in such patients is fluid overload, a condition amenable to timely dialysis. Other problems seen at a rate greater than in patients not on dialysis include pneumonia and bleeding.

19. The answer is C. Measure of <2 g/dL is one of the definitions of severe malnutrition. Others are a recent weight loss of >20 lb (9 kg); transferrin <100 mg/dL; prealbumin <7 mg/dL; and absolute lymphocyte count <1,000 cells/mm³. A serum albumin level <3.5 (>3) g/dL is considered mildly malnourished and a level of ≤3 but >2 is considered moderately malnourished, assuming no special circumstances to account for the measurement as an isolated finding.

20. The answer is A. Measure of 35 kcal/kg, of which 20% should be protein, is the minimum caloric (and per-

centage protein) oral intake criterion that the physician should expect from the patient before ruling out at least oral supplementation given preoperatively.

21. The answer is A. Lymph node biopsy in the neck area is considered a "clean" procedure as long as it does not involve entering the foregut or other part of the gastrointestinal tract. Any procedure that enters the gastrointestinal tract, the urinary tract, the respiratory tract, or biliary tract, or any procedure that involves operating on an inflamed area, requires prophylactic antibiotics.

22. The answer is C. Surprisingly, patients with hypertrophic cardiomyopathy warrant preoperative antibiotic prophylaxis against bacterial endocarditis. *In none of the other conditions is prophylactic antibiotic indicated.* Other indications (not presented as choices here) are not surprising and include the presence of prosthetic cardiac valves, previous bacterial endocarditis, rheumatic and other valvular dysfunction, and the presence of significant congenital cardiac malformations, even if they have been repaired.

References

Adler JS, Goldman L. Preoperative evaluation and perioperative management. In: Tierney LM, McPhee SJ, Papadakis MA, eds. *Current Medical Diagnosis and Treatment.* 45th ed. New York: McGraw-Hill/Appleton & Lange; 2006:35–49.

Friedman LS. Liver, biliary tract and pancreas. In: Tierney LM, McPhee SJ, Papadakis MA, eds. *Current Medical Diagnosis and Treatment.* 45th ed. New York: McGraw-Hill/Appleton & Lange; 2006:649–701.

Vanderhoff BT. Preoperative clearance and preparation. In: Rudy DR, Kurowski K, eds. *Family Medicine: House Officer Series.* Baltimore: Williams & Wilkins; 1997:617–636.

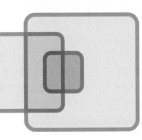

chapter **38**

Obesity and Dyslipidemia

Examination questions: *Unless instructed otherwise, choose the ONE lettered answer or completion that is BEST in each case.*

1 Each of the following is a disadvantage of the weight loss drug Orlistat (xenical) except for which one?

(A) Side effect of diarrhea
(B) Hypoglycemia
(C) Caution when combined with an antidiabetic agent
(D) Cholelithiasis as a side effect
(E) Side effect of reduction of high-density lipoprotein cholesterol (HDL-C)

2 The 3-hydroxy 3-methylglutaryl coenzyme A (HMG-CoA) inhibitors (also called "statins") are extremely useful drugs because they lower low-density lipoprotein cholesterol LDL-C and triglycerides and raise HDL-C as well as inhibit the inflammatory process that plays a role in atherosclerosis. A disadvantage is the risk of the side effect rhabdomyolysis that occurs in susceptible patients in proportion to dosage. In addition to the dosage, each of the following is risk factor for rhabdomyolysis in patients taking statins except for which one?

(A) Diabetes mellitus
(B) Renal insufficiency
(C) Concomitant drugs including amoxicillin
(D) Age
(E) Small frame

3 Regarding rhabdomyolysis associated with statin therapy, the most significant sequela is acute renal failure. Which of the following defines the syndrome in someone known to be taking one of the drugs in the statin family?

(A) Myalgias
(B) The occurrence of renal failure
(C) Elevation of creatine phosphate (CK)
(D) Tenfold elevation of CK levels
(E) Onset of symptoms within 6 months of institution of the medication

4 A 45-year-old man sees you for a "checkup," having not seen a physician since the age of 35. His older brother died recently after a myocardial infarction at the age of 49 and his father died at the age of 55 of heart disease. The patient has smoked for 25 years but quit after the death of his brother. His weight is 165 lb (74.8 kg) at a height of 5 ft, 9 in. (1.75 m). His blood pressure is 135/88. You measure his lipids and find the following: total cholesterol (TC), 240 mg/dL; HDL-C, 37 mg/dL; LDL-C, 155 mg/dL; triglycerides, 300 mg/dL. Which of the following is the best therapeutic plan for this patient?

(A) Advise weight loss to the ideal, 160 lb (72.5 kg), and repeat lipid screen after 2 months
(B) Start a lipid-lowering agent and repeat the lipid screen after 1 month
(C) Start the patient on a low-carbohydrate diet to prevent diabetes
(D) Start the patient on a low-fat diet and repeat the lipid screen in 2 months
(E) Reassure the patient that because he has stopped smoking, he need not be further concerned about his cardiovascular status

5 If drug therapy were chosen for the patient in Question 4, which of the following would be the best selection?

(A) Nicotinic acid
(B) Fibric acid derivative
(C) Metformin
(D) An HMG-CoA inhibitor
(E) Cholestyramine

6 A 23-year-old man weighs 180 lb (81.5 kg) at a height of 5 ft, 10 in. (1.78 m). The patient has no family history of cardiovascular disease, and there is no dyslipidemia in his family's history. He has never smoked. He is concerned about his weight because his mother is significantly overweight and his father is modestly overweight, neither of whom has diabetes or cardiovascular disease. His TC is 240 mg/dL; his HDL-C is 53 mg/dL; his LDL-C is 110 mg/dL;

and his triglyceride level is 130 mg/dL. His blood pressure is 128/78 ± 5/2 mm Hg. What is your best advice regarding this patient's weight?

(A) Reassure the patient that he has no weight-related health problem
(B) Place the patient on a diet consisting of 1,300 calories, with 175 g of carbohydrate, 50 g of fat, and 50 g of protein
(C) Place the patient on a very-low-calorie diet (VLCD)
(D) Start sibutramine for appetite control
(E) You cannot formulate a plan based on the information given.

7 A young mother brings to you her 18-month-old boy who weighs 30 lb (13.6 kg). This is at the 95th percentile for his height and sex. She is concerned because her family has many members who are overweight, and she worries that the child's future health is at risk. Your best advice is which of the following?

(A) She should commit the child to a weight-reduction program forthwith.
(B) The child's weight-related health is not an issue until he reaches adolescence.
(C) The child should be committed to a weight-loss program but not before he reaches the age of 2 years.
(D) A child's obesity-related health issues involve vascular disease, diabetes, and joint health only, and these problems do not begin until adulthood.
(E) Obesity in early childhood is not a health issue.

8 A 50-year-old woman consults you for weight loss. She weighs 200 lb (91 kg) at a height of 66 in. (1.68 m). Her body mass index (BMI) is 31; she is well into the obese range and 48% above the ideal weight. She says she has tried on her own for several years to lose weight but has never consulted a physician, and recently, she was told of the health risks attendant to her status. Which of the following is a workable program *for her*?

(A) Reassure the patient that she is not in a health risk status as a result of her weight
(B) Refer her to Overeaters Anonymous
(C) Place the patient on a VLCD
(D) Start fluoxetine
(E) Enroll the patient in a commercial weight-loss program

9 A 40-year-old mother of a teenaged daughter complains to you that her daughter is significantly obese and that her own parents and two sisters are obese and have diabetes mellitus type 2. She asked you to brief her as to what caveats she might point out to her daughter so as to persuade her to take seriously her obesity as a health risk and to stimulate her to commit herself to a weight-loss program. You answer that each of the following occurs at increased incidence in obese individuals, except which one?

(A) Breast cancer
(B) Uterine cancer
(C) Chronic obstructive pulmonary disease
(D) Osteoarthritis of the knees
(E) Gallstones

10 Regarding the patient in Question 7, what is his calculated BMI?

(A) 22
(B) 24
(C) 34
(D) 44
(E) 55

11 Regarding the patient in Question 7, which of the following is true regarding his status compared with that of nonobese people?

(A) He probably consumes more calories than nonobese individuals.
(B) He has a 30% chance of having a binge-eating disorder.
(C) His rate of energy expenditure is probably the same as that of nonobese individuals.
(D) His rate of physical activity is likely the same as that of nonobese individuals.
(E) He is expected to have a greater likelihood of psychological problems even when not dieting.

12 A 45-year-old man has a family history of diabetes mellitus, is 25% overweight, has a pretreatment blood pressure of 145/92 averaged over three determinations, an LDL-C level of 160 mg/dL, and an HDL-C level of 35 mg/dL. You placed him on aspirin, 81 mg, daily and atorvastatin (Lipitor) eventually at a dosage of 80 mg once daily. His LDL-C has fallen to 130 mg/dL and his HDL-C has risen only to 38 mg/dL. He has not been able to lose weight. Which of the following changes in the treatment regimen is the most logical?

(A) Increase the atorvastatin to 120 mg/dL
(B) Add niacin at an initial dosage of 100 mg daily
(C) Add gemfibrozil (Lopid) at an initial dosage of 600 mg daily
(D) Change to lovastatin (Mevacor) starting at a dosage of 40 mg daily
(E) Change to colestipol (Colestid) starting at 5 mg daily

13 A 45-year-old man weighs 180 lb (81.5 kg) at a height of 5 ft, 11 in. (1.8 m). His TC is 180 mg/dL; his HDL-C is 35 mg/dL and his LDL-C is 105 mg/dL; and his serum triglyceride level is 220 mg/dL. The patient's father died of coronary artery disease at the age of 55 years. Neither the patient nor his father ever smoked cigarettes. He has followed your diet of limited saturated fats, limited cholesterol content, and net calories balance for the past year, and the foregoing lipid profile represents a 10% improvement in the HDL-C and triglycerides. Which of the following pharmacological approaches to his dyslipidemia would be the most effective?

(A) Nicotinic acid
(B) Simvastatin
(C) Gemfibrozil
(D) A bile sequestrant
(E) Atorvastatin

14 Assume a patient is already following a low-fat, low-cholesterol diet. Also, assume this test was done with the patient fasting. Which of the following lipid profiles would be most appropriate for treatment with gemfibrozil?

(A) TC of 200 mg/dL, HDL-C of 40 mg/dL, triglyceride level of 200 mg/dL
(B) TC of 230 mg/dL, HDL-C of 30 mg/dL, triglyceride level of 1,000 mg/dL
(C) TC of 290 mg/dL, HDL-C of 40 mg/dL, triglyceride level of 150 mg/dL
(D) TC of 290 mg/dL, HDL-C of 40 mg/dL, triglyceride level of 280 mg/dL
(E) TC of 320 mg/dL, HDL-C of 50 mg/dL, triglyceride level of 300 mg/dL

15 A 22-year-old woman is 5 ft, 6 in. (1.68 m) in height and weighs 148 lb (67 kg) and is asking you about pharmacologic approaches to weight loss. You calculate her ideal weight to be 130 lb, or 61 kg (100 lb at 60 in. or 5 ft, plus 5 lb/in. for every inch over 5 ft). Which of the following plans best fits her weight status?

(A) Reassure the patient that she is not in a health risk status as a result of her weight
(B) Place the patient on a diet consisting of 1,300 calories, with 175 g of carbohydrate, 50 g of fat, and 50 g of protein
(C) Place the patient on a VLCD
(D) Start fluoxetine
(E) You cannot formulate a plan based on the information given.

16 A 33-year-old man weighs 350 lb (159 kg) at a height of 5 ft, 10 in. (1.78 m). He has lost up to 100 lb (45 kg) on various diets but has always regained his lost weight after 1 to 2 years. He has been morbidly obese since he was 25 years old. He wishes to discuss bariatric surgery (e.g., gastric bypass surgery). You reply that each of the following is true, except for which one?

(A) This patient is more than 110% above ideal weight.
(B) Indications for bariatric surgery include being 100 lb (45 kg) overweight.
(C) Indications for bariatric surgery include a BMI of ≥40.
(D) Indications for bariatric surgery include a BMI of 35 to 40 when associated with sleep apnea.
(E) Indications for bariatric surgery include osteoporosis.

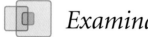

Examination Answers

1. The answer is E. That is, the incorrect statement is that a side effect of xenical (Orlistat) is reduction of HDL-C. This weight loss drug functions by inhibiting lipase, thus rendering exogenous triglycerides unabsorbable. To the extent weight loss is achieved, lipids are improved on average, and thus, HDL-C is increased. As exogenous triglycerides would be less absorbed, diarrhea would be expected to occur; hypoglycemia, as expected, is more likely when the drug is combined with antidiabetic agents. Cholelithiasis may be a side effect of any aggressive weight loss program.

2. The answer is C. Amoxicillin is not listed among those drugs that increase the risk of rhabdomyolysis. However, calcium channel blockers, erythromycin, amiodarone, and niacin do increase the risk of rhabdomyolysis in patients taking HMG-CoA inhibitors. Diabetes, renal insufficiency, age, and small frame are indeed risk factors, the latter perhaps related to the fact that a given dosage is increased per unit weight of the patient in a smaller person.

3. The answer is D. The definition of rhabdomyolysis in a patient who is taking a statin is 10-fold elevation of CK levels. Myalgias may occur, but in the absence of elevation of CK, 10 times normal, the drug need not be discontinued. It occurs in less than 1% of cases. When rhabdomyolysis occurs, it may take place early in the course but usually after the patient has been on the drug for an average of 6 months, but that period does not define the syndrome. It will subside over a course of several days. Acute renal failure occurs due to myoglobinuria. If acted upon promptly, rhabdomyolysis rarely will result in acute renal failure.

4. The answer is B. The patient is within 5 lb (2.27 kg) of his ideal weight (at 69 in. or 1.75 m, ideal weight is 106 + 6 lb for each inch over 5 feet in height = 160 lb, or 72.5 kg). Therefore, even if the patient were very sensitive to the relationship between weight and hypertension, dyslipidemia, and prediabetes (metabolic syndrome), this man cannot be expected to change his vascular risk profile to a significant degree by losing less than 5% of his present weight. Thus, specific methods of weight loss, such as low carbohydrate or low fat, are equally inapplicable at this time, although low-fat maintenance is always advisable. Most authorities have moved to the position of advising pharmacologic therapy for virtually anyone with preexisting heart disease or with strong family history of atherosclerotic vascular disease and present significant risk factors, including a significant recent history of smoking.

5. The answer is D. Of all the agents presented, an HMG-CoA inhibitor ("statin") addresses this patient's profile the best. The patient has abnormally elevated TC and LDL-C levels, and the ratio of TC to HDL-C is 6.5; for men, an acceptable ratio is 4.5 or lower. In addition, his triglyceride level is markedly elevated. Statins reduce TC and LDL-C levels as well as triglyceride levels, and they elevate HDL-C. Metformin is an excellent drug for reducing insulin resistance and, as such, improves lipids in the face of insulin resistance. However, it is not established that this patient has insulin resistance. In any event, metformin's effect is modest compared with that of the statin drugs in this type of case.

6. The answer is A. The only risk factor known to this patient is obesity in his parents. The fact that neither parent has diabetes may mean that both his parents had hip–thigh obesity rather than the central obesity that is associated with the metabolic syndrome. Obesity is defined as a weight 20% above ideal. This patient's weight of 180 lb (81.5 kg) at a height of 70 in. (1.78 m) is calculated as a BMI of 25.8, which is overweight but not obese (top normal limit for men is 24 kg/m^2). Because his lipids are within normal limits for a man (TC to HDLC ratio is 4.5), there is no evidence that his overweight status is in his case a risk factor. Thus, the diet, although well designed for weight loss, is not clinically indicated nor certainly the radical VLCD. Sibutramine (Meridia) is an appetite suppressant and by definition of limited value for long-range control of weight.

7. The answer is C. Obesity in early childhood conveys a risk of obesity in adulthood with all the attendant risks of diabetes, hypertension, dyslipidemia, and vascular disease, as well as osteoarthritis. In addition, there is an association between childhood obesity not only with the adult organic health risks mentioned but also with poor psychological health and decreased economic well-being. For a child to be neurologically equipped for participation in a weight-loss program, he or she must have attained the age of 2 years.

8. The answer is E. Enroll the patient in a commercial weight loss program. The most well-known commercial programs are Weight Watchers, Jenny Craig, and Nutrisystems. This is a good approach for a patient who appears to need social support. Nevertheless, weight regain is common if patients are followed for years after a commercial program was instituted. Nutritional assessment and program modifications can be done by the physician, trained nursing staff, or a dietitian. Patients typically lose 11 to 22 pounds, but attrition is high. Commercial programs tend to be very expensive. Overeaters Anonymous is one of the group self-help programs and is not commercial. They do not appear to achieve as much weight loss, and they exhibit a high attrition rate. Reassurance is inappropriate because the patient is moderately obese. VLCDs and pharmacotherapy such as fluoxetine are not to be applied until these more conservative measures have been tried.

9. The answer is C. Chronic obstructive pulmonary disease. Obesity is associated with an increased incidence of sleep apnea and restrictive lung disease, but not chronic obstructive pulmonary disease. Obesity is a risk for breast cancer and uterine cancer, perhaps based on the storage of estrogens in adipose tissue. Breast and uterine tissues are responsive to circulating estrogen. Osteoarthritis of the knees and hips are in greater incidence in obesity as a result of the increased load bearing required of the joints. Gallstones, especially cholesterol stones, occur in greater incidence in obesity, most likely because of the higher cholesterol levels found in obesity; for uterine cancer, the risk is for unknown reasons.

10. The answer is C. The BMI is 34. BMI is defined as weight in kilograms divided by height in meters squared. This man's BMI is 34, because 240 lb/(2.2 kg/lb) = 109 kg; 70 in. × 2.54 cm = 178 cm, or 1.78 m; and 109 kg/$(1.78 \text{ m})^2$ = 34. A BMI above 24 is considered overweight. Above 27, health problems begin to accumulate in proportion to the degree that the individual is overweight.

11. The answer is B. About 30% of patients with moderate or severe obesity have a binge-eating disorder. Obese people consume more calories than needed for maintenance of a stable body weight, but the amount is typically less than that found in age-, height-, and sex-comparable nonobese controls. (That generalization does not apply to bulimic, non-purging, non-emesis-inducing individuals.) Physical activity and energy expenditure are lower than in nonobese patients, but caloric consumption is not on average higher. Psychological problems associated with obesity are a complicated area to consider. Most adults who succeed in weight-loss programs experience an increase in self-esteem, although relapses are frequent and with relapses, a greater possibility of reversal of self-esteem.

12. The answer is B. Combining niacin with a statin drug may increase HDL-C and certainly adds its effect to lower LDL-C. Atorvastatin is already at the maximum allowable dosage. Addition of gemfibrozil is contraindicated while a statin is in place because of the increased risk of myolysis, a known side effect of the statins. Changing to the bile sequestrant colestipol is a valid option but does not hold any particular promise in the present situation.

13. The answer is C. Gemfibrozil (Lopid) is very effective in raising HDL-C and reducing triglyceride levels. The statins (i.e., here, simvastatin and atorvastatin) are effective in both these areas but not as effective as fibric acid derivatives such as gemfibrozil in raising HDL-C levels. Nicotinic acid is effective in reducing triglycerides but not in raising HDL-C. Bile sequestrants are most effective in reducing TC and LDL-C.

14. The answer is B. TC is 230 mg/dL, which is mildly elevated, but HDL-C is 30, significantly low. The triglyceride level of 1,000 mg/dL is in the monogenic category of dyslipidemia (i.e., Fredrickson type IV), assuming the blood specimen does not show the triglycerides as chylomicrons. Gemfibrozil does raise HDL and has a dramatic effect to lower triglyceride levels. The best candidate would be a patient with only modest TC elevations, but low HDL-C and a marked hypertriglyceridemia.

15. The answer is A. The definition of obesity requires that the patient be 20% overweight. At 148 lb (67 kg), she is 18 lb (5.89 kg) or <14% over ideal body weight, and thus, she is not an appropriate candidate for pharmacotherapy, in particular because she is female. Her weight of 148 lb or 67 kg corresponds to a BMI of 24, which is quite in the acceptable range. As stated earlier, BMI is calculated by the formula of weight in kilograms divided by height in meters squared. By body mass criteria, moderate obesity for women is defined as 30 to 40; severe obesity as ≥40. A diet of 1,300 calories, with 175 g of carbohydrate, 50 g of fat, and 50 g of protein, would be a well-designed modest weight-reduction diet; 1,300 calories meets a guideline for the maintenance needs of a 130-lb (59 kg) woman; 175 g of carbohydrate approximates 55% of total calories, and 50 g of fat provides less than 30% of the total calories. This meets American Heart recommendations and would satisfy the requirements for managing diabetes. A VLCD is defined as 800 calories and is normally reserved for more severe cases, such as morbid obesity (100% above ideal weight). Fluoxetine, likewise, is reserved for severe cases (e.g., ≥40% above ideal weight).

16. The answer is E. Indications for bariatric surgery include being 100 lb (45 kg) overweight; having a BMI ≥40; or having a BMI of 35 to 40 in the presence of sleep apnea, Pickwickian syndrome, obesity-related cardiomyopathy, severe diabetes mellitus, and obesity-induced physical problems that are interfering with lifestyle (e.g., precluding or severely interfering with employment, family function, and ambulation). Osteoporosis is not associated with obesity as being overweight is in fact a protective factor against osteoporosis. Thus, it does not enter into the decision for bariatric surgery.

References

American Society of Bariatric Surgery Web site: www.asbs.org/html/rationale/rationale.html

Family Medicine Review. Kansas City, Missouri; May 3–10; 2009.

McPhee SJ, Papadakis MA. *Current Medical Diagnosis and Treatment 2010*, 49th ed. New York/Chicago: Lange; McGraw-Hill; 2010.

Smith PO, Noble SL, Johnson WG. Obesity and dyslipidemias. In: Rudy DR, Kurowski K, eds. *Family Medicine: House Officer Series*. Baltimore: Williams & Wilkins; 1997:637–648.

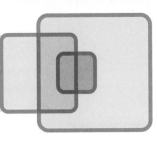

chapter 39

Smoking Cessation

Examination questions: Unless instructed otherwise, choose the ONE lettered answer or completion that is BEST in each case.

1 A 45-year-old two-pack-per-day cigarette smoking woman with diabetes and taking metformin 500 mg twice daily obtained a prescription for varenicline (Chantix) to assist her in smoking cessation. Her dosage was 0.5 mg daily for 3 days followed by 0.5 mg daily for the balance of 1 week; after the first week she followed the instructions to increase dosing to 1 mg twice daily. After a week of the definitive dosing, she requested a visit and complained of a side effect sufficient to cause the drug to be discontinued. Which of the following is the most likely side effect that forced the discontinuation of the prescription?

(A) Hypoglycemia
(B) Uncontrolled diabetes
(C) Nausea
(D) Disturbance in attention span
(E) Anxiety and depression

2 A 35-year-old male worker who was employed for the past 3 years in the field for a company that specializes in asbestos abatement in structures built 60 to 80 years ago is now complaining of dyspnea and cough. He is atopic, subject to allergic rhinitis, and he has smoked cigarettes for 20 pack-years. As smoking is known to increase asbestosis and asbestosis multiplies the risk of lung cancer, which of the following is the least likely cause of the recent onset of dyspnea in this patient?

(A) Asthma
(B) Mesothelioma
(C) Carcinoma of the lung
(D) Chronic bronchitis
(E) Emphysema

3 A 25-year-old woman in her first trimester of pregnancy is seeing you for a prenatal visit. She smokes one pack of cigarettes per day. In advising her to stop smoking, you tell her that her baby will be at increased risk for which of the following, if she continues to smoke?

(A) Preterm birth
(B) Macrosomia
(C) Transient tachypnea of newborn
(D) Spinal cord defects
(E) Neonatal hypoglycemia

4 You are designing a program for your office to encourage patients to stop smoking. Which of the following is correct with respect to physician office efforts to encourage smoking cessation?

(A) It may be assumed that smokers have already been told of the adverse effects of smoking if they have seen other physicians recently.
(B) Smoking in the physician's office should only be allowed in partitioned, ventilated smoking areas.
(C) Counseling to cease smoking should await a time when a detailed, lengthier discussion of smoking cessation can occur.
(D) Smoking should be listed on the problem list of anyone who smokes and on the child's chart of any child in a smoking household.
(E) If the dangers of smoking are pointed out vigorously, cessation can usually be accomplished in one office visit.

5 A family consisting of mother, father, a 1-year-old boy, and a 3.5-year-old girl are under your care. Both parents smoke. The incidence of which of the following childhood diseases is increased in households with smokers present?

(A) Reactive airway disease
(B) Epiglotitis
(C) Sudden infant death syndrome
(D) Lymphatic leukemia
(E) Wilms tumor

6 A 33-year-old man who has smoked a pack per day for 15 years since his first year in college (15 pack-years) has discovered that his uncle who smoked 30 pack-years has been diagnosed with lung cancer. He is seriously considering quitting but asks your advice as to whether it is too late to reduce his risk of lung cancer. Which of the following is the best response to this patient in answer to the question?

(A) It is too late to reduce his risk of lung cancer, as the cumulative maximum smoking volume for reversibility of the odds for lung cancer is 10 pack-years of smoking.

(B) It is too late for practical purposes because one must quit smoking for at least 40 years before the risk of lung cancer is significantly reduced.

(C) Actually, the risk of lung cancer begins to subside significantly at 10 years after cessation of smoking, and the vast majority of lung cancer patients have smoked for more than 20 years before contracting the disease.

(D) One must quit for 20 years and have smoked for fewer than 15 years to benefit from cessation to reduce risk of lung cancer.

(E) If the man stops smoking, he need not fear lung cancer after a period of 5 years.

7 You are counseling a 50-year-old man who has been smoking for 20 years. He has decided to quit smoking. In which of the following situations would he be the best candidate to benefit from a nicotine withdrawal program such as a patch or varenicline (Chantix) to assist in smoking cessation?

(A) He has his first cigarette before breakfast.

(B) He smokes approximately a half-pack, in social situations such as while at clubs or parties, once or twice per week and not at other times.

(C) He smokes for solace or reward, usually at work, but seldom on weekends.

(D) He relapsed after being exposed to a situation that made him want to smoke.

(E) He clearly has a psychological but not a physiological addiction.

8 Which of the following represents a contraindication to the use of a nicotine patch in the previous patient?

(A) He would sometimes note pruritus at the patch site when he tried the patches 5 years ago.

(B) He has a history of hypertension and poorly controlled diabetes mellitus.

(C) He is currently being treated with oral sustained-release buproprion for smoking cessation.

(D) He had some erythema at patch sites when he used the patches 5 years ago.

(E) He suffered a myocardial infarction 2 weeks ago.

9 A 45-year-old man who smokes a pack per day tends to smoke most heavily at his office, where he is a senior architect. His first cigarette of the day is usually midmorning, after he has completed a phase of a design and is ready to present it to colleagues (or after he becomes discouraged and must start again at a different point in a project). On weekends he relaxes by playing golf or fishing at a local river, during which times he seldom smokes more than 10 cigarettes per day. He wishes to quit. Because you consider him not to be addicted, you discuss with him forgoing nicotine replacement therapy in favor of buproprion therapy. Which of the following would constitute a contraindication to bupropion in this patient?

(A) History of symptomatic coronary insufficiency

(B) History of asthma

(C) History of chronic obstructive pulmonary disease

(D) History of seizures

(E) History of peptic ulcer disease

10 A heavily smoking 45-year-old woman stops smoking and starts on the nicotine patches. She is applying a new patch each day. How long must she wait before she reuses a skin site where she had previously applied a patch?

(A) 1 day

(B) 2 days

(C) 3 days

(D) 1 week

(E) 2 weeks

Examination Answers

1. The answer is C. Nausea is the most common side effect of varenicline, and it was reported in 40% of patients over a one-year study. Although disturbance in attention span, anxiety and depression have garnered much attention they arise in only 1% to 2% of patients. The metabolism of metformin is not affected by Chantix; therefore, chances of either hypoglycemia or hyperglycemia are no more likely in this diabetic patient while taking the varenicline than would be the case if she were not taking the drug. Varenicline functions as an acetyl-choline agonist, resulting in decreased urge to smoke during withdrawal.

2. The answer is B. Mesothelioma does not become symptomatic until at least 15 years after the original exposure to asbestos. Each of the other choices could be causes of symptoms and each of which in turn is accelerated in progression if not precipitated outright by smoking, particularly at the duration and intensity of smoking exhibited by the patient depicted.

3. The answer is A. Smoking during pregnancy carries the risk of preterm birth. Smoking during pregnancy is associated with smaller, premature newborns, but not with tachypnea, specific birth defects, hypoglycemia, or macrosomia.

4. The answer is D. Smoking should be listed on the problem list of anyone who smokes and on the child's chart of any child in a smoking household. Surveys may demonstrate to patients how important the physician views the impact of smoking on their health and quantifies the habit. Some smokers say that their physicians never told them to quit and some will respond to brief interventions, but almost never in one session. Smoke-free offices are necessary without exception. One need not wait for a "propitious" or adequate length of time for initiating conversation about the desirability of smoking cessation. Even 5 minutes devoted to the subject has been shown statistically to have eventual long-term success, compared with never mentioning smoking dangers and the wisdom of cessation at all.

5. The answer is A. Reactive airway disease and exacerbations of known asthma are more likely in children of households with smokers living in the abode than those without smokers. Ear and upper respiratory infections decrease if the smoking is stopped. Although cigarette smoking by the parents is not known to cause childhood asthma, the smoke can serve as a respiratory irritant that precipitates the asthma. In addition, otitis media is more likely in smoking households. No causal relationship between parental cigarette smoking and sudden infant death syndrome or childhood malignancies has been established.

6. The answer is C. The risk of lung cancer begins significantly to subside at 10 years after cessation of smoking, and it approaches the expected risk of non-smokers by about 13 years. This estimate is on less secure ground with the passage of time due to the increasing proportion of lung cancers found in non-smokers. Still, the vast majority of lung cancer patients have smoked heavily (≥ 1 pack per day) for more than 20 years before contracting the disease.

7. The answer is A. He has his first cigarette before breakfast (i.e., "before his feet hit the floor"). This patient is among the 30% or so of smokers who are truly addicted, as opposed to those whose impulses to smoke occur in certain situations, such as after dinner, in times of "stress" or when out with friends rather than "on the clock."

8. The answer is E. If he suffered a myocardial infarction 2 weeks ago, the vasoconstrictive effects of nicotine are a clear danger. Recent myocardial infarction, unstable angina, cardiac dysrhythmia, or true hypersensitivity reaction to the patch (not just local erythema or pruritus) are the only real contraindications. The length of the critical period after a myocardial infarction is generally not given in the literature. However, following perioperative guidelines for elective surgery, and allowing for somewhat more leeway for smoking versus an assumed compelling case for even elective surgery, 3 months would be a good estimate.

9. The answer is D. Bupropion is contraindicated where there is history of seizures. Most suitable in situations where the compulsion to smoke appears to be psychological rather addictive, bupropion is contraindicated in the presence of a history of seizures, bulimia, presence of monoamine oxidase inhibitors, headache, nausea, or recent head trauma.

10. The answer is D, 1 week. The 1-week delay before reusing a site in rotation is recommended so that contact irritation can be avoided.

References

Bope ET. Smoking cessation. In: Rudy DR, Kurowski K, eds. *Family Medicine: House Officer Series.* Baltimore, MD: Williams & Wilkins; 1997:649–656.

Family Medicine Board Review 2009. Kansas City, MO; May 3–10, 2009.

McPhee SJ, Papadakis MA. *Current Medical Diagnosis and Treatment*, 49th ed. New York, Chicago: Lange, McGraw-Hill; 2010.

Okoyemi KIS, Nollen ML, Ahluwahlia JS. Interventions to facilitate smoking cessation. *Am Fam Physician.* 2006; 74:262–271, 276.

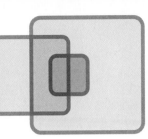

chapter 40

Exercise and Health

Examination questions: Unless instructed otherwise, choose the ONE lettered answer or completion that is BEST in each case.

1 An obese 45-year-old male wishes to inaugurate an exercise program and asks for advice as to what precautions he should observe. Each of the following is a contraindication for prescribed exercise except for which one?

(A) Compensated congestive heart failure
(B) Complex ventricular dysrhythmias
(C) Unstable angina
(D) Significant aortic stenosis
(E) Significant aortic aneurysm

2 Each of the following statements is correct regarding principles in the language of exercise physiology except for which one?

(A) Isometric exercise involves exertion against a fixed load without moving it.
(B) Isotonic exercise involves exertion against a constant load through movement in space.
(C) In eccentric exercise, muscle tension is increased along with its lengthening.
(D) In concentric exercise, objects of graduated weights are moved toward the body.
(E) Power lifting by children should not occur until the child has attained Tanner stage V.

3 Which of the following is the definition of basal energy expenditure (BEE)?

(A) The amount of energy expended per unit time by a person at rest, who has not eaten for 2 hours
(B) The amount of energy expended per unit time by a person at rest, who has not eaten for 12 hours
(C) The amount of energy expended by a person doing normal wakeful activity, not involving pulse-raising exercise
(D) The amount of energy expended per unit time by a person during sleep
(E) The amount of energy expended by a person in performing basic activities of daily living

4 A 45-year-old man weighs 240 lb (109 kg) at a height of 5 ft 10 in. (1.77 m) and is now seriously contemplating weight loss. You feel you can exploit this teaching moment. How much time for exercise can you tell the patient is recommended for American adults by the Center for Disease Control and Prevention?

(A) 15 minutes of mild-intensity physical activity 3 days a week
(B) 15 minutes of moderate-intensity physical activity 3 days a week
(C) 15 minutes of moderate-intensity physical activity 5 to 7 days a week
(D) 30 minutes of moderate-intensity physical activity 3 days a week
(E) 30 minutes of moderate-intensity physical activity 5 to 7 days a week

5 In helping the patient to recognize moderate exercise in his individual case, what pulse rate would this 45-year-old patient need to achieve to be reaching at least moderate physical activity?

(A) 70 beats per minute
(B) 104 beats per minute
(C) 122 beats per minute
(D) 154 beats per minute
(E) 170 beats per minute

6 Regarding the patient who is inaugurating a weight loss program, you tell the patient that each of the following benefits accrue to a person who exercises except for which one?

(A) Prevention and control of type II diabetes are improved in regular exercise, even controlling for weight.
(B) Osteoporosis of aged individuals is retarded or prevented by regular exercise.
(C) Risk of colon cancer is lessened by regular exercise.
(D) Blood pressure control in hypertension is facilitated by regular exercise.
(E) Risk of rectal cancer is reduced by regular exercise.

7 A 35-year-old man weighs 210 lb (95 kg). His height is 5 ft, 10 in., or 70 in. (1.78 m). Thus, his ideal weight, 106 lb plus 6 lb for each inch over 5 ft, is 166 lb (75.2 kg). You point out that he is 44 lb or about 20 kg overweight. You advise him to begin walking 1 mile every day. How many kilocalories will he burn, regardless of his pace or pulse rate while walking?

(A) 50 kcal
(B) 100 kcal
(C) 140 kcal
(D) 200 kcal
(E) 240 kcal

8 In walking, the 210 adult takes 20 minutes to travel a mile and maintains a pulse of 100 while walking at that pace. How many calories will he burn if he is doing fast cycling for 1 hour, maintaining a pulse rate of 150 beats/minute?

(A) 110 cal
(B) 210 cal
(C) 320 cal
(D) 430 cal
(E) 630 cal

9 Which of the following best applies to the "cooldown period" component of an exercise program?

(A) During this component there is a net clearing of lactic acid from the muscles.
(B) It has four characteristics described by the mnemonic FITT (frequency, intensity, type, and time).
(C) It is only necessary for patients in vigorous-intensity programs.
(D) It represents the aerobic phase of the workout.
(E) It increases peripheral blood pooling in muscles.

10 Which of the following is a valid reason to terminate an exercise session?

(A) The systolic blood pressure rises and the diastolic pressure falls during strenuous exercise.
(B) The pulse rate doubles during strenuous exercise.
(C) The patient experiences persistent headache during exercise.
(D) The patient is fatigued during strenuous exercise.
(E) Patient develops tachypnea.

Examination Answers

1. The answer is A. *Compensated* congestive heart failure is not a contraindication to prescribed physical exercise. Complex ventricular dysrhythmias, unstable angina, significant aortic stenosis, significant aortic aneurysm are the most commonly mentioned contraindications to prescribed physical exercise. Be that as it may exercise programs by any adult who has not been physically active for a period of years or who has a history of supervention of changing health history for any period of time since being active should be instructed to graduate the volume and load and intensity of activity after starting modestly.

2. The answer is D. The incorrect statement as, "In concentric exercise objects of graduated weights are moved toward the body." Concentric exercise refers to the process in which the activated muscle shortens with the exertion, as occurs in the biceps with curling. Each of the other statements is correct. Concentric exercise overlaps with isometric exercise because in the former activity the movement is less significant than is the constant resistance encountered. In both cases the constructive application is in strength building. Isotonic exercise involves exertion against a constant load through movement in space and applies best to cardiovascular conditioning. In eccentric exercise muscle tension is increased along with its lengthening, as in the "exertional letdown" by the quadriceps femori in the act of squatting. Power lifting by children should not occur until the child has attained full sexual maturity, that is, Tanner stage V.

3. The answer is B. BEE is the amount of energy expended per unit time by a person at rest, who has not eaten for 12 hours. The basis of the 12-hour fast is that food intake adds energy consumption attached to it (i.e., the thermic effect of food). The third factor in energy consumption, of course, is that attendant to physical activity. For practical purposes it is too difficult to obtain subjects in a 12-hour fasting state. Therefore, a compromise is usually accepted for standardization, which is measurement of energy expenditure during a 2-hour fast. This adds about 10% to the BEE.

4. The answer is E, 30 minutes of moderately intense physical activity 5 to 7 days a week, preferably 7 days per week.

5. The answer is C, 122 beats per minute. Moderate activity produces about 70% of the predicted maximum pulse; thus, a functional definition of moderate exercise is that which produces a heart rate equal to 70% of the predicted maximum, in a patient with no heart disease. The maximum pulse is 220 minus the age, in this case 45 years. Thus, 220 minus $45 = 175$; then, 175×0.7 (or 70%) ≥ 122 beats per minute.

6. The answer is E. The risk of rectal cancer is *not* reduced by regular exercise, in contrast to colon cancer. All the other statements regarding the benefits of exercise are true.

7. The answer is C, 140 kcal is the estimated caloric consumption for the 210-lb (95-kg) person in walking 1 mile at any pace. This is based on a rule of thumb that is easy to memorize: Weight in pounds multiplied by two-thirds.

8. The answer is E, 630 cal. It is assumed that calories consumed in exercise are directly proportional to the pulse during such exercise and to the time involved in such exercise, using as a baseline the calories consumed in walking 1 mile and the pulse in beats per minute during the normal walking pace:

$$Cx = Cw \times (Px/Pw) \times (Tx/Tw),$$

where
Cw is the calories consumed in locomotion of 1 mile at any pace (140 for this 210-lb man)Px is the pulse during exercise
Pw is the pulse during a 1-mile walk (100 in this example)
Tx is the time spent at new exercise (150 in this example)
Tw is the time spent walking 1 mile (60 minutes in the example)

$$140 \times (150/100) \times (60/20)$$

Thus, $Cx = 140 \times (150/100) \times (60/20) = 630$ kcal for this individual to pedal a bicycle for 1 hour, raising his pulse to 150 bpm. Thus, it is shown how to calculate a pulse-raising activity.

9. The answer is A. The cooldown period is the voluntary deceleration of the exercise activity over several seconds to 1 minute. During this component, there is a net clearing of lactic acid from the muscles as a result of resumption of normal venous return. Lactic acid contributes to muscle soreness during the early phase of conditioning; the cooldown period decreases the peripheral blood pooling in muscles. This return to normal venous circulation serves also to minimize light-headedness and nausea as circulation returns to the head and to the splanchnic bed. The FITT mnemonic refers to the defining characteristics of an exercise program: frequency, intensity, type of activity, and time invested in the activity. The aerobic phase applies to the activity phase of the workout, not the cooldown period.

10. The answer is C. Persistent headache during exercise may be indicative of a metabolic abnormality or anemia; in any event, it is not a desirable concomitant of exercise. Doubling the heart rate is within normal limits for stress testing. Rising systolic and falling diastolic pressure during exercise is a physiological response. A rising diastolic pressure may be a sign of a pathological cardiovascular response to exercise.

References

Coleman MT. Exercise and health. In: Rudy DR, Kurowski K, eds. *Family Medicine, House Officer Series.* Williams and Wilkins; 1997:657–667.

Family Medicine Board Review 2009. Kansas City, MO; May 3–10, 2009.

Hay WW, Levin MJ, Sondheimer JM, Deterding RR, eds. *Current Diagnosis & Treatment Pediatrics.* New York, Chicago: McGraw-Hill/Lange; 2009.

McPhee SJ, Papadakis MA. *Current Medical Diagnosis and Treatment,* 49th ed. New York, Chicago: Lange, McGraw-Hill; 2010.

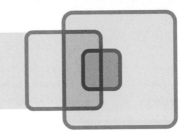

chapter 41

Concepts in Epidemiology and Research Method

Examination questions: *Unless instructed otherwise, choose the ONE lettered answer or completion that is BEST in each case.*

1 A study to investigate a new drug for primary prevention of colorectal cancer enlisted 400 subjects with histories of adenomatous polyps by colonoscopy in the treatment group and 400 subjects with histories of adenomatous polyps in a placebo group, matched for age, sex, geography, and other variables. They were followed for 10 years, and the treatment group had a 3% incidence of colorectal cancers, whereas the control group a 5% incidence. Assuming the study was valid and results were statistically significantly different in the two groups, how many patients, matched with the study group for age, sex, and risk factors for colorectal carcinoma would you have to treat for 10 years to prevent one colorectal cancer?

(A) 25
(B) 50
(C) 100
(D) 200
(E) 400

2 Which of the following is an example of secondary prevention?

(A) Salt restriction to prevent onset of hypertension
(B) Pap smears to prevent carcinoma of the cervix
(C) Aspirin 80 mg daily to prevent vascular thrombotic disease
(D) Angioplasty of the right coronary artery to prevent recurrence of angina pectoris
(E) Prescription of simvastatin to correct dyslipidemia in a patient who has had a myocardial infarction

3 Smoking cessation to prevent lung cancer is an example of which type of prevention?

(A) Primary
(B) Secondary
(C) Tertiary

(D) Quaternary
(E) Common sense

4 Which of the following is an example of tertiary prevention?

(A) Resection of a carcinoma of the colon, found to be in Duke's stage A in a patient who presented with hematochezia.
(B) Finding an elevated thyroid stimulating hormone (TSH) in a patient whose T-4 and T-3 are within normal limits and who has no symptoms or a palpable goiter.
(C) Removal of an adenomatous polyp during screening colonoscopy
(D) Voluntary weight loss in a 50-year-old man with central obesity to prevent diabetes.
(E) Carotid endarterectomy in a 57-year-old man with an incidental finding of 80% stenosis of the right carotid artery.

5 A new test for colorectal cancer is based on detecting carcinoma DNA in stool. 1,000 subjects with first degree relative who had manifested either adenomatous colon polyp or colorectal carcinoma were followed to test for the development of colorectal cancer. Annual colonoscopy by endoscopists who were blinded to results of the new testing served as the "gold standard" for appearance in 1,000 subjects of average risk followed over a period of 10 years. Over the 10-year period there were 65 cases of cancer diagnosed by colonoscopy. Of these 63 tested positive to the new stool test and 110 tested positive for the test who did not have colorectal cancer upon colonoscopy. Which of the following figures represent the sensitivity of the new stool test (chances of a cancer of the colon being diagnosed by the new test)?

(A) 63%
(B) 89%
(C) 90%
(D) 36%
(E) 100%

6 In the foregoing problem what is the calculated specificity of the new test for colorectal cancer (chances of patients without cancer for testing negative by the new test)?

(A) 63%
(B) 88%
(C) 90%
(D) 36%
(E) 100%

7 In the problem presented which of the following is the positive predictive value (PPV) which is the chance of a patient with a positive test having the disease colorectal cancer?

(A) 63%
(B) 88%
(C) 99%
(D) 36%
(E) 0%

8 In the problem presented in Question 5, which of the following is the negative predictive value (NPV) of the test, that is, the chances of a patient with a negative result on the new test, actually not having the disease?

(A) 63%
(B) 88%
(C) 90%
(D) 99%
(E) 0%

9 Which of the following is the descending order of the five cancer *incidences* listed in the United States, both sexes?

(A) Lung, prostate, breast, colorectal, invasive cervix
(B) Prostate, colorectal, breast, lung, invasive cervix
(C) Breast, invasive cervix, prostate, colorectal, lung
(D) Invasive cervix, prostate, colorectal, lung, breast
(E) Colorectal, lung, breast, invasive cervix, prostate

10 Which of the following is the descending order of cancer *mortality* in the United States of the five cancers listed?

(A) Lung, prostate, breast, colorectal, invasive cervix
(B) Prostate, colorectal, breast, lung, invasive cervix
(C) Breast, invasive cervix, prostate, colorectal, lung
(D) Lung, Colorectal, breast, prostate, invasive cervix
(E) Colorectal, lung, breast, invasive cervix, prostate

11 The greatest advantage of a case–control study over a retrospective or prospective cohort study is:

(A) It facilitates the calculation of an odds ratio.
(B) It facilitates the calculation of a relative risk.
(C) It is a prospective study.

(D) Bias is generally less of a factor.
(E) For rare diseases, it allows study of risk factors, given known cases rather than cases, given suspected risks.

12 Incidence of *invasive* cervical cancer in the United States was 14,500/year in 1996 and 13,700/year in 1998. Disease-specific mortality in 1998 was 4,900. Each of the following conclusions *from the above data* may be drawn except:

(A) Overall case mortality rate from invasive carcinoma of the cervix is about 36%.
(B) A significant number of lives are saved by preventive care in this formerly fatal cancer.
(C) Inference of case mortality from the above data requires assumption of fairly stable incidence and death rates over time.
(D) The incidence of precancerous lesions and cervical cancer *in situ* may be falling.
(E) Incidence of invasive cancer may have fallen between 1996 and 1998.

13 In a population of 2,000 people 600 are cigarette smokers. Of these, 120 develop disease X. Of the 1,400 non-smokers 140 develop disease X. The relative risk of disease X for cigarette smoker in this population is:

(A) 0.2
(B) 0.1
(C) 0.857
(D) 2.0
(E) 3.33

14 Which of the following would tend to result in a low disease prevalence:

(A) High disease incidence
(B) Natural history characterized by slow progression to death
(C) Low rate of cure
(D) High disease specific mortality
(E) Short disease latency period, and long symptomatic period

15 Which of the following is an example of incidence:

(A) 11 million Americans have type II diabetes.
(B) 10% of Americans have type II diabetes.
(C) Invasive cervical cancer strikes 11.6/100,000 U.S. females per year.
(D) 30 of 100 cases of cervical cancer are fatal.
(E) The number of cases of AIDS in the U.S. population now stands at 0.8 to 1.2 million.

16 The advantages of a cross-sectional study include which one of the following:

(A) Incidence can be calculated.
(B) Cause and effect can be evidenced.
(C) Effectiveness of intervention(s) can be inferred.
(D) Associations of possible risk factors and disease can be postulated.
(E) It is useful in investigating a rare disease.

17 An article in *J.A.M.A.* reported on two groups of women with known coronary artery disease (CAD) assigned randomly and blindly to the investigators to take hormone replacement therapy (HRT) or not (control group). The two groups were followed for 3 years and compared for rates of coronary events. Subjects were excluded if they had complicated heart disease or uncontrolled hypertension. Both groups were followed for 21 years and those taking HRT had a statistically similar number of cardiac events as the control group. The authors concluded and the media announced that HRT therefore does not prevent CAD. This was an example of what type of study:

(A) Case–control study
(B) Prospective interventional study
(C) Prospective observational study
(D) Ecological study
(E) Cross-sectional study

Examination Answers

1. The answer is B. A treatment group of 50 would prevent one colorectal cancer case employing the new preventive regimen in 10 years. As a simple matter of mathematics, one method of arriving at this conclusion is as follows: the difference of incidence between the treatment group (3%) and the control group (5%) is 2%. Thus, the treatment is assumed to prevent colorectal cancer in 2% of the population as defined in the body of the question. Two percent of the population in the treatment group is eight subjects. Thus, to prevent colorectal cancer in one patient, the group size needed is 1/8 of 400 or 50.

2. The answer is B. Papanicoulau smears are examples of secondary prevention. The malignant disease process of carcinoma of the cervix will have been underway if or when the pap smear has become positive, leading to an intervention such as conization of the cervix. Salt restriction to prevent hypertension is primary prevention, if it is effective; if the hypertension is established, salt restriction may alleviate the process, effectively preventing progression of hypertension, thus being a form of secondary hypertension if there be no symptoms, such as headaches, precipitation of angina, etc. In the latter events, prevention is tertiary in type because not only is the disease process underway but it is symptomatic. Aspirin to prevent platelet aggregation is a form of primary prevention, assuming that no vascular events have occurred. Angioplasty to alleviate angina and prevent future events is a form of tertiary prevention since the disease process is present and symptomatic. Simvastatin to correct dyslipidemia is a form of tertiary prevention in the patient who has experienced a vascular event.

3. The answer is A, primary. Cigarette smoking cessation prevents the vast majority of lung cancers from developing if embarked upon early enough. Thus, a disease process not underway and prevented from developing is an example of primary prevention.

4. The answer is A. Resection of a carcinoma of the colon, found to be in Duke's stage A in a patient who presented with hematochezia is definitely tertiary prevention. The cancerous disease process is underway and symptomatic with bright red blood in the stool. Finding an elevated TSH in a euthyroid patient without goiter and correcting the metabolic status by prescribing exogenous thyroid hormone is an example of secondary prevention, interruption of an asymptomatic disease process. Removal of an adenomatous polyp during screening colonoscopy is primary prevention of colon cancer. Voluntary weight loss in a centrally obese man with family history of type II

diabetes is primary prevention of diabetes, assuming the patient would have been destined to contract the disease. Medically indicated carotid endarterectomy in an asymptomatic person is an example of secondary prevention.

5. The answer is C, 90%. 63 cancers were discovered and 70 cancer occurred in the study group (Table 41–1).

TABLE 41–1 Presentation of Data from Which the Shown Functions Can Be Calculated from Questions 5 and 8

	Subjects with +Tests	Subjects with −Tests	Totals of Cases (Columns 2 and 3)
Cancer present	63	7	70
Cancer absent	110	820	930
Totals	173	827	1,000

Sensitivity = 63/70 = 0.9 × 100 = 90%
Specificity = 820/930 = .88 × 100 = 88%
PPV = 63/173 = .36 × 100 = 36%
NPV = 820/827 = 0.991 × 100 = 99.1%

6. The answer is B. The specificity of the test is 88%, that is, the chances of a patient who is negative for the test not having the disease (Table 41–1).

7. The answer is D. The PPV is 36%, that is, the chances of someone with a positive test actually having the disease. This illustrates the fact that the value of a screening test is heavily dependent on the proportion of the population who will be positive. Such tests must be evaluated on the basis of cost and discomfort attendant to the test and the cost, both emotional and financial, of the false-positive tests that will occur, and of the subsequent testing that must be done to rule out the false positives and avoid chronic and terminal care avoided (Table 41–1).

8. The answer is D. 99% is the chance of actually not having the disease if the test is negative (Table 41–1). Several observations should be apparent from the foregoing problems. First might be that even with an impressive sensitivity (e.g., 90%) when testing for a disease with low incidence or prevalence in the population, the predictive power of a positive test may be less than 50%. Conversely, in that situation even a modest specificity may convey a very high negative predictive power simply because of the paucity of patients who have the disease.

9. The answer is A. Lung, prostate, breast, colon, invasive cervix, the descending order of incidence of the five cancers mentioned. Left out are cancers of the skin and blood and blood forming tissues. For the individual sexes, the order is breast, lung, colorectal and for men prostate, lung, colorectal.

10. The answer is D. Lung, colorectal, breast, prostate, invasive cervix is the descending order of cancer mortality among the five significant cancers listed. For the individual sexes, the descending order of mortality is lung, breast, colorectal; for males it is lung, prostate, colorectal. The obvious message of this and the previous question and text is the low case mortality of lung cancer, about 75% in 2008 if the incidence was not falling rapidly (by forming the proportion of case mortality to incidence for a given disease).

11. The answer is E. For rare diseases, it allows a study of risk factors, given known cases rather than cases given suspected risks. The latter requires much more expense than the former and especially so for a disease as uncommon as, for example, amyotrophic lateral sclerosis. In that instance, absent the discovery of a clear-cut cause not found in any normal people, causes to be investigated will be partial in causation present in a vast majority of the normal or unaffected population; a huge denominator would be required to prove statistical significance of a risk factor to arrive at conclusions.

12. The answer is D. One *cannot* conclude from the data given in the body of the question that the incidence of precancerous lesions and cervical cancer *in situ* may be falling, as the figures given relate only to invasive cancer. In fact, most evidence suggests that precancerous lesions and carcinoma *in situ* are still increasing in incidence, but the utilization of the pap smear has prevented a great majority from progressing to invasive cancer.

13. The answer is D. Relative risk is calculated by forming the ratio between the expected incidence (rate of disease X in the case given) in the *at risk* group or exposed group (smokers) and the *non-at risk* group (non-smokers). Thus, 120 of 600 smokers developed disease X or 20%, a rate of 0.2 and the rate of disease X in the non-smokers is 140 of 1,400 for a rate of 0.1. The ratio of the rate of disease X in smokers, 0.2 to the rate in non-smokers, 0.1 is 0.2:0.1, or 2.0. By the same token if the factor to which the "exposed" is protective, then the relative "risk" could be <1.

14. The answer is D. High disease-specific mortality results in low prevalence of that disease. Prevalence is defined as either the proportion of disease expressed as a rate or percentage or the absolute number of cases in the population expressed as the number of cases per unit population, e.g., 2,500/100,000. Thus, diseases with short fatal courses, such as pancreatic carcinoma will have low prevalence, whereas those with long courses such as diabetes will have high prevalence (11% in that example). Higher disease incidence *per se*, other things being equal, favors higher prevalence (e.g., increasing incidence of tuberculosis). Slower progression to death produces higher prevalence. A short latency period (i.e., disease becoming apparent sooner) and long symptomatic period, another way of defining chronicity, produces higher prevalence.

15. The answer is C. The statement "Invasive cervical cancer strikes 11.6/100,000 U.S. females per year" is an expression of incidence. Both statements regarding the numbers of cases of diabetes (types I and II) are expression of prevalence; similarly the statement of the estimated number of AIDS cases in the United States is an expression of prevalence. That 30% of invasive cervical cancer die of the disease is an expression of disease-specific mortality, more often expressed on a larger scale, such as 3,710 of 10.370/U.S. population (2005).

16. The answer is D. Associations of possible risk factors and disease can be ascertained in a cross-sectional study. A cross-sectional study is a "snapshot" in time, effected typically by a survey of a population for the presence or absence of one or more suspected risk factors, causes perhaps inferred thereby but not assumed without an interventional or observational study. Both the latter study types are prospective and employ the passage of time. The interventional study entails a treatment group and a control group, matched as closely as possible for all factors except the treatment intervention. Conclusions in that case can include strong evidence (or not) in favor of cause and effect. A prospective observational study allows calculation of incidence, within the population at large or in a population perhaps defined by exposure to a postulated risk factor and compared to a demographically matched population except for the possible risk factor.

17. The answer is B. Prospective interventional study. The intervention is the HRT group, and in this case, both treatment and control group were (attempted to be) matched for (absence of other) atherosclerotic risk factors.

References

Cancer statistics, 2005. *CA Cancer J Clin.* 2005; 55(1).

Cancer statistics, 2008. *CA Cancer J Clin.* 2008; 58(2).

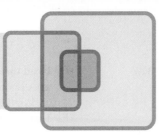

chapter 42

Newborn and Infant Care and Prevention, Birth to Age 1

Examination questions: Unless instructed otherwise, choose the ONE lettered answer or completion that is BEST in each case.

1 A 15-year-old girl without prior medical care turns up the emergency department complaining of mild malaise and a rash. She manifests a mild generalized morbilliform eruption. Examination reveals readily palpable retroauricular and suboccipital lymph nodes as well as erythematous palatal spots. If the pregnancy is carried to term and delivered the newborn will be at risk for each of the following except:

(A) Cataracts
(B) Sensorineural deafness
(C) Jaundice
(D) Small for gestation
(E) Koplik spots

2 A primiparous Hispanic woman who has had no prenatal care delivers at 36 weeks, 20 hours after premature rupture of her membranes. On the third day of extra-uterine life, the baby exhibits bouts of apnea and "floppiness." There are rales heard upon auscultation of the lung fields. There is no rash, and the pharynx is unremarkable nor are there cardiac auscultatory abnormalities. Which of the following is the most likely diagnosis?

(A) Beta hemolytic Group A streptococcus infection
(B) *Staphylococcus aureus* infection
(C) Group B streptococcus infection   GBS
(D) Rubeola
(E) Erythema infectiosa

3 A full-term male infant is born cyanotic without apparent dyspnea. Each of the following is within the differential diagnosis of the condition except for which one?

(A) Transposition of the great vessels
(B) Anomalous pulmonary return
(C) Truncus arteriosus
(D) Critical pulmonary stenosis
(E) Coarctation of the abdominal aorta

4 Each of the following statements regarding routine circumcision of the male newborn is true except for which one?

(A) Circumcised males have fewer urinary tract infections.
(B) Phimosis is prevented.
(C) Circumcision reduces the chances of carcinoma of the cervix in future female partners.
(D) Circumcision is contraindicated in the presence of hypospadias.
(E) Circumcision reduces the lifetime risk of penile cancer.

5 A healthy newborn boy, weighing 7 lb 6 oz (3.34 kg), has been accepted for well baby care. In regard to hydration and renal function, which of the following is an accepted indication of adequate urine output in the first 24 hours of life?

(A) Moist mucosae
(B) Good skin turgor
(C) Nonsunken eyeballs
(D) One wet diaper
(E) Normal pasty stools

6 A full-term newborn boy was born to a gravida 3, para 3 woman who had not committed to regular prenatal care. There is a history of neonatal jaundice in her second baby caused by a minor blood group incompatibility. Assuming this baby exhibits jaundice in the first few days of life, which of the following cutoff points is satisfactory for alerting the primary care physician to the likely need for phototherapy?

(A) Bilirubin level ≥15 mg/dL at 10 hours of age
(B) Bilirubin level ≥10 mg/dL at <12 hours of age
(C) Bilirubin level ≤15 mg/dL at 18 hours of age
(D) Onset of clinical jaundice
(E) Bilirubin level at ≥18 mg/dL at ≤48 hours of age

7 What is the average caloric requirement for a new-born infant?

(A) 50 kcal/kg/day
(B) 120 kcal/kg/day
(C) 150 kcal/kg/day
(D) 500 kcal/day
(E) 700 kcal/day

8 Each of the following is a risk factor for sudden infant death syndrome (SIDS) in the United States, except for which one?

(A) Low socioeconomic status
(B) Minority ethnicity
(C) Maternal smoking
(D) Sleeping in the prone position
(E) Family history of atopic disease

9 Which of the following immunizations should be given in the newborn period?

(A) Diphtheria, tetanus, pertussis (DTaP), first dose
(B) *Hemophilus influenzae* type B (Hib), first dose
(C) Inactivated polio vaccine (IPV), first dose
(D) Pneumococcal vaccine (PCV), first dose
(E) Hepatitis B (HepB), first dose

10 At birth, a full-term female infant has received silver nitrate ointment 1%. Five days later she exhibits conjunctivitis. Which of the following is the most significant likely possible etiologic origin?

(A) *S. aureus*
(B) Group A beta-hemolytic streptococci
(C) Gonococcus
(D) *Chlamydia trachomatis*
(E) *H. influenzae*

11 In counseling a first-time mother regarding normal growth and development of her baby, which of the following do you outline as the normal course of developmental milestones?

(A) Head up and controlled at 2 weeks, sit unsupported at 3 months, crawl at 6 months, and walk at 9 months
(B) Head up and controlled at 2 months, sit unsupported at 4 months, crawl at 6 months, and walk at 9 months
(C) Head up and controlled at 3 months, sit unsupported at 6 months, crawl at 9 months, and walk at 12 months

(D) Head up and controlled at 4 months, sit unsupported at 8 months, crawl at 10 months, and walk at 14 months
(E) Head up and controlled at 6 months, sit unsupported at 10 months, crawl at 12 months, and walk at 18 months

12 In advising the mother referred to in Question 9, which of the following rules of thumb do you suggest regarding body weight for her infant?

(A) The child should weigh 15 lb (6.8 kg) by 6 months and 22 lb (10 kg) by 1 year.
(B) The child should weigh 10 lb (4.5 kg) by 6 months and 15 lb (6.8 kg) by 1 year.
(C) The child should double the birth weight by the age of 6 months and increase it three times by the age of 1 year.
(D) The child should double the birth weight by 6 months and triple it by 1 year.
(E) Weight does not matter as long as the child has a normal appetite.

13 You are counseling an expectant couple regarding the many benefits of breast feeding. Which of the following is a recognized beneficial effect?

(A) It decreases neonatal jaundice.
(B) It increases weight gain in the infant relative to those who are fed formula.
(C) Breast milk supplies IgG antibodies.
(D) The uterus returns to normal size faster in mothers who breast feed.
(E) Term babies who are breast fed do not need fluoride supplementation.

14 Besides prematurity, certain situations predispose a child to iron deficiency. Which of the following children may have this problem?

(A) An infant who is breast fed
(B) An infant born at term, now 4 months old, who has been on Enfamil formula
(C) A postdate newborn, now 3 months old, who has been on Isomil formula
(D) A 10-month-old infant who has an allergy to cow's milk protein
(E) An infant started after 6 months on solid foods that are rich in vitamin C

Examination Answers

1. The answer is E. Koplik spots are associated with and diagnostic of rubeola. The clinical picture in the vignette is typical of rubella, and the palatal exanthem consists of Flourscheimer spots, quite different in number and distribution from Koplik spots that occur on the buccal mucosae approximately opposite the upper second molars, one on each side. The list of neonatal conditions, affecting 50% to 80% of fetuses when maternal rubella occurs in the first trimester includes the other choices, cataract, sensorineural hearing loss, hepatitis and smallness for gestational age as well as several congenital cardiac anomalies, micophthalmia, glaucoma, retinitis, chronic encephalitis, and blood disorders.

2. The answer is C. Group B streptococcus infection occurs more often after premature labor and prolonged rupture of membranes. This serious infection with a high case mortality if untreated must be suspected in any systemic illness occurring within the first week of life. Delayed cases may appear after 1 to 16 weeks. Pneumonitis and apnea are typical and progress rapidly to sepsis and meningitis. Failure to diagnose may have grave medicolegal implications. Beta strep infection is rare during the neonatal period. *S. aureus* usually is localized and pointing. Rubeola manifests a classic morbilliform rash and otherwise is entirely different in expression. Finally, the mother's immunity covers the newborn for several months. Erythema infectiosa, "fifth disease" appears nearly always in the age range of 5 to 15 years.

3. The answer is E. Coarctation of the abdominal aorta. This condition of course does not cause cyanosis. Perhaps surprising is that congenital critical pulmonary stenosis may result in cyanosis, on the basis that at birth, the foramen ovale and the ductus arteriosis will remain open as a mechanical response to the increased right ventricular pressure, to maintain a right to left shunting. Each of the other choices is a condition that results in unoxygenated blood shunting into the left ventricular outflow circulation by its permanent anatomical nature.

4. The answer is C. The incorrect statement is that circumcision reduces the chances of carcinoma of the cervix in future female partners. However, the presence of the foreskin does appear to be associated with a greater risk of penile cancer. It is true that uncircumcised males have a greater risk of urinary tract infections, compared with circumcised males; circumcision is contraindicated in newborns with hypospadias because the foreskin may be invaluable in plastic repair of the deformity, most specifi-cally to reconstruct the urethral orifice. Obviously, phimosis is not possible in the absence of a foreskin.

5. The answer is D. One wet diaper in the first 24 hours should be adequate to ensure normal hydration and kidney function. Normal alimentation is not sensitive enough, whereas all the other signs listed, that is, waiting for dry mucosae, poor skin turgor, and sunken eyeballs, which are quite valid for clinical dehydration, are later in development than optimum care dictates. By day 2, there should be a wet diaper two to three times per 24 hours, and by day 5 there should be a wet diaper six to eight times per 24 hours.

6. The answer is B. A bilirubin level ≥10 mg/dL at <12 hours of age is an appropriate signal that the indirect-acting bilirubin may reach the level of 20 mg/dL by the third or fourth day, setting the stage for kernicterus. Other cutoff points are bilirubin levels of ≥14 mg/dL between 12 and 24 hours and ≥15 mg/dL at >24 hours of age. Jaundice that is due to a pathological as opposed to a physiological cause appears on the first day of life, and bilirubin levels can rise by more than 5 mg/dL/day. Peak bilirubin levels in physiologic jaundice rarely exceed 12 mg/dL but pathologic jaundice peaks at a much higher level, as stated. Exchange transfusion may be necessary if phototherapy does not obviate that need.

7. The answer is B, 120 kcal/kg/day is the average caloric requirement for a newborn infant.

8. The answer is E. Family history of atopic disease is not mentioned in the literature as a risk factor for SIDS. The two strongest (and remediable) risk factors are a smoking mother and prone sleeping position. Minority ethnicity and low socioeconomic status are risk factors but are not specific enough to be helpful.

9. The answer is E. Hep B (hepatitis B) is the only routine immunization recommended for infants in the newborn period (≤1 month of age) and should be given at birth. It may await the first or second month if the mother is negative to hepatitis B surface antigen. DTaP, Hib, IPV, and PCV are each given at 2, 4, and 6 months.

10. The answer is D, *C. trachomatis.* The two most significant causes of neonatal conjunctivitis (ophthalmia neonatorium) are gonorrhea and *C. trachomatis.* Gonorrheal conjunctivitis is prevented by routine neonatal treatment with silver nitrate. Presently the approach to chlamydial conjunctivitis is diagnosis by culture or rapid antigen detection followed by the treatment with erythromycin.

11. The answer is C. The timing is head up and controlled at 3 months, sit unsupported at 6 months, crawl at 9 months, and walk at 12 months. These are good screening guidelines and serve the family doctor or pediatrician well, not only in educating parents, but also in reviewing to establish a database for a new pediatric patient. Many children, especially those from families of higher socioeconomic status, will walk before 1 year and some as early as 6 months. Also, children may take longer than 6 months to sit unsupported. If only one of these mile markers is a departure from the normal rules of thumb, it may be explained by factors unique to the child's personality or family living status. Nevertheless, such a departure should trigger a more detailed examination for development. Delay in walking may be based on neurological, orthopedic, or cerebral development. Such refinements of developmental evaluation include grasp progressing from ulnar palm to radial, including the thumb at 3 to 4 months; using the thumb in opposition to pick up objects at 7 months.

12. The answer is C. The child should double the birth weight by the age of 6 months and increase three times by the age of 1 year. Choice A is virtually the same rule for a child of average birth weight. Many children will exceed this rate of growth, which is acceptable as long as the child is not becoming obese (i.e., simply growing bigger and faster is alright). Obesity should be addressed when it appears and prescribed for by the age of 2.

13. The answer is D. The uterus returns to normal size more rapidly in mothers who breast feed. Breast-fed babies also have decreased weights relative to formula-fed babies during the initial months, but this does not affect their final stature or weight. Breast milk supplies secretory IgA and macrophages but not IgG. One disadvantage of breast feeding is that some infants develop jaundice. The neonatal jaundice produced by breast feeding is felt to be benign and is not believed to produce kernicterus.

14. The answer is D, a 10-month-old who has an allergy to cow's milk protein. The reaction to the ingested protein causes inflammation in the intestine and resultant chronic low-grade gastrointestinal blood loss, which predisposes to iron deficiency. The iron in breast milk, though not high in concentration, is very well absorbed because of the effect of lactoferrin in breast milk to enhance absorption. Vitamin C increases intestinal iron absorption. Term and postdate babies are not at increased risk, as even "standard" formulas are iron fortified.

References

Family Medicine Board Review 2009. Kansas City, MO; May 3–10, 2009.

Gegas BG. Preventive care and triage of the infant and newborn. In: Rudy DR, Kurowski K, eds. *Family Medicine: House Officer Series.* Baltimore, MD: Williams & Wilkins; 1997:669–688.

Thilo EH, Rosenberg AA. The newborn infant. In: Hay W Jr, Levin MJ, Sondheimer JM, Deterding RR, eds. *Current Pediatric Diagnosis and Treatment,* 19th ed. New York/Chicago/San Francisco: McGraw-Hill; 2005.

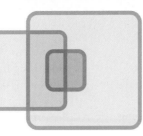

chapter 43

Care and Prevention, Ages 1 to 5 Years

Examination questions: *Unless instructed otherwise, choose the ONE lettered answer or completion that is BEST in each case.*

1. A 4-year-old otherwise healthy boy is brought to the family physician's office with an 8-day history of non-specific malaise and low grade fever as he begins to feel better now manifests a red maculopapular rash on the cheeks that on the day he is brought in appears to be coalescing to produce a diffuse red color now involving the chin and area behind the ears as well as the trunk and buttocks, sparing the circumoral zone. There is no palpable lymphadenopathy and the oral examination is not remarkable for descriptive abnormality. Which of the following is the likely diagnosis?

   (A) Rubella
   (B) Rubeola
   (C) Erythema infectiosum
   (D) Roseola infantum subitum
   (E) Atopic dermatitis

2. A 4-year-old boy is brought to a physician by a foster parent who believes the boy has had no well child immunization. There is coryza for 2 weeks of and now cough is developing, which increasingly is characterized by inspiratory stridor. The WBC is 20,000 with 80% lymphocytes. Chest x-ray reveals bronchial thickening and a "shaggy" heart border. While further evaluation proceeds, which of the following empiric treatments is most appropriate?

   (A) Amoxicillin
   (B) Cephalexin
   (C) Symptomatic treatment pending culture result
   (D) A macrolide
   (E) Penicillin V-potassium

3. A first-time mother brings her 18-month-old male child in for routine well care. His birth weight was 7 lb 8 oz (3.4 kg). His weight at 1 year was 22 lb 6 oz (10.13 kg). Today's weight is 25 lb 8 oz (11.55 kg). The boy walked at 11 months and is able to make known two "wants" and occasional two-word sentences. The mother is concerned regarding his apparent cessation in growth and notes that he eats less now than he had been eating at the age of 1 year. Your response is appropriately which of the following?

   (A) Plan to track calorie intake for 30 days and reevaluate
   (B) Draw blood for thyroid functions tests
   (C) Place the child on a high-calorie diet
   (D) Draw blood for growth hormone and testosterone levels
   (E) No action needed at this time; reassure the parent that the child is growing normally

4. A child should have at least four of each of the following immunizations by the age of 5 years, except for which one?

   (A) Diphtheria, tetanus, pertussis (DTaP)
   (B) Pneumococcal vaccine (PCV)
   (C) Varicella
   (D) *Hemophilus influenzae* type B (Hib)
   (E) Inactivated polio vaccine (IPV)

5. Which of the following patients, according to opinions among the American Academy of Pediatrics (AAP), the American Academy of Family Physicians (AAFP), and the Advisory Committee on Immunization Practices (ACIP), should receive influenza vaccine on an annual basis?

   (A) Infants from birth to 1 year of age
   (B) Children from 1 to 5 years of age
   (C) Children from 5 to 12 years of age
   (D) All persons older than 6 months of age
   (E) All adults only

6. Well examination of a 5-year-old child reveals that he speaks only six-word sentences but they are intelligible. The parents are concerned. Which of the following responses is most appropriate?

   (A) Refer the child for specialized evaluation of growth and development

(B) Arrange a conference with the child's teacher
(C) Order a magnetic resonance image of the child's brain
(D) Reassure the parents that the child is developing within normal limits
(E) Review the milestones of growth and development in this child

7 Which of the following measures is the most effective to prevent drowning among children who are between 1 and 5 years of age?

(A) Providing consistent discipline in teaching children safety policies
(B) Teaching children to swim at the earliest possible age before allowing them to swim in private pools
(C) Requiring children to play in pairs (i.e., the "buddy system")
(D) Using high (4 ft or 1.8 m) fences with self-latching gates around swimming pools
(E) Outlawing private swimming pools

8 A 4-year-old girl is brought to a family doctor for her preschool checkup. She has had unremarkable growth and development. The family members are Italian-American (father) and Anglo-American (mother) and were born in the United States; the father is a worker in a factory that manufactures batteries, and the family lives in a house built in 1945. Which of the following has the highest priority as to routine testing at this point?

(A) Blood lead level
(B) Thyroid-stimulating hormone
(C) Tuberculosis skin testing
(D) Complete blood cell count·
(E) Urinalysis for protein and sugar

9 Which of the following accounts for the largest number of deaths in children?

(A) Motor vehicle accidents
(B) Infectious diseases
(C) Acute abdominal emergencies
(D) Violence (gunshots, knife wounds, strangulation)
(E) Drowning

10 You are evaluating a 1-year-old child who is short (less than fifth percentile on growth curves), even when you correct for midparental height. There are multiple potential causes for short stature. Which of the following is *not* among them?

(A) Parental deprivation
(B) Intrauterine growth retardation
(C) Human immunodeficiency virus (HIV) infection
(D) Klinefelter syndrome
(E) Familial short stature

Examination Answers

1. The answer is C. Erythema infectiosum or fifth disease. The "slapped cheek" look is like none of the other choices. Rubella has a much shorter course, a typical morbilliform rash and suboccipital and post auricular adenopathy. Rubeola manifest a seriously toxic illness, the harder and more severe morbilliform rash and the buccal mucosal Koplik spots opposite the lower second molar; roseola is the well-known rash that appears as a prolonged highly febrile phase abates.

2. The answer is D. A macrolide. The description is classic for pertussis, which has been making a comeback, due in great part to hysteria over vaccine side effects. The typical aspects mentioned, besides the "whoop" of inspiratory stridor are the prolonged prodromal catarrhal stage; the whoop (which if untreated, may last for another 4–6 weeks); the absolute lymphocytosis and the "shaggy heart border" on x-ray. An acceptable application of a macrolide antibiotic would include the standard dosages of erythromycin for 7–14 days.

3. The answer is E. No action is needed at this time; reassure the parent that the child is growing normally. Although babies should double the birth weight by 6 months and many babies triple their birth weights by the age of 1 year, growth rate decelerates rapidly after the first year. The average boy gains about 5 lb (2.26 kg) during the period from 1 year to 2 years of age. In this situation, there is neither indication for endocrinological testing nor any need for force feeding.

4. The answer is C. Varicella vaccine requires only one dose, when the child is between 12 and 25 months of age. It may be given at any time through the years of youth to anyone who has not received it. The child receives DTaP at 2, 4, 6, and 12 to 15 months, and then a booster at 4 to 6 years. PCV is given at 2, 4, 6, and 12 to 15 months. Hib vaccine is given at 2, 4, 6, and 12 to 15 months. IPV is given at 2, 4, and 6 to 15 months and at 4 to 6 years.

5. The answer is D. All persons older than 6 months of age should receive the influenza vaccine on an annual basis. The AAP and AAFP agree that all children between the ages of 6 months and 18 years should receive the vaccine, and the ACIP states that all adults should receive influenza vaccine yearly.

6. The answer is D. Reassure the parents that the child is developing within normal limits. A fair rule of thumb in evaluating language development is two-word sentences at age 2; four-word sentences at age 3; five-word sentences at age 4; and six- or seven-word sentences at age 5. Review of growth and development milestones is not a matter reserved for addressing a genuine concern. It is something that should take place at each well child visit.

7. The answer is D, high (4 ft or 1.8 m) fences with self-latching gates around swimming pools. Each of the other choices merits attention and would be an effective supplement to fencing the swimming pools, but the choices are unproven in effectiveness to prevent drowning. Choice E, outlawing private swimming pools, has not been tried and tested; such a law would not likely be passed in any community. Blood lead level should be <10 mcg/dL. Even exposures to levels in the 10–15 mcg/dL range if prolonged can produce behavioral and cognitive effects. Ongoing studies have resulted in steady reduction of lead level cutoff points over the past 30 years. All the other choices are appropriate periodically but not annually if the child is healthy. The child need not be screened for thalassemia despite the half Italian parentage. Both α and β thalassemias would be picked up on a CBC with attention to the MCV that would show microcytosis out of proportion to an anemia.

8. The answer is A. Lead-based paint was used in houses built before 1960. Nearby industry that places children at high risk includes lead smelting and battery manufacturing. Routine screening starts when the child reaches the age of 1 year, with checks at 6 months only for those children at high risk. Some physicians apply a written questionnaire for risk factors instead of automatic level checks in neighborhoods where lead toxicity is rare. Children should be checked with serum lead levels at any age if they have symptoms of lead poisoning or exhibit a lot of hand-to-mouth activity.

9. The answer is A, motor vehicle accidents. Motor vehicle accidents (with children as a vehicle occupant or pedestrian) account for about 47% of injury deaths in children. In 1998, 57% of children 15 years of age and younger who died in motor vehicle accidents were unrestrained.

10. The answer is D, Klinefelter syndrome. Klinefelter syndrome is associated with tall stature with disproportional increases in long bones. All the other mentioned diseases result in growth retardation of a child. Parental deprivation leads to starvation, sometimes through anorexia; intrauterine growth retardation, by definition, is characterized by the child's starting life in a growth-retarded state; HIV infection exerts a nonspecific affect of failure to thrive; familial short stature has its effects from birth and could account for short stature in a 1-year-old child.

References

Family Medicine Board Review 2009. Kansas City, MO; May 3–10, 2009.

Hay WW, Levin MJ, Sondheimer JM, Deterding RR, eds. *Current Diagnosis & Treatment Pediatrics,* 19th ed. New York, Chicago: McGraw-Hill/Lange; 2009.

Kurowski K. Preventive care of the preschool child (1–5 years). In: Rudy DR, Kurowski K, eds. *Family Medicine: House Officer Series.* Baltimore, MD: Williams & Wilkins; 1997: 689–702.

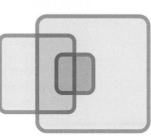

chapter 44

Care and Prevention, Ages 6 to 12 Years

1 A 6-year-old boy is diagnosed with attention deficit/hyperactivity disorder and the family doctor decides to prescribe methylphenidate (Ritalin). In explaining the treatment to the parents the doctor points out that each of the following may be a side effect except for which one?

(A) Growth retardation
(B) Aggravation of certain psychotic symptoms if they pre-exist
(C) Precipitate seizures
(D) Addiction
(E) Precipitate motor tics

2 A 7-year-old girl has complained of sore throat, headache, and productive cough. A chest x-ray shows patchy bilateral lower lobe infiltrates. The family doctor suspects mycoplasma pneumonia. Which of the following treatment would be appropriate?

(A) Penicillin V-K
(B) Cephalexin
(C) Cefadroxil
(D) Clarithromycin
(E) Cipro

3 A conscientious couple, a 25-year-old mother and 26-year-old father of three children, wish to discuss preventive health care for their eldest, a 6-year-old boy. Which of the following, against the background of current preventive measures already in place, is the area that presents the greatest opportunity of saving him from an earlier than average death?

(A) Practice safety in automobile travel
(B) Take measures to prevent fires
(C) Screen for lipids
(D) Teach proper care of firearms
(E) Enforce pneumonia vaccination

4 A 30-year-old mother brings her 12-year-old son for a routine well child visit. He has had four doses of diphtheria, tetanus, and pertussis (DTaP), four of *Hemophilus influenzae* type B (Hib), four of inactivated polio vaccine (IPV), and two of varicella vaccine. Which of the following immunizations is specially indicated at this time?

(A) Varicella
(B) DTaP
(C) IPV
(D) Booster of tetanus toxoid and a smaller dose of diphtheria toxoid (Td)
(E) Hib

5 Children who have had significant social contact with people with acquired immunodeficiency syndrome (AIDS), who are human immunodeficiency virus (HIV) positive, or are prisoners, migrant farm workers, or illicit drug users are considered at risk for which of the following diseases?

(A) HIV disease
(B) Hepatitis B
(C) Infectious mononucleosis
(D) Syphilis
(E) Tuberculosis

6 Which of the following forms of hypertension is found in children in a lesser proportion of hypertensive cases than in adults?

(A) Essential hypertension
(B) Pheochromocytoma
(C) Coarctation of the aorta
(D) Renal artery stenosis
(E) Chronic renal failure

7 Which of the following is the accepted mode for screening for tuberculosis in a child?

(A) Tuberculosis tine test
(B) Chest x-ray
(C) Mantoux test

(D) Pulmonary sputum culture

(E) Throat culture

8 Parents, both 30 years old, are together in a family physician's office to support their 6-year-old boy at his well child visit. They ask what rate of growth can be expected over the years, between now and the boy's adolescence. What is the general rate of growth they can anticipate throughout this period?

(A) 0.5 to 1 in. (1.27 to 2.54 cm) per year

(B) 1 to 2 in. (2.54 to 5.08 cm) per year

(C) 2 to 2.5 in. (5.08 to 6.35 cm) per year

(D) 3 to 3.5 in. (7.62 to 8.89 cm) per year

(E) 4 to 5 in. (10.16 to 12.70 cm) per year

9 A 19-year-old young woman exhibits scoliosis of 20 degrees in the thoracic spine (convexity) with compensating lumbar curvature. What is the best approach for following this patient?

(A) Follow with x-rays for the next several years

(B) Refer to a spine surgeon

(C) Evaluate for bracing

(D) Evaluate for spinal fusion

(E) Reassure the patient that the degree of curvature is benign and bears no further attention

10 Which of the following may be constitutionally associated with scoliosis (part of the primary syndrome as opposed to being secondary to the disease)?

(A) Cerebral palsy

(B) Poliomyelitis

(C) Slipped femoral capital epiphysis

(D) Neurofibromatosis

(E) Constrictive lung disease

Examination Answers

1. The answer is C. Precipitate seizures methylphenidate does not do. Each of the other side effects listed does in fact occur in susceptible individuals. Growth retardation occurs in 15% of cases but will be made up, provided the drug is discontinued before the end of adolescence. Abuse and addiction obviously may occur as well as motor tics and Tourette syndrome but eliciting family histories for these conditions can avoid the vast majority of these cases. Dextroamphetamine has the exact same profile as methylphenidate.

2. The answer is D, Clarithromycin, the antibiotic of choice among those presented; any other macrolide and any tetracycline-based antibiotic would do as well and in the latter group the most commonly used is doxycycline. The helpful historical hints are very much the same as in dealing with adults to diagnose mycoplasma. The same would also hold for chlamydia pneumonia (and psittacosis, also caused by a chlamydia) as would the choice of antibiotics and the infrequent occurrence in young children. Mycoplasma pneumonia is rare under the age of 5 years. The cough is non-productive at first. Otitis media and also bullous myringitis may be complications – the latter is not unique to mycoplasma. Neither of the two pneumonia types respond to any of the other listed antibiotics among the choices.

3. The answer is A. Motor vehicle accidents are the leading cause of death in children. Assuming that the parents maintain recommended immunizations in the first 5 years of life and the required immunization schedules after the age of school matriculation, the best thing they could do for this child is to protect him from automobile accidents, the chief cause of mortality in children of all ages. Fires and burns are in second place. Bicycle accidents are statistically significant as well; 85% of injuries sustained by children in bicycle accidents involve head injuries. Therefore, bicycle helmets worn by children (and adults) should be routine practice.

4. The answer is D, Td vaccine. The other vaccines mentioned here have been completed by the time the child reaches the age of 5 to 6 years (see chapter 41). From the age of 12, all individuals should receive the Td vaccine every 10 years for the remainder of life.

5. The answer is E. Tuberculosis is contagious through close social contact and has a high prevalence in the groups mentioned, that is, people with HIV, prisoners, migrant farm workers, and illicit drug users, as well as people from countries with highly endemic tuberculosis.

All the other choices in the question are diseases that require closer association than social (i.e., airborne) contact, except for infectious mononucleosis. The latter is not particularly contagious and is not particularly prevalent in the groups mentioned.

6. The answer is A, essential hypertension. Although hypertension in children is defined the same as in adults (i.e., blood pressure consistently in the 95th percentile or higher), the causes are more likely to be secondary rather than primary in children as compared to the distribution of hypertension in adults; 28% in children, whereas in adults only about 5% of hypertension falls into that category.

7. The answer is C, the Mantoux test, the intradermal injection of five units of purified protein derivative, followed by inspection for palpable induration in 48 to 73 hours. The tine test should not be used because it is lacking in sensitivity. A chest x-ray is not practical from the cost standpoint. The sputum culture is not ordered except in symptomatic cases.

8. The answer is C, 2 to 2.5 in. (5.08 to 6.35 cm) per year. The period begins with a growth rate of 2.5 in. or 6.35 cm per year and subsides to about 2 in. or 5.08 cm per year by the time the child reaches the age of 10, before the growth spurt that occurs at puberty.

9. The answer is A, observe for the next several years, following with plain x-rays. Twenty percent of curvature is nearly always asymptomatic and most cases will not progress. The longer the patient manifests no progression of the curvature, the less likely it will ultimately require correction. The male-to-female ration is 1:4 for affliction with scoliosis. This disorder has its onset when the child is between 8 and 10 years of age. The most serious degrees of scoliosis will occur before the child reaches the age of 16 (i.e., before the closure of the epiphyses). Only with progression should consultation be resorted to, with consideration of aggressive methods of prevention. At 40 to 60 degrees of curvature, bracing is indicated. At 60 degrees, fusion may be indicated to prevent respiratory deficiency in the future. However, the latter is a very serious undertaking and entails the better part of a year of nearly total disability in the patient.

10. The answer is D. Neurofibromatosis may be constitutionally associated with scoliosis. Cerebral palsy, poliomyelitis, and muscular dystrophy may predispose the patient to scoliosis on the basis of asymmetrical forces bearing on the spinal column. Constrictive lung disease may occur secondary to the scoliosis because of impedance of expansion of the lung fields. Slipped femoral capital epiphysis is not known to be associated with scoliosis.

References

Family Medicine Board Review, 2009. Kansas City, MO; May 3–10, 2009.

Hay WW, Levin MJ, Sondheimer JM, Deterding RR, eds. *Current Diagnosis & Treatment Pediatrics,* 19th ed. New York, Chicago: McGraw-Hill/Lange; 2009.

Welker MJ. Preventive care of the child through the latent years (5–12). In: Rudy DR, Kurowski K, eds. *Family Medicine: House Officer Series.* Baltimore, MD: Williams & Wilkins; 1997:703–712.

chapter 45

Care and Prevention, Ages 13 to 20 Years

Examination questions: *Unless instructed otherwise, choose the ONE lettered answer or completion that is BEST in each case.*

1 In growing children, there are unique issues attendant to trauma to the growth plates (physes) of the growth plates of long bones. Which of the following is most likely to result in growth deformity, even with correct treatment?

(A) Psalter
(B) Psalter II
(C) Psalter III
(D) Psalter IV
(E) Psalter V

2 A 16-year-old male suffers a fracture of her right tibia as she steps down off her deck that entailed an 18-in. drop. She admits that previously she had had pain in the limb and that others had noticed a limping gait favoring the right leg. Without initial studies, which of the following is the most likely diagnosis?

(A) Fibrous dysplasia
(B) Osteomyelitis
(C) Ewing tumor
(D) Osteosarcoma
(E) Enchondroma

3 A family physician is concerned that a thin 17-year-old female may be anorectic (nervosa). Each of the following is compatible with that diagnosis except for which one?

(A) Elevated Follicle stimulating hormone (FSH)
(B) Refusal to allow weight to go above barely minimal for height
(C) Unreasonable and intense fear of obesity
(D) Distorted body image
(E) Secondary amenorrhea

4 Parents visit a family doctor with their 15-year-old son who is unhappy because he feels he is not as tall as his classmates. Which of following would constitute an indication for proceeding with an endocrinological evaluation?

(A) Growth 4 cm (2 in.) per year
(B) Bone age delayed 1 year behind the mean normal for his age
(C) Disproportionate lower segment length
(D) Decreased sense of smell
(E) Elevated alkaline phosphatase

5 Members of which of the following groups are most likely to *attempt* suicide (without succeeding)?

(A) Black men who are 20 to 30 years old
(B) White boys or men who are 15 to 24 years old
(C) White girls or women who are 15 to 24 years old
(D) Black women who are 20 to 30 years old
(E) White women who are 20 to 30 years old

6 Members of which of the following groups are most likely to *commit* suicide?

(A) Black men who are 20 to 30 years old
(B) White boys or men who are 15 to 24 years old
(C) White girls or women who are 15 to 24 years old
(D) Black women who are 20 to 30 years old
(E) White women who are 20 to 30 years old

7 Parents of a 13-year-old boy believe their son, who is demonstrating a growth spurt, is not drinking enough milk and ask you about calcium-intake requirements. What do you tell them are the current daily recommendations for calcium intake?

(A) Between 300 and 500 mg/day
(B) Between 600 and 1,000 mg/day
(C) Between 1,200 and 1,500 mg/day
(D) Between 1,500 and 2,000 mg/day
(E) Between 2,000 and 2,500 mg/day

8 You are deciding on preventive screening for a young woman who began menarche at age 13. Her cycles are every 30 days, with 4 days of moderate flow. Her last menstrual period was 2 weeks ago. She denies ever being sexually active. She denies any vaginal discharge or pelvic area pain. At what age should Pap smears be performed on her?

(A) At age 13
(B) At age 15
(C) At age 20
(D) At the age of first sexual activity
(E) At the age of regular sexual activity

9 A 19-year-old sexually active female college student has recently married and has been taking oral contraceptive medication for 3 months. She complains of headaches since starting "the pill." Her blood pressure is 132/78; she weighs 120 lb (54.4 kg) at a height of 5 ft, 4 in. (1.63 m). Which of the following alterations in her regimen would be the most appropriate?

(A) Reduce the estrogen component of her birth control pill (BCP)
(B) Reduce the progestational component of her BCP
(C) Investigate the androgenic effects of her BCP
(D) Prescribe a 5-hydroxytryptamine agonist (e.g., sumatriptan)
(E) Discontinue the BCP

10 Regarding the tolerability of oral contraceptive medications, each of the following is a side effect of the estrogenic component of BCPs, except which one?

(A) Increased breast size
(B) Enlargement of leiomyomas
(C) Hepatocellular adenomas
(D) Cyclic weight gain
(E) Oily skin

11 A 16-year-old female patient visits her family doctor for treatment of a viral upper respiratory tract infection. She appears to have lost weight since the last visit of 6 months ago. The doctor inquires regarding her menstrual history and finds she has missed the last two periods. Pregnancy testing is negative. Suspecting anorexia, the doctor checks her weight against the ideal for her age and sex. Which of the following weight criteria satisfy the minimal definition of anorexia nervosa (AN)?

(A) Weight <100 lb (45 kg) in a female individual
(B) Weight <100 lb plus 5 lb for every inch over 60 in. (5 ft or 1.52 m)
(C) Ideal body weight (IBW) <60th percentile for age and sex
(D) Weight <85% of IBW
(E) Caloric intake <500 kcal/day

12 A 16-year-old is undergoing a routine health maintenance examination. He has had five immunizations of diphtheria, tetanus, and pertussis (DTaP; three in the first year, one at 2 years, and one at 5 years); four shots of *Hemophilus influenzae* type B (Hib); four shots of inactivated polio vaccine (IPV); two shots of measles, mumps, and rubella (MMR) vaccine; a varicella vaccine; three shots of pneumococcal vaccine (PCV); three doses of hepatitis B vaccine (HBV); and yearly influenza vaccines. Besides the yearly influenza vaccine, which of the following vaccines is due at this time?

(A) DTaP, sixth dose
(B) MMR, third dose
(C) Diphtheria and tetanus booster (Td)
(D) IPV, fifth dose
(E) Varicella, second dose

Examination Answers

1. The answer is E. Psalter V fracture of the growing long bone refers to crush injury of the physis or growth plate, itself. Surgery is usually indicated. The Psalter classification is invoked frequently by radiologists and orthopedic surgeons. Psalter I involves simply the growth plate or physis without deformity and can easily be missed on x-ray as this cartilaginous growth area is radiolucent, of course. Psalter II fractures extend from the physis into the metaphysis (the widened end of the adjacent shaft of long bone). Psalter III breaks the other way, extending from the physis into and through the epiphysis, or boney cap interposed between the growth plate, into the joint space beyond. Psalter IV involves a combination of Psalters II and III, that is, from the physis into both the metaphysis and epiphysis. This fracture may require internal fixation as well.

2. The answer is D, Osteosarcoma. This is a case of pathologic fracture in a young person. Osteosarcoma is the most common malignancy of bone in adolescents and young adults, comprising 60% of bone cancers in that group. Typically, there has been pain and dysfunction in the affected site. Ewing tumor is the second most common. Ewing's sarcoma is in distant second place for cancers in this group, often presents with metastases in the lungs or spine. Fibrous dysplasia and enchondroma are benign conditions of preadolescent children that can lead to pathologic fractures but usually are asymptomatic beforehand. They have similar appearances on plain x-ray and can be treated by surgical curettage and bone grafting on occasion. Osteomyelitis is noted for pain but not pathologic fractures. Hematogenous osteomyelitis occurs more often in younger children, and exogenous infection occurs by contiguous spread from a surface wound.

3. The answer is A. In AN elevated FSH does not occur. As opposed to the case of ovarian failure, the cause of secondary amenorrhea (cessation after normal menarche and menstrual periods for an extended period) in AN is pituitary, and FSH is lower than normal. Other criteria for diagnosis of AN are refusal to allow weight to go above barely minimal for height; unreasonable and intense fear of obesity; distorted body image and the afore mentioned secondary.

4. The answer is D. Decreased sense of smell may indicate pituitary pathology. For growth delay of any cause, height attainment is defined as inadequate if growth rate is less than 3.7 cm (1.5 in.)/year or bone age is more than 1.5 years behind expected for age. If this occurs, it cannot be attributed to other than constitutional growth delay or

familial short stature if the review of systems is normal; nutrition is appropriate; upper to lower body segment ratio is appropriate (longer lower segment does not occur in growth insufficiency); sella tursica is of normal size by scanning techniques; and the following laboratory studies are within normal limits: count (CBC), erythrocyte sedimentation rate (ESR), urinalysis (UA), tetraiodothyronine (T4), lactic dehydrogenase (LH), FSH. Elevated alkaline phosphatase is normal for adolescent growth at any rate.

5. The answer is C. White female individuals who are between 15 and 24 years of age attempt suicide at a rate three times that of male individuals in the same age group. For all groups, the ratio between suicide threats and successful suicide ranges from 50:1 to 100:1.

6. The answer is B. White male individuals who are between 15 and 24 years of age, which is a high-risk age group, are five times as likely to commit suicide as women. This age group produces the greatest number of both attempts and completed suicides.

7. The answer is C, between 1,200 and 1,500 mg/day. The new adolescent recommendations are close to the 1,500 mg/day recommended for adults to help prevent osteoporosis.

8. The answer is D, at the age of first sexual activity. Officially, most authorities maintain that Pap smears should begin when sexual activity starts but, in any event, no later than at age 18.

9. The answer is B. Reduce the progestational component of her BCP. Progestational agents in BCPs may cause side effects consisting of breast tenderness, hypertension, headaches, and, rarely, myocardial infarction (the latter presumably related to the androgenic effects of progestational agents that include reduced high-density lipoprotein cholesterol and elevated low-density lipoprotein cholesterol and increased insulin resistance). This patient's blood pressure appears to be elevated for her age. Although it is true that many people experience migraine headaches when they begin oral birth control medications, manipulating the progesterone agent may address both the headaches and the possible hypertension lurking in the wings with this patient, although hypertension may be caused by the estrogenic effects as well.

10. The answer is E. Oily skin as a change in someone who has started the BCP is caused by androgenic effects, which are due to the progestational agent. Related to that is exacerbation of acne, depression, and fatigue. The other effects mentioned among the distracters are due to estrogenic effects, in addition to which are thromboembolic phenomena (rare), cervical ectasia (cervical ectopy), and rise in biliary cholesterol.

11. The answer is D, weight <85% of IBW. This corresponds approximately to the definition of malnutrition, which is less than fifth percentile for body mass index. Use of percentile and percent of ideal may cause confusion: 85% of ideal weight refers to the spectrum of people who are living at less than ideal weight, only 5% of whom would be expected to weigh less than 85% of ideal. Thus, the choice of 60% of ideal weight may hardly exist in a living person, except in a prison camp situation. A weight of <100 lb (45 kg) in a female individual may well be within normal limits for a small person. There is no direct relationship between caloric intake and anorexia. However, anorectics may take in as little as 100 to 200 kcal/day. The formula of 100 lb plus 5 lb for every inch of height over 60 in. is simply a rough formula for *ideal* weight estimation. There are two forms of anorexia: The "classic" is the type wherein the individual, ostensibly in unreasonable fear of weight gain, simply overrides her appetite and refuses to take in more than a minimal amount of food. The other form applies to those who vomit or purge following food intake, often prodigious amounts (i.e., bulimia). These people often experience deterioration of teeth, particularly the upper incisors, from frequent vomiting. In both cases, amenorrhea occurs after a critical level of weight loss, which is the result of homeostatic mechanisms that result in hypothalamic hypofunction in response to malnutrition, especially when it occurs in association with stress. This can be thought of as a redirecting of energy resources in favor of survival.

12. The answer is C. Vaccines of Td, a tetanus booster with an attenuated dose of diphtheria, should be administered every 10 years, starting when the child reaches the age of 11 or 12. Each of the other choices mentioned is up to date and completed at this point.

References

Centers for Disease Control: Adult Immunization Schedules, endorsed by ACIP, AAP, and AAFP.

Family Medicine Board Review, 2009. Kansas City, MO; May 3–10, 2009.

Hay WW, Levin MJ, Sondheimer JM, Deterding RR, eds. *Current Diagnosis & Treatment Pediatrics,* 19th ed. New York, Chicago: McGraw-Hill/Lange; 2009.

Kurowski K. Preventive care of the preschool child (1–5 years). In: Rudy DR, Kurowski K, eds. Baltimore, MD: Williams & Wilkins, 1997:689–702.

Rudy DR. Endocrinology. In: Rakel RE, ed. *Textbook of Family Practice,* 6th ed. Saunders; 2002.

Sternback M, Lipsky MS. Preventive care of the dolescent (12–20 years). In: Rudy DR, Kurowski K, eds. *Family Medicine: House Officer Series.* Baltimore, MD: Williams & Wilkins; 1997:713–720.

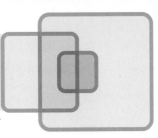

chapter **46**

Care and Prevention, Ages 21 to 40 Years

Examination questions: Unless instructed otherwise, choose the ONE lettered answer or completion that is BEST in each case.

1 In screening for obesity which of the following is the definition of obesity by body mass index (BMI):

(A) 22
(B) 25
(C) 30
(D) 35
(E) 40

2 The U.S. Preventive Services Task Force takes a very conservative approach to screening for diabetes mellitus. Which of the following is a valid criterion for routine screening for type 2 diabetes in asymptomatic adults according to the US Preventive Services Task Force (USPSTF)?

(A) BMI > 30
(B) BMI > 35
(C) Obese people who have first degree family history of diabetes
(D) Blood pressure >135/80
(E) Abdominal obesity

3 What category among the following accounts for the largest proportion of deaths in the age group of 25 to 40 years?

(A) Homicide
(B) Accidental injuries
(C) Cancer
(D) Suicide
(E) Human immunodeficiency virus (HIV) infection

4 Cancers are the third leading cause of death in the age group of 25 to 44 years. In this age group, which cancer is the leading cause of cancer death?

(A) Lung
(B) Breast
(C) Prostate
(D) Colorectal
(E) Cervix

5 A 30-year-old man who weighs 170 pounds at a height of 5 ft 10.5 in. has a repeatable blood pressure in the 110–130/70–75 range. His family history reveals that his parents are living and well at 50 and 55 years of age. He wishes to know when he should be screened for "cholesterol." You reply that according to the U.S. Preventive Services Task Force that should begin at what age?

(A) 25 years
(B) 30 years
(C) 35 years
(D) 45 years
(E) 50 years

6 A 35-year-old woman is sent for a pre-employment physical examination but had all scheduled immunizations to the age of 20. She has not seen a doctor or other health care professionals for 15 years. Which of the following immunizations should she have, assuming no special occupational risk factors and compliance with recommendations for immunizations at earlier ages?

(A) Measles, mumps, rubella (MMR) vaccine
(B) Pneumococcal vaccine
(C) Influenza vaccine
(D) Tetanus booster
(E) Hepatitis B vaccine

7 Which of the following is the least statistically important condition for which to screen in a 30-year-old woman who has no known special risk factors or family history and presents for an annual physical examination?

(A) Breast cancer
(B) Papanicolaou smear
(C) Blood pressure
(D) Complete blood cell count
(E) Presence of a smoke detector in the home

8 What are the three leading causes of death in the age group of 35 to 44 years?

(A) Malignant neoplasms, heart disease, accidents
(B) Suicide, homicide, accidents
(C) Acute lower respiratory disease, liver disease
(D) Kidney diseases, diabetes mellitus, chronic lung disease
(E) Cerebrovascular disease, influenza, chronic lung disease

9 Suicide and suicide attempts may take many turns. Which of the following statements is not true regarding suicide, the fifth-leading cause of death in the age group of 25 to 44 years and the third-leading cause of death in the age group of 25 to 34 years?

(A) Victims have often been in contact with medical services in the period just before suicide.
(B) Firearms are a significantly prevalent method in male individuals, young adults, and adolescents.
(C) Persons who have histories of previous suicidal "gestures," often dramatic, are at low risk for suicide.
(D) HIV infection and acquired immunodeficiency syndrome (AIDS) constitute significant risk status.
(E) Suicidal persons often leave subtle hints of their intentions.

For Questions 8 through 12, match the numbered immunization with the lettered condition under which it should be offered. A choice may be correct for more than one item.

10 Tetanus booster, in combination with an attenuated dose of diphtheria (Td)

11 MMR vaccine

12 Hepatitis B vaccine

13 Pneumococcal vaccine

14 Influenza vaccine

(A) Those with chronic medical conditions
(B) Those individuals born after 1956 who lack evidence of immunity
(C) Health care workers, or recipients of blood products
(D) All adults every 10 years
(E) One dose per year for ≥50 years

Examination Answers

1. The answer is C. 30, the BMI at or above which defines obesity. 25 or above is overweight; 35 or above is morbid obesity as defined for risk of obstructive sleep apnea in truck drivers. BMI is calculated as weight in Kg/height in meters squared; that is, Kg/m^2.

2. The answer is C. Obese people with first degree family histories of diabetes. Each of the other choices constitutes a significant risk factor for diabetes but does not rise to the level of an indication for screening in the eyes of the Task Force. Though now, the USPSTF is a living document published on the Net, its basic approach has not changed.

3. The answer is B. Accidental injuries is the most common cause of death in the age group of <45 years.

4. The answer is B. Breast cancer is the leading cause of cancer death in the 25–44 year group. This is astounding since the statistic applies to both sexes. In fact, for *all ages,* breast and prostate cancers are virtually tied for third ranking causes of death in causation, well behind lung cancer and the second cause, colorectal cancer. Be that as it may, the ages of onsets of the four most incident cancers in the U.S. population lend a perspective. Lung cancer is the greatest killer, but, while the cause of that cancer is laid down in the period between 16 and 40, the cancer does not generally strike until the 50s and 60s. Colorectal cancer is the second leading cause of cancer deaths and, like lung cancer, strikes nearly equally each sex but not until the 50s or later except in unusual cases. Prostate cancer also does not strike until the 50s in the most aggressive cases and most often well into the 60s and 70s.

5. The answer is C. Begin at 35 years of age screening men for cholesterol and other lipids, assuming no increase in risk for atherosclerotic disease (previous heart disease, hypertension, diabetes); USPSTF recommends lipid measurement in women beginning at age 45. Most practitioners consider this to be overly conservative and would favor such screening in the early adult years before setting out a recommended frequency of testing for each patient individually.

6. The answer is D. A tetanus booster, usually given as a Td vaccine, should be administered every 10 years.

7. The answer is A. Breast cancer is the least likely among the listed screenings to be positive in a 30-year-old woman with no particular personal or familial risk factors. Breast cancer, though the second-ranking cancer killer of women, is not screened routinely until a woman reaches the age of 40, or at an age 10 years younger than a first-degree relative who has or has had breast cancer. This question is a matter of intuition to an experienced practitioner but has not been posed in the literature in this manner. The Pap smear is recommended annually in a woman who is sexually active, reduced to every 3 years after three negative smears. Blood pressure is recommended by the USPSTF for all patients at all visits. A complete blood count has a higher chance of revealing an iron-deficiency anemia in a menstruating female than discovery of breast cancer at this age. Physicians are expected to become involved in environmental risk factors, thus, asking about smoke detector. The same with carbon monoxide detectors in a gas heated. Some physicians, particularly some psychiatrists and pediatricians, feel patients should be asked about guns being kept in the home and how they might be stored safely. Drug or alcohol abuse should also be explored in all adult patients.

8. The answer is A. Malignant neoplasms, heart disease, and accidents easily comprise the ranking causes of death in the decade of life from 35 to 44, averaging 36.8, 31, and 29.7, respectively, over the 3 years of 1999, 2000, and 2001. These data present a stark contrast to those of the previous decade and portend a significant change in the risks of life over that 10-year period. In fourth place is homicide at 14 deaths per 100,000. Thus, cancer and vascular disease virtually burst upon the scene, whereas accidents remain significant, but markedly decreased, as causes of death.

9. The answer is C. The incorrect statement is that those who have made previous ostensible attempts are at no more risk for suicide than the population at large. Although the suicidal "gesture" has become notorious in emergency rooms, anyone who makes such a gesture or attempt falls along a spectrum of attention getting at one end and determination at the other. Virtually no one in that group who has gone so far as to "rehearse" the act is without a level of intent or serious consideration for suicide.

Matching the numbered immunizations with the lettered conditions

10. Td booster: **The answer is D,** all adults every 10 years.

11. MMR vaccine: **The answer is B,** those born after 1956 who lack evidence of immunity.

12. Hepatitis B vaccine: **The answer is C,** health care workers or recipients of blood products.

13. Pneumococcal vaccine: **The answer is A,** those with chronic medical conditions.

14. Influenza vaccine: **The answer is E,** one dose per year for ≥50 years.

References

Arias E, Anderson RN, Kung H-C. Deaths: Final data for 2001. Centers for Disease Control. *Natl Vital Stat Rep.* 2003; 52(3):1–116.

Ferrante JM. Preventive care of the young adult (20–40 years). In: Rudy DR, Kurowski K, eds. *Family Medicine: House Officer Series.* Baltimore, MD: Williams & Wilkins; 1997:721–728.

U.S. Preventive Services Task Force. Screening for high blood cholesterol and other lipid abnormalities. In: *Guide to Clinical Preventive Services: Report of the U.S. Preventive Services Task Force.* Baltimore, MD: Williams & Wilkins; 1996:39–53.

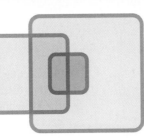

chapter 47

Care and Prevention of the Middle-Aged Adult, Ages 41 to 65 Years

Examination questions: Unless instructed otherwise, choose the ONE lettered answer or completion that is BEST in each case

1. A 65-year-old man had smoked for 40 pack years until the age of 60. He has become aware of 7 of his high school classmates who have died or are under treatment for lung cancer over the previous 5 years. All were cigarette smokers, three of whom had stopped smoking more than 10 years before diagnosis. The patient asks about lung cancer screening tests. After telling the patient that lung cancer screening is far from adequate, he explains that (which of the following screening methods) is the most sensitive?

(A) Chest x-ray PA and lateral
(B) Sputum cytology
(C) Low dose computed tomography (LDCT)
(D) Bone scan
(E) positive emission tomography (PET) scan

2. You are consulting with a 50-year-old man at the time of his first comprehensive physical examination in 15 years. You have on hand a baseline electrocardiogram (EKG) taken when he had his last examination 15 years ago, read as normal (another was unchanged during an emergency department visit for atypical chest pain 1 year ago). He expresses a desire to begin preventive health care under your guidance. Along the way, you elicit information that he smokes one pack of cigarettes per day, weighs 208 lb (94.2 kg) at a height of 5 ft 10 in. (1.78 m), and has a history of "high cholesterol." Which of the following is the most appropriate combination of screening tests for this person, in addition to routine physical examination?

(A) EKG, complete blood cell (CBC) count, and lipid screen
(B) EKG stress test, CBC count, and liver and kidney function studies

(C) Chest x-ray, EKG, and comprehensive chemical profile
(D) Prostate-specific antigen (PSA) test, lipid screen, fecal occult blood test (FOBT), and blood sugar test
(E) Chest x-ray, pulmonary function studies, lipid screen and routine chemistries, and CBC count

3. A 45-year-old white woman returns to you for routine preventive care, having not seen you except for episodic problems for the past 6 years. Her family history is unremarkable except for the mention of colon polyps in her sister, who is 10 years older than she is. Her weight is 120 lb (54.4 kg) at a height of 5 ft 5 in. (1.65 m). She is a nonsmoker. Which of the following, in addition to a routine physical examination, is the most appropriate combination of screening tests for this patient?

(A) EKG stress test, CBC count, and liver and kidney function studies
(B) Papanicolaou smear (Pap smear), mammogram, colorectal cancer (CRC) screening, CBC count, and comprehensive chemical profile
(C) Chest x-ray, Pap smear, EKG, and comprehensive chemical profile
(D) Lipid screen, FOBT, mammogram, and blood sugar
(E) Chest x-ray, pulmonary function studies, lipid screen and routine chemistries, and CBC count

4. The patient in Question 3 returns for her routine examination on schedule for the following 2 years. Her Pap smears have all been normal and adequate for evaluation. She is in a monogamous relationship. She asks how frequently she should have Pap smears in the future. What is your answer?

(A) Every 6 months
(B) Annually
(C) Every 2 years

(D) Every 3 years

(E) Every 5 years

5 A 55-year-old woman is being followed for her type 2 diabetes. She takes metformin 500 mg thrice daily and glyburide 2.5 mg twice daily, and the diabetes control has been fair, but she has been somewhat careless in complying with the recommended frequency of visits. The glycohemoglobin was 7.1 on her last visit 2 weeks ago. Each of the following is recommended by the American Diabetes Association (ADA) in monitoring this diabetic's progress except for which?

(A) Annual examination by an ophthalmologist

(B) Glycohemoglobin level check every 3 months

(C) Annual EKG

(D) Annual check of blood urea nitrogen and creatinine levels

(E) Examination of the feet on each visit

6 A 48-year-old male municipal bus driver is 40 lb (18 kg) overweight. In counseling him to lose weight, you allude to all of the following problems as aggravated by obesity except for which one?

(A) Coronary heart disease

(B) Diabetes

(C) Osteoporosis

(D) Osteoarthritis

(E) Hypertension

7 A 41-year-old black man comes to you for his first comprehensive physical examination. Of the following, which screening procedures merit attention not accorded to white men, otherwise matched for age, weight, and other risk factors?

(A) Prostate cancer and glaucoma

(B) CRC and lung cancer

(C) Diabetes and dyslipidemia

(D) Coronary artery disease and mitral valve prolapse

(E) Hypertrophic cardiomyopathy

8 In selecting out special guidelines for management of certain diseases in certain ethnic groups, in which of the following groups should you adjust therapeutic targets to tighter control of hypertension and diabetes?

(A) Mexican Americans

(B) Ashkenazi Jews

(C) South Asians (Indians and Pakistani)

(D) Chinese Americans

(E) African-Americans

9 A 45-year-old man, a new patient, visits the office for a complete physical examination. You discover while eliciting the family history that his father died of colon cancer, contracted at the age of 60. He has no other first-degree relatives with colon cancer. On the basis of the American Cancer Society recommendations, you recommend that this patient have CRC screening by what modalities?

(A) Digital rectal examination (DRE), FOBT, and flexible sigmoidoscopy every 2 years

(B) DRE and FOBT annually

(C) DRE and colonoscopy now and every 3 years if negative

(D) Colonoscopy annually

(E) Flexible sigmoidoscopy and barium enema every 5 years

10 The Guide to Preventive Services notwithstanding, what is the community standard for screening for prostate cancer in men of average risk?

(A) DRE annually for all males starting at 40 years of age

(B) Serum PSA for males starting at age 50

(C) BUN and creatinine at age 40 and above

(D) PSA and DRE starting at age 50

(E) Urinalysis, BUN, and creatinine at age 40

Examination Answers

1. The answer is C. LDCT is 4 times more sensitive than that of a chest x-ray. However, the specificity is not satisfactory, and an LDCT brings with it the serious problem of expense and emotional trauma entailed in following up false-positive studies. Sputum cytology has not yielded evidence of effectiveness as a screening method. Bone scan is not a screening tool nor is PET scan.

2. The answer is D. PSA, lipid screen, FOBT, and blood sugar. This smoking, overweight man first should have certain screening examinations that begin at the age of 50 years in individuals of average health risk status. These include prostate cancer screening (which, in addition to the PSA, requires a digital rectal examination for prostate cancer) and CRC screening. The minimal level of CRC screening is the FOBT (two sites on each of three random stools, annually). In addition, a lipid screen should be obtained (at the least, total cholesterol level, but ideally the total spectrum of total, high-density lipoprotein, and low-density lipoprotein cholesterol levels, as well as serum triglyceride level). Comprehensive chemistries including hepatic and renal function studies serve a commonsense purpose in a 50-year-old man who has not had a complete examination in years; however, the U.S. Preventive Services Task Force, an ultraconservative organization, is not assertive on this issue. An EKG, especially in light of two previous baseline traces, has limited value and is not recommended on a routine basis, although often done in consultation with the patient. Chest x-ray in an asymptomatic patient has no screening value, even in a smoker, as lung cancers diagnosed on x-ray are at too advanced a stage for cure. Pulmonary function studies and EKG stress testing are also not recommended for routine screening.

3. The answer is B. Pap smear, mammogram, CRC screening, CBC count, and comprehensive chemical profile. There are three critical points to be made here. First, a Pap smear is essential in a sexually active woman. Second, a mammogram should be performed annually, beginning when the woman reaches the age of 40 years. Third, CRC screening, starting at 50 years of age in people of average risk, should begin annually in a person's 40s when there is a first-degree family history of either adenomatous polyps or CRC. The CBC count and chemical profile are reasonable in a patient who has not had a comprehensive examination for 6 years. Chest x-ray has no place as a screening tool. The EKG is not important but has some value to provide a baseline datum.

4. The answer is D. Pap smears can be performed at the reduced frequency of every 3 years after three consecutive benign readings (i.e., no precancerous or malignant changes), provided the patient has no significant risk factors. The reasons for this are first, that the 60% to 80% sensitive Pap smear becomes 94% on the third smear; second that "most" invasive disease occurs in women who have either never had Pap smears or have had none in 5 years (Guide, 2009). This is in accord with most medical organizations with the possible exception of the American College of Obstetrics and Gynecology.

5. The answer is C. An annual EKG is not one of the recommendations of the ADA. Each of the other parameters should be checked according to the ADA in the frequencies noted. In addition, lipids should be checked annually; home blood sugars should be recorded upon every visit, along with blood sugar levels at the times of visits with the physician; and, of course, blood pressure and weight should be recorded at each visit as well. An annual ophthalmologic examination is done to diagnose early retinopathy of the proliferative type that extends into the vitreous body, which is treatable by laser. Renal function deteriorates at an accelerated pace in the face of poor blood sugar (and blood pressure) control. Thus, in addition to blood urea nitrogen and creatinine, urine for microalbumen should be investigated annually as well. Feet should be examined for light touch, sharp and dull perception, skin nutrition, and pulses, as well as for nonhealing ulcers and other sores.

6. The answer is C. Osteoporosis is the least aggravated by obesity among those conditions listed. Sedentary lifestyle predisposes one to all the others listed. Sedentary lifestyle is characterized by a tendency for obesity that may precipitate diabetes, aggravate hypertension, increase total cholesterol, and decrease high-density lipoprotein cholesterol. In addition, through an increase in weight bearing, obesity promotes osteoblastic in excess of osteoclastic activity (thus protecting against osteoporosis). All but osteoporosis and osteoarthritis are in turn risk factors for coronary artery disease.

7. The answer is A. Prostate cancer and glaucoma are two conditions that merit screening at the age of 40 in black men, whereas in the rest of the male population, otherwise matched for weight, family history, and other risk factors, these conditions are not addressed until the age of 50.

Although diabetes is more prevalent in African-Americans, it is not so when matched for weight and age with white individuals. The same can be said for coronary heart disease and dyslipidemia. Mitral valve prolapse and hypertrophic cardiomyopathy are not discussed meaningfully in epidemiologic terms.

8. The answer is E. African-Americans with hypertension suffer earlier onset and a greater incidence of cerebrovascular disease (strokes) and renal failure as complications than do other group with matched levels of average blood pressure. Therefore, the therapeutic target for control of hypertension is set at 125/75 rather than simply settling it for statistically normal blood pressure, ≤140/≥90. Similarly, diabetes mellitus exacts a greater price in accelerated decremental renal failure for given levels of blood sugar control. Although Mexican Americans and indigenous Americans have a far greater risk of diabetes for a given body mass index, their complication rates are not out of proportion to their levels of blood sugar control.

9. The answer is C. Colonoscopy now and every 3 years if negative. A family history of colon cancer in a first-degree relative (father at age 60) multiplies the lifetime risk of colon cancer, normally about 2.5%, 3 times, so this patient now has a 7.5% chance of colon cancer. Most of the risk in this circumstance is telescoped into the decades of the 50s and above. Thus, this patient's chances are higher than 7.5%. Colonoscopy, if negative, need not be repeated for 3 years because of the long "dwell time" for that cancer.

10. The answer is D. Serum PSA and digital rectal examination starting at age 50 is the community standard. The reason the Guide to Preventive Services, published by the USPSTF, makes no commitment as to screening for prostate cancer is that the PSA is not as specific as would be desired, given the costs of working up false positives. However, in primary care practice, the great sensitivity of the test in a population with low to average risk allows peace of mind in a vast number of cases for any false positives that may emerge, leading to emotional and financial expense. Moreover, many of the "false positives" who are thus subjected to worry and uncomfortable procedures such as needle biopsy of the prostate eventually show up with prostate cancer after long follow-up.

References

Jennifer O. Assistant Professor Chicago Medical School. Personal communication.

Kerlikowske K, Grady D, Barclay J, et al. Effects of age, breast density, and family history on the sensitivity of first screening mammography. *JAMA.* 1996; 276:33–38.

Marwick C. Other voices weigh in on mammography decision. *JAMA.* 1997; 277:1027–1028.

Miller KE. Preventive care of the middle-aged adult (40–65 years). In: Rudy DR, Kurowski K, eds. Baltimore: Williams & Wilkins, 1997:729–740.

The Guide to Preventive Services 2009. Recommendations of the U.S. Preventive Services Task Force. Agency for Healthcare Research and Quality.

chapter 48

Care and Prevention of the Older Adult, Age 65 and Older

Examination questions: Unless instructed otherwise, choose the ONE lettered answer or completion that is BEST in each case.

1 Which of the following statements best supports the position of the Guide to Preventive Services of the U.S. Preventive Services Task Force regarding screening for cutaneous melanoma?

(A) Patients over 65 years of age should undergo total body skin examination by a physician on an annual basis.

(B) Patients should carry out total body skin self-examination on a regular basis.

(C) Patients over 65 years of age with more than 50 moles should be examined on a regular basis for melanoma.

(D) Dark complexioned people over the age of 65 should see a physician annually for total body skin examination.

(E) Any mole that is asymmetrical, variegated in color, or greater than 6 mm in diameter should be referred for excision.

2 A 78-year-old woman has seemed difficulty to follow in conversation. In interviewing her, the doctor sometimes wonders if her mind had wandered because she cannot discern a coherent message in her conversation. Otherwise, she manifests no neurological symptoms or signs. A comprehensive metabolic profile reveals both alanine aminotransferase and aspartate aminotransferase levels to be elevated by about 50% of their normal values. Suspecting alcoholism, you (the doctor) contemplate which strategy you should use to confirm this fact. Which of the following would be the most sensitive?

(A) Ask the patient how much she drinks

(B) Check the patient's cerebellar function on physical examination

(C) Ask the patient standardized screening questions for alcoholism, such as those from the CAGE questionnaire

(D) Palpate for ascites

(E) Look for spider angiomas on the patient's skin

3 A 65-year-old female is being seen for a general physical examination. She is active and without complaints. She had a complete hysterectomy 20 years ago for benign uterine fibroids. Two months ago, she had a negative mammogram as ordered by her gynecologist. She has no family history of colorectal cancer (CRC). She had a flu vaccination two months ago and a pneumonia vaccination five years ago. She had a normal mammogram last year. She had a normal cholesterol level 2 years ago. Her physical examination is unremarkable. Her lungs are clear. Her breasts have no masses. There are no abdominal masses. Her rectal examination is negative. She is concerned regarding the cost. Which of the following preventive measures is clearly indicated for her?

(A) Repeat pneumonia vaccination

(B) CRC screening

(C) Mammogram

(D) Pap smear

(E) Lipid profile

4 A 55-year-old female of mixed English and Scottish descent is undergoing her annual pelvic examination, Pap smear, and breast examination. The subject of her cigarette smoking comes up, as it does each year. Again, the doctor takes time to point out the dangers of smoking, hoping for the "teachable moment." For each of the following items, smoking is a significant risk, except for which one?

(A) Bladder cancer

(B) Bulimia nervosa

(C) Hip fracture

(D) Lung cancer

(E) Peptic ulcer disease

5 Of the following persons, who is most likely to be an abuser of an elderly individual in the United States?

(A) A spouse
(B) A hired caretaker
(C) A son
(D) A daughter
(E) A stranger who has broken into the home

6 Which of the following hypertensive blood pressure readings is most likely to be found particularly in a patient over the age of 65 years?

(A) 210/110
(B) 190/100
(C) 120/95
(D) 160/80
(E) 140/90

7 A 75-year-old man is in good health and mentally competent to care for himself. He underwent a complete examination 5 years ago that included a normal screening colonoscopy, and he has submitted fecal occult blood test (FOBTs) in the intervening years. He lives alone and wishes to undergo a routine health maintenance examination. Which of the following would be least fruitful as a screening test?

(A) Flexible sigmoidoscopy and FOBTs
(B) Thyroid-stimulating hormone test
(C) Urinalysis
(D) Blood pressure reading
(E) "Up-and-go test"

8 A 50-year-old patient brings in her dependent mother, aged 81. The elderly woman has been forgetting things recently, but she is able to subtract sevens from 100 (she is a retired math teacher). She is well groomed and socially adept. The daughter wishes for her to be screened for Alzheimer disease (AD). Which of the following would be the most relevant reason for screening for early diagnosis of AD?

(A) Improve the intelligence quotient of the patient
(B) Stop the progression of AD
(C) Reverse the course of AD
(D) Prepare caregiver(s) and family for management and socioeconomic issues
(E) Prevent strokes

9 A family doctor chooses to screen for AD with the Folstein Mini-Mental State Examination, of which the sensitivity is known to be 87%. What approximate percentage of those tested will exhibit a false-positive result?

(A) 10%
(B) 20%
(C) 40%
(D) 50%
(E) 60%

10 Each of the following statements regarding falls in "older elderly" persons (>75 years of age) is true, except for which one?

(A) Most falls occur outside of the home environment.
(B) The risk of falls is directly related to the number of medications the elderly patient is taking.
(C) Alcohol is a contributing risk factor for falls.
(D) The most common injuries incurred in falls among elderly individuals are wrist, hip, and vertebral fractures.
(E) Falls often occur in mentally competent elderly people.

11 An elderly couple ask several questions about living wills while you are updating their health history. Which of the following statements is correct with respect to living wills?

(A) They are not usually honored by courts.
(B) They are only appropriate for the terminally ill individual to communicate desires regarding specific life-support measures.
(C) The wishes of immediate family members take legal precedence over the living will of the individual.
(D) They allow the individual to communicate desires for or against specific life-support measures toward the time when health status makes him or her unable to do so.
(E) They must be prepared by attorneys.

Examination Answers

1. The answer is C. Patients over 65 years of age with more than 50 moles should be examined on a regular basis for melanoma. Even that conclusion is an inference, not a definite position statement in the 2009 Guide. Such an inference could be drawn as well from the Guide's acknowledgment that other high-risk categories include (65 years old) fair skinned people, those with histories of frequent sun burning in the past, and family histories of melanoma. The Guide acknowledges the high-risk status of moles' shapes (asymmetrical), colors (variegated), and sizes (>6 mm) but implies that these characteristics are criteria for treatment, not screening. Their general position is that they cannot, based on "the balance of benefits and harms," recommend for or against total body professional or self-examination for basal cell and squamous cell carcinomas and cutaneous melanomas.

2. The answer is C. Ask standardized screening questions for alcoholism such as the CAGE questionnaire. Sets of standardized alcoholic screening questions are a more sensitive indicator than just asking about alcohol consumption. Cerebellar function impairments may be subtle and only manifest with acute intoxication. Patients vary in their propensities to develop alcoholic hepatitis and telangiectasias, even for a given amount and duration of alcohol consumption. An elevated aspartate aminotransferase level is a nonspecific indicator of hepatocellular damage, which is not necessarily present in alcoholism. The other choices yield positive results but at a much later stage of alcoholism than the CAGE questionnaire, assuming it is done with a low threshold for suspicion. (CAGE is an acronym taken from the following items: C, cutting down; A, annoyed by criticism of others; G, guilty about drinking; E, (need) eye opener.)

3. The answer is B. CRC screening is indicated in this hypothetical 65-year-old patient. The lifetime incidence of CRC in people of average risk is 2.5%. It is safe to say that for a cancer whose incidence in the population accelerates with age and that the over 60 age group has survived heart disease, accidents, and so on, the incidence of CRC would be expected to be significantly higher than 2.5% in this cohort. There are at least five methods approved by the American Gastroenterology Association with the gold standard being colonoscopy. Mammogram should be done yearly beginning at the age of 40 years until at least the age of 65 as has occurred in this patient. The pneumococcal vaccine is generally indicated once or twice in the adult lifetime. Her hysterectomy was for benign disease and she does not need Pap smears. A favorable lipid profile on a postmenopausal female need not be repeated frequently unless there has been a material change in the patient's living style and weight.

4. The answer is B. Bulimia nervosa. Pure bulimia is an overeating disorder, without, in its pure form, purging or vomiting. Thus, weight loss is not a part of the syndrome. Actually, part of the addiction, if it occurs at all, is due to a stimulant effect of nicotine. This results in an amphetamine-like effect so that one of the complications of *smoking cessation* is weight gain. All the other diseases mentioned in the choices occur at significantly greater incidence in smokers as compared to nonsmokers. For the slender postmenopausal woman of Celtic origin, osteoporosis is a significant risk, multiplied 1.5 to twofold in a cigarette smoker.

5. The answer is A. A spouse. Relatives, especially spouses, are most likely to be the abusers. They may be actively or passively abusive.

6. The answer is D. 160/80, if in a steady state, fits the definition of isolated systolic hypertension (ISH). This is more likely in the older age group. Thiazide diuretics are most effective in salt/water retention conditions; namely, the low renin end of the hypertensive spectrum. Implied is that ISH is a low renin state. It is well known that if beta-adrenergic blocking agents are used in the oldest age group, a greater dosage is required. Thus, being anti-renin agents, they are less effective because renin played a less significant part in ISH as compared to the broad spectrum of the remainder of hypertension.

7. The answer is A. Flexible sigmoidoscopy and FOBTs are the least likely to prevent disease in a patient who has a life expectancy of 5 to 10 years. Blood pressure control can prevent strokes; thyroid-stimulating hormone can unearth hypothyroidism in the absence of typical symptoms, especially in an elderly person; urinalysis can reveal subclinical urinary tract infection. The up-and-go test can rule out the possibility that the patient may be physically unable to care for himself alone. The test consists of asking the patient to arise from a sitting position without the use of his or her hands, walk 10 ft (3 m), and return to the originally sitting site and position. If the patient can perform this satisfactorily in ≤10 seconds, then he or she is assumed to be physically able. If the activity requires more than 30 seconds, then the patient very likely will require physical assistance at home.

8. The answer is D. Preparing caregiver(s) and the family for management and socioeconomic issues for a patient with imminent AD is worthwhile in the view of most clinicians. Early diagnosis of AD alerts the primary care physician to avoid anticholinergic medications, as these are agents that worsen dementia. Among the serious mental illnesses to be found in elderly individuals, dementia is the most prevalent, with the others being depression, delirium, schizophrenia, and bipolar disorder. Another good reason for early diagnosis of dementia is the unearthing of reversible causes of dementia in elderly persons, such as anemia, urinary tract infection, chronic pain, and, sometimes, simply radical change of environment.

9. The answer is C. 40%. Actually, the official figure for the false-positive rate in the Folstein Mini-Mental State Examination is 39.4%, that is, somewhere in the range of 30% to 50% of elderly persons older than the age of 85 years, they suffer from a degree of dementia, but the vast majority do not qualify for a diagnosis of AD. This should lend a note of sobriety to the administration of the Folstein test. Elderly persons may fail the test because of fatigue, motivation, or anxiety. Dementia, of which AD is the most common form among elderly individuals, involves (a) at least one language-impairment problem (word finding, later difficulty following a conversation, or mutism); (b) apraxia (inability to perform certain previously learned manual tasks, such as cutting a loaf of bread by using both hands despite manifesting no sensory or motor abnormalities); and (c) impaired organization (sometimes called executive ability) such as poor mental flexibility, planning, and judgment. Subsets in screening regarding the foregoing categories are in play. In the verbal category, including attention and concentration, the patient may be asked to recite name, address, and phone numbers; to recall three unrelated words such as "tulip, umbrella, scar" or parts of objects such as lapel and cuff; and follow a mildly complex command such as "point to the ceiling before you point to the floor." A corollary to praxis functioning is visuospatial organization such as drawing a clock with a prescribed time indicated. Regarding organizational ability, there may be questions involving logic, such as "how is a peach like a pear?"

10. The answer is A. The incorrect statement is that most falls among elderly persons occur outside of the home environment. Thus, most falls among elderly persons occur in or around the home. Falls in the home may be indirectly caused by conditions that would be viewed as relatively benign for agile and mentally competent people, such as slippery or warped floors, shag carpet, or thick rugs, which present opportunities for elderly individuals to trip. Risk of falls is directly related to the number of medications the elderly patient is taking, obviously especially those involving sedatives, antihypertensives, alcohol, antidepressants, or neuroleptics, or overdosage with beta-adrenergic blocking agents. The most common injuries incurred in falls among elderly individuals are wrist, hip, and vertebral fractures. Hip fractures will occur in one-third of women and one-sixth of men in the "old elderly" age group. Hip fractures carry a 20% first-year mortality rate. Another significant risk from trauma in elderly individuals is subdural hematoma. Falls often occur in mentally competent elderly people. These are the frail elderly, often victims of osteoporosis or malnutrition, the former more often among women and the latter among men.

11. The answer is D. They allow the individual to communicate the desire for or against specific life-support measures in the event that the individual's health status at some point makes him or her unable to do so. Living wills have been honored by courts and do not require the use of an attorney. Catastrophic illness, which leaves the individual unable to communicate wishes, can occur with anyone, but particularly with elderly persons. Living wills give them a mechanism to convey their wishes.

References

Bross MH, Tryon AF. Preventive care of the older adult (>65 years). In: Rudy DR, Kurowski K, eds. *Family Medicine: House Officer Series*. Baltimore: Williams & Wilkins; 1997:741–750.

Dickman R. Care of the elderly. In: Rakel RE, ed. *Textbook of Family Practice*. Philadelphia: WB Saunders; 2002.

Family Medicine Review. Kansas City, Missouri; May 3–10; 2009.

McPhee SJ, Papadakis MA. *Current Medical Diagnosis and Treatment*. 49th ed. New York/Chicago: Lange, McGraw-Hill; 2010.

Rudy DR. Endocrinology. In: Rakel RE, ed. *Textbook of Family Practice*. 6th ed. Philadelphia: WB Saunders; 2002.

The Guide to Preventive Services 2009. Recommendations of the U.S. Preventive Services Task Force.

chapter 49

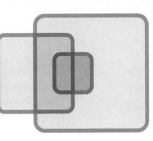

Travel Medicine

Examination questions: Unless instructed otherwise, choose the ONE lettered answer or completion that is BEST in each case.

1 What is the minimal age at which an infant should be allowed to share in commercial travel?

(A) One day
(B) One week
(C) One month
(D) Six months
(E) One year

2 At which of the following regions of the world is the drug of choice to treat travelers diarrhea likely to be azithromycin?

(A) Mexico
(B) Guatemala
(C) Kenya
(D) Thailand
(E) Republic of South Africa

3 Which of the following diseases is encountered most commonly among travelers?

(A) Diarrhea
(B) Pneumonia
(C) Malaria
(D) Skin rashes
(E) Viral hepatitis

4 Which of the following is the most significant (i.e., serious as well as frequent) medical problem of those related to travel?

(A) Diarrhea
(B) Pneumonia
(C) Sunburn
(D) Skin rashes
(E) Viral hepatitis

5 Which of the following drugs is the first choice for malaria prophylaxis in an area of the world in which the plasmodium is known to be resistant to multiple drugs?

(A) Hydroxychloroquine
(B) Doxycycline

(C) Halofantrine
(D) Mefloquine
(E) Pyrimethamine

6 Your patient, a 25-year-old married woman who is pregnant, solicits your opinion as to advisability of travel. Which of the following statements is true regarding travel during pregnancy?

(A) Travel is best done in the first trimester.
(B) Most airlines require a physician's permission for air travel by a pregnant woman.
(C) Travel to areas of high risk for malaria should be avoided.
(D) For treatment of upper respiratory tract infections in the first trimester, for example, in covering symptoms as well as the possibility of beta-hemolytic streptococcal disease, ampicillin may be used, along with astemizole (Hismanal) or terfenadine (Seldane).
(E) For diarrhea during the first or second trimester, sulfamethoxazole, erythromycin, and loperamide (Imodium) should be avoided.

7 Alveolar PO_2, normally about 100 mm Hg in a healthy person at sea level, falls to what level at an altitude of 10,000 ft (3,048 m)?

(A) 47 mm Hg
(B) 79 mm Hg
(C) 61 mm Hg
(D) 46 mm Hg
(E) 88% saturation

8 A 25-year-old male patient is mountain climbing. On the 2nd day, he develops nausea, headache, inability to concentrate, and 1 to 2+ ankle edema. What is the altitude above which, it can be said, these symptoms begin to occur in significant number of travelers who have not accommodated to altitude in advance?

(A) 2,000 ft (610 m)
(B) 6,500 ft (1,981 m)
(C) 8,000 ft (2,438 m)
(D) 12,500 ft (3,810 m)
(E) 15,000 ft (4,572 m)

9 Regarding the patient in Question 8, which of the following measures would be most reasonable and beneficial, assuming descent is not a practical solution and relief seems necessary at this time?

(A) Acetazolamide (Diamox) administration
(B) Dexamethasone in a tapering course
(C) Oxygen administration
(D) Pressure tent
(E) Diltiazem

10 The most serious symptoms that may occur with high-altitude sickness (HAI) are pulmonary edema, that is, high-altitude pulmonary edema (HAPE), and cerebral edema, that is, high-altitude cerebral edema (HACE). At what altitude do they become significant possibilities for travelers who are unaccommodated to altitude?

(A) 2,000 ft (610 m)
(B) 6,500 ft (1,981 m)
(C) 8,000 ft (2,438 m)
(D) 12,500 ft (3,810 m)
(E) 15,000 ft (4,572 m)

11 An 18-year-old man, who lives on the east coast, flies to Cuzco, Peru (11,152 ft, or 3,399 m) and immediately pursues his plan to hike to 2,000 ft (610 m) above the town, joining a group of high-altitude hikers. On the morning of the 2nd day, the group has reached 12,000 ft (3,658 m) of altitude en route to the Fortress of Sacsayhuaman. He begins to complain of coughing and shortness of breath, eventually producing a frothy pink sputum. Each of the following would be appropriate except for (which) one?

(A) Rapid descent of 500 ft (152 m), if possible
(B) Furosemide
(C) Oxygen 1 to 2 L/minute
(D) Acetazolamide
(E) Hyperbaric tent

12 A 45-year-old female patient reveals that a friend has offered to take her on a transcontinental flight in his private unpressurized aircraft. The patient has a history of HAI at 13,500 ft (4,114 m) during a mountain hiking expedition. She has had numerous benign experiences at altitudes of 10,000 ft (3,048 m) or lower. Otherwise, she is healthy. Which of the following is appropriate advice for her regarding the prospective flight and her health?

(A) She should not make the flight because of her history of HAI.
(B) She should postpone the trip until she has undergone blood gas studies.
(C) She may take the trip and will require no special preparations or treatments compared with other people on the plane.

(D) She is safe but should undergo electrocardiogram testing before making the final decision.
(E) She may go on the trip as long as she takes oxygen throughout the flight.

13 What cabin altitudes (terrestrial altitudes equivalent in atmospheric pressure to pressures in cabins of pressurized aircraft) would the patient in Question 11 expect to encounter in pressurized commercial jet aircraft?

(A) Sea level (cabin pressure encountered at sea level)
(B) 500 ft (152 m)
(C) 2,000 ft (610 m)
(D) Up to 5,000 ft (1,524 m)
(E) Up to 10,000 ft (3,048 m)

14 Many immunizations are recommended before travel simply for the general principle of the traveler remaining current for all routine immunizations. Others are recommended for reasons more specific to the country to be visited. Which of the following immunizations is recommended in the period of 1 to 3 months before travel to any developing country?

(A) A tetanus booster with an attenuated dose of diphtheria (Td)
(B) Influenza
(C) Polio
(D) Rabies
(E) Japanese encephalitis

15 A 36-year-old woman with a history of atopic diseases consisting of seasonal rhinitis (in the spring and fall), but without asthma, consults you in August after a week of rhinitis symptoms because she is planning a trip by commercial air travel to Nova Scotia. Once, while recovering from a cold, she had suffered severe ear pain. Which of the following statements is true regarding secretory otitis media of flight ("barotitis" or "aerotitis")?

(A) It occurs most frequently during ascent in flight.
(B) The proximate cause of barotitis media is *Streptococcus pneumoniae.*
(C) It can be prevented if the patient is able to force air into the middle ears through the Eustachian tube during descent by means of the modified Valsalva maneuver.
(D) The physical evidence of this form of secretory otitis media is a bulging tympanic membrane seen at otoscopy.
(E) The same problem may occur during scuba diving, requiring the diver to delay ascent to control symptoms and to "clear the ears."

16 Your patient consults you regarding travel abroad. Eventually, you introduce the topic of typhoid because you know he is planning a trip into a country for which typhoid vaccination is recommended. To which of the following regions is he planning to travel?

(A) Canada
(B) Indian subcontinent
(C) Europe
(D) Australia
(E) New Zealand

17 Which of the following is true regarding "jet lag"?

(A) Rapid west-to-east travel across time zones often results in somnolence that is inappropriate to local time at the destination.
(B) Rapid east-to-west travel often results in difficulty in sleep onset relative to local time at the destination.
(C) Anti-jetlag diets have proven effective in preventing jetlag symptoms.
(D) Paradoxical hypovolemia in the face of fluid retention plays a significant part in the pathophysiology of jetlag.
(E) Cabin altitudes of 5,000 ft (1,524 m) play a significant part in the pathophysiology of jetlag.

18 An emerging concept in travel medicine is that of post-travel evaluation. Which of the following would be checked for logically in an *asymptomatic* returning traveler who had been to a tropical location?

(A) Giardiasis
(B) Tuberculosis skin testing
(C) Hepatitis screen
(D) Sigmoidoscopy for schistosomiasis
(E) Malarial smear

19 Which of the following patients should be denied medical approval for travel?

(A) A 55-year-old white man with stable angina pectoris
(B) A 62-year-old African-American man with nocturnal dyspnea and orthopnea
(C) A 58-year-old white woman whose status is 5 weeks after uncomplicated myocardial infarction
(D) A 57-year-old man with chronic lung disease who is unable to climb two flights of stairs or to walk for two blocks
(E) A 35-year-old woman who is 7 months into an uncomplicated pregnancy

Examination Answers

1. The answer is B. At less than 1 week of age, the lower cabin pressure brings a lower partial pressure of oxygen. This may be insufficient for the cardiorespiratory system of the newborn as it adapts to extra-uterine life. This applies to full-term babies without congenital heart disease resulting in desaturation such as right to left shunting lesions.

2. The answer is D. In Thailand, travelers diarrhea is more likely to be caused by a fluoroquinolone-resistant invasive bacterium such as *Campylobacter pylori*. Azithromycin is thus the drug of choice at this point in time. Latin America where toxin-producing bacteria are the most likely cause of travelers diarrhea, the malady is best treated with something like loperamide titrated to dose responsiveness and perhaps a single dose of ciprofloxacin, levofloxacin, or fluoroquinolone. If that approach fails, then 100 mg azithromycin is appropriate.

3. The answer is A. Diarrhea is the most common medical problem in travelers. Those who spend at least 1 month in the other country face a 60% chance of becoming ill and a 1% chance of being admitted to hospital. Antibiotic/antibacterial prophylaxis against travelers diarrhea is best employed in anticipation of short stays, presence of diabetes, or chronic diarrhea, and, in those situations, is 90% successful. Prophylactic antibiotics are generally *not* recommended except in the above situation. Bismuth subsalicylate is about 65% effective in preventing travelers diarrhea, but salicylate contraindications must be observed. For travel to South Asia, the best regimen is a quinolone, such as norfloxacin 400 mg/day, ciprofloxacin 500 mg/day, or ofloxacin 200 mg/day.

4. The answer is E. Viral hepatitis, of those mentioned in the question, is the most serious common medical problem encountered in travel. Not only is it commonly encountered, but it is also likely to be particularly disabling to a traveler. Unless the traveler has participated in parenteral illicit drug use or risky sexual practices, any hepatitis encountered will be hepatitis A or E, contracted from water or uncooked raw vegetables in an underdeveloped country.

5. The answer is D. B. Doxycycline is *presently* the first choice for malaria prophylaxis in areas known to harbor multiple drug resistance.

6. The answer is C. Travel during pregnancy to areas of high risk for malaria should be avoided, especially in areas noted for chloroquine resistance. Malaria has a more malignant course in pregnancy and the alternative therapies in event of chloroquine resistance are more toxic, even in nonpregnant patients. Air travel is best done in the *second* trimester. Most airlines require a physician's permission for air travel by a pregnant woman only after she has reached 35 or 36 weeks of gestation. Although ampicillin is safe in pregnancy, astemizole and terfenadine should not be used in the first trimester. For diarrhea during pregnancy, trimethoprim/sulfamethoxazole, erythromycin, and loperamide are safe to use.

7. The answer is C. A measure of 61 mm Hg is the *alveolar* PO_2 at an altitude of 10,000 ft (3,048 m). Remember, the alveolar PO_2 is, at best, the ambient PO_2 minus the partial pressure of alveolar CO_2 and H_2O, the latter constant at 47 mm Hg; 47 mm Hg is the constant partial pressure of water vapor at all *ambient* pressures. Note that 79 mm Hg is the *ambient* PO_2 at 18,000 ft (5,486 m), the altitude beneath which lies half the atmosphere; 46 mm Hg is the *alveolar* PO_2 at an altitude of 15,000 ft (4,572 m); 88% represents the arterial blood saturation, normally 95%, in a healthy person at 7,500 ft (2,286 m).

8. The answer is B. Height of 6,500 ft (1,981 m) is the altitude above which it can be said that symptoms of mountain sickness occur in 25% of travelers. This degree of illness is called acute mountain sickness. The incidence increases to 50% as altitude rises to 10,000 ft (3,048 m). These symptoms are likely to be classified as mild, consisting of headache, dysphoria, nausea, peripheral edema, unexpected sighing, and nocturnal Cheyne–Stokes breathing. Nearly always, resting at altitude for 1 to 2 days will result in abatement of mild symptoms of altitude sickness. Wrong advice would be to exercise strenuously during the first 2 days at altitude to prevent altitude sickness. All others are correct. The saying is "climb high, sleep low," especially at higher altitudes, to avoid HAPE and HACE.

9. The answer is A. Acetazolamide (Diamox) administration, one 750-mg tablet, perhaps repeated, or 250 mg every 6 hours, will probably be enough to treat the symptoms in the scenario presented. The other measures are generally not needed for acute mountain sickness.

10. The answer is D. Height of 12,500 ft (3,810 m). Pulmonary HAPE and cerebral HACE are the most serious symptoms that may occur with mountain sickness. Both are emergencies. HAPE symptoms, which are more likely and worse if ascent is rapid, consist of tachycardia, tachypnea, severe dyspnea, frothy or blood-tinged sputum, and weakness. HACE symptoms and signs consist of undue drowsiness, unsteadiness, irritability, hallucinations, and neurologic focal symptoms and signs.

11. The answer is B. Furosemide would not be appropriate in this patient who has HAPE. The pulmonary edema is not due to passive congestion as in congestive heart failure with significant hypervolemia. Rather, it is caused by porosity of the alveolar capillary bed, caused by relative hypoxia. The man lives at sea level and should have taken a day or more to accommodate to 11,000 ft (3,353 m) of altitude before embarking and physically exerting on a hike to yet a higher altitude. His youth in itself is not an advantage in the avoidance of HAI. Not only would remaining at 11,000 ft or 3,353 m have allowed him to acclimatize, but the resting period of a day would also in itself make him more resistant to altitude sickness. Acetazolamide is a first-line drug; rapid descent is always a good idea, if it is possible, then oxygen therapy and a hyperbaric tent are effective, if available, and if all else fails and the situation becomes urgent.

12. The answer is C. Height of 10,000 ft (3,048 m) is the altitude limit for normal passenger conveyance in unpressurized aircraft, a safe altitude for this patient. Above that level, oxygen supplementation must be supplied. However, this patient need not have oxygen throughout the trip unconditionally any more than any other person. Above 10,000 ft or 3,048 m, oxygen should be supplemented at increasing concentrations for all passengers and for the pilot. At 20,000 ft (6,096 m), supplemental oxygen must be given at 100% concentration. At 40,000 ft (12,192 m), oxygen must be applied under pressure exceeding the atmosphere. In commercial travel, the foregoing are effected by cabin pressurization.

13. The answer is D. Up to 5,000 ft (1,524 m) is supposedly the maximum cabin pressure encountered in commercial pressurized aircraft. In practice, some probably will go as high as 8,000 ft (2,438 m; equivalent to that found at Machu Picchu) but never more.

14. The answer is B. Influenza vaccination is recommended in the period of 1 to 3 months before travel to every developing country. Td immunization is also recommended to be *current* before travel to these countries, but one may be current for up to 10 years before travel, as long as the person has not had a skin wound in the country when the Td booster was last given more than 5 years previously.

15. The answer is C. Secretory otitis media of flight (aerotitis media) can be prevented if the patient is able to force air into the middle ears through the Eustachian tube ("clear the ears") during descent by the modified Valsalva

maneuver. Naturally, this presupposes that the underlying cause (e.g., viral upper respiratory tract infection or atopic symptoms) is not so severe as to preclude this preventive measure, wherein the Eustachian tube may be so obstructed even before descent in flight that it cannot be opened. Thus, barotitis in flight occurs most frequently during *descent.* Bacterial organisms are not involved in barotitis media. The physical evidence of this form of secretory otitis media is a retracted tympanic membrane seen at otoscopy. This entity occurs during scuba diving, likewise during descent, but the definitive treatment is simply to return to the surface, along with clearing the ears.

16. The answer is B. The Indian subcontinent (both India and Pakistan), still considered to be underdeveloped, is the one region mentioned among the choices where typhoid vaccination is recommended. On the contrary, Canada, Europe, Australia, and New Zealand are among the very few regions of travel for which typhoid vaccination is not recommended. Examples of other countries that present significant risk of typhoid fever are all of Latin America, all of Africa, all of Asia and India; in short, all countries except for all of western Europe, the United States, Canada, Australia, and New Zealand. Recommended pretravel immunizations change from year to year and destination to destination and too voluminous for this work. They are best tracked by consulting the CDC web site, http://www.cdc.gov/nip.

17. The answer is D. Paradoxical hypovolemia in the face of fluid retention plays a significant part in the pathophysiology of jetlag. Rapid east-to-west travel often results in difficulty in staying awake appropriate to the local time, whereas west-to-east travel results in sleep onset relative to the local time at destination (the opposite to the statements as presented in the question). Anti-jetlag diets have not proven effective in preventing jetlag symptoms. Cabin altitudes of 8,000 ft (2,438 m) for prolonged periods may play a significant part in the pathophysiology. Resting in a seat at 5,000 ft (1,524 m), the altitude of Denver, has little effect on healthy persons.

18. The answer is E. Only a malarial smear, among those items mentioned, should be checked for in an asymptomatic returning traveler who had been to a tropical location. All the others are aimed at symptomatic conditions, except for tuberculosis. In the latter case, although conversion may occur without symptoms, we recommend skin testing only in symptomatic cases. The only hepatitides to be acquired in travel are A and E, neither of which causes chronic disease and need not be screened for in the absence of symptoms.

19. The answer is B. A 62-year-old African-American male with nocturnal dyspnea and orthopnea should be denied air travel, along with those having other symptoms of congestive heart failure. Allow the 55-year-old Caucasian male with *stable* angina pectoris to travel. Approve 58-year-old Caucasian female 5 weeks post-uncomplicated myocardial infarction – but not if there has only been 4 weeks or less since the event. Approve the 57-year-old male with chronic lung disease, unable to climb two flights of stairs nor walk for two blocks, so long as he can climb one flight of stairs and walk one block or if he belongs to the "50/50" club, that is, with $PAO_2 \leq 50$ and $PCO_2 \geq 50$. Approve the 35-year-old woman 7 months into an uncomplicated pregnancy. The only squeamishness by the commercial airlines is that they prefer women do not fly with them near their due dates. The other caveat is that pregnant women should not travel to areas where the risk of malaria is significant.

References

Gross Z, Rudy DR. Travel medicine. In: Rudy DR, Kurowski K, eds. *Family Medicine: House Officer Series.* Baltimore: Williams & Wilkins; 1997:751–770.

Health Information for International Travel. Updated regularly on http://www.cdc.gov/nip.

McPhee SJ, Papadakis MA. *Current Medical Diagnosis and Treatment.* 49th ed. New York/Chicago: Lange, McGraw-Hill; 2010.

Rakel ER, Bope ET, eds. *Conn's Current Therapy 2009.* Philadelphia: Saunders; 2009.

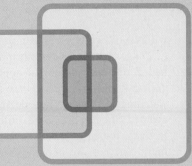

SECTION **XIV**

Behavior and Psychology in Primary Care

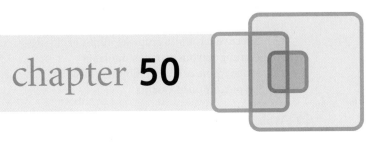

chapter **50**

Depression

1 If present for at least two weeks, each of the following is a criterion among those comprising a diagnostic basis for major depression, except for which one?

(A) Insomnia
(B) Anhedonia
(C) Feeling of guilt
(D) Suicidal ideation
(E) Depressed mood worse as the day progresses

2 Each of the following antidepressant medications may effective as single drug therapy in a primary care practice except for which one?

(A) Buspirone (buproprion)
(B) Zoloft (sertraline)
(C) Prozac (Fluoxetine, Sarafem)
(D) Pamelor (nortriptyline)
(E) Effexor (venlafaxine)

3 A 45-year-old man has been treated by his family doctor in conjunction with a psychiatrist for classic bipolar disorder (manic depression) with lithium (lithium carbonate 300 mg 3 times per day with trough levels tested regularly). Each of the following is true regarding lithium treatment except for which statement?

(A) Polydipsia is an expected side effect.
(B) Hypothyroidism is a common side effect.
(C) Manic symptoms will recur sooner than depression if lithium is discontinued.
(D) Organic hypoglycemia is a side effect.
(E) Sodium loss makes diuretics relatively contraindicated.

4 The highest incidence of depression occurs in which of the following age groups?

(A) 5 to 14 years
(B) 15 to 24 years
(C) 25 to 34 years
(D) 35 to 55 years
(E) >65 years

5 A 28-year-old woman reports feeling depressed after her 18-year-old younger sister died after an illicit drug overdose 1 month earlier. She does not feel like participating in her usual social activities, but she has continued to work and take care of her family without difficulty. She has unintentionally lost 5 lb (2.27 kg) over the last month and admits that she has had a relatively depressed appetite. She expresses guilt that maybe if she had been spending more time watching her sister, her death could have been avoided. She has had some difficulty initially falling to sleep, but once she does she sleeps through the night. She has not noted episodes of inflated self-esteem and has not been going on spending sprees. She has been on no medication (including no street drugs), and she has no medical condition to explain these symptoms. She denies suicidal ideation, hallucinations, or delusions. She has no personal or family history of psychiatric illness. How would you best classify her symptoms according to the criteria listed in the fourth edition of the *Diagnostic and Statistical Manual of Mental Disorders*?

(A) Mixed episode
(B) Dysrhythmic disorder
(C) Major depressive episode
(D) Cyclothymic disorder
(E) Adjustment disorder with depressed mood or bereavement

6 A 55-year-old woman complains of inability to sleep through the night, although she falls off to sleep relatively easily. You note that you have seen her for several falls at home leading to contusions, and on one occasion for a laceration of the scalp requiring sutures in repair. She admits that she has lost the ability to enjoy occasions that, in the past, were fulfilling to her. You notice vascular ectasias about the face and upper trunk anteriorly. Laboratory studies show elevated serum glutamic pyruvate transaminase and gamma-glutamyl transpeptidase levels. You suspect she is alcoholic and also that she is depressed. Which of the following is the wisest strategic approach to this patient?

(A) Because she is female, the chances of her being both depressed and alcoholic are slight. Therefore, you should choose one or the other and treat accordingly.
(B) Alcoholic depressed patients fail at abstinence unless the depression is treated first.
(C) The alcoholism should be arrested before the depression is treated.
(D) Suicide is of low probability because patients with the two diagnoses are less likely to attempt suicide.
(E) Antidepressants are to be avoided in alcoholics, even if their depression persists after months of abstinence.

7 A 35-year-old woman has suffered from rheumatoid arthritis for 3 years and exhibits symptoms of Sjogren syndrome as well. She visits monthly and

more frequently when she runs through pain medication, which is oxycodone, ahead of schedule. Rarely has she pressed for increased dosage and frequency but complains of dysphoria and sleep problems that do not always appear to be related to her nocturnal pain. What are the odds that this patient suffers from depression?

(A) About one in five
(B) About one in four
(C) About one in three
(D) About two in three
(E) About three in four

8 To which category of antidepressant medications does each of the following belong: citalopram, escitalopram, and enantiomeer?

(A) Tricyclic antidepressants (TCAs)
(B) Selective serotonin reuptake inhibitors (SSRIs)
(C) Central nervous system stimulants
(D) Monoamine oxidase inhibitors (MAOIs)
(E) Atypical antidepressants

9 Which of the following categories of antidepressants is associated with the side effects of headache, nausea, tinnitus, insomnia, and akathisia?

(A) TCAs
(B) SSRIs
(C) Central nervous system stimulants
(D) MAOIs
(E) Atypical antidepressants

10 Which of the following classes of antidepressants are associated with the side effects of anticholinergic effects, including cardiac dysrhythmias, sedation, and orthostatic hypotension?

(A) TCAs
(B) SSRIs
(C) Central nervous system stimulants
(D) MAOIs
(E) Atypical antidepressants

11 Which of the following classes of antidepressants is associated with hypertensive crises when combined with certain sympathomimetic drugs and meperidine and dextromethorphan when followed by foods with tyramine?

(A) TCAs
(B) SSRIs
(C) Central nervous system stimulants
(D) MAOIs
(E) Atypical antidepressants

12 With respect to postpartum depression, which of the following statements is correct?

(A) It lasts on average as long as major depressive episodes not occurring in association with childbirth.
(B) It affects about 3% of new mothers.
(C) It takes longer for a spontaneous remission to occur than in major depressive episodes not associated with childbirth.
(D) The depression is more severe and suicide attempts are more common in postpartum depression.
(E) It is sometimes considered an adjustment disorder with depressed mood.

13 A 45-year-old male patient unknown to you has been brought in by his sister's family, whom he has been visiting from out of town. He was observed to have what was described as a grand mal seizure. In inquiring about his medications, you find he has been treated with a medication for depression, the identity of which the patient cannot recall. He has history of neither head trauma nor seizure disorder in the past. Which of the following is the most likely drug he may have been taking?

(A) Fluoxetine (Prozac)
(B) Amitriptyline (Elavil)
(C) Trazodone (Desyrel)
(D) Bupropion (Wellbutrin)
(E) Phenelzine (Nardil)

14 You are selecting an antidepressant for a 35-year-old man. Which of the following antidepressants carries the highest incidence of the side effect of priapism?

(A) Trazodone
(B) Nefazodone
(C) Escitalopram
(D) Sertraline
(E) Fluoxetine

15 You are concerned about the potential for suicide in an 18-year-old patient you are treating for depression. Which of the following increases this patient's risk for suicide?

(A) The patient is felt to have dysrhythmic disorder.
(B) The patient has a moderate bout of depression that improves after the patient has been on SSRIs for 1 month.

(C) The patient fulfills criteria for a major depressive episode.
(D) The patient is an African-American living in an inner-city environment.
(E) The patient is frequently asked if he has suicidal thoughts or plans.

16 Venlafaxine (Effexor) and duloxetine (Cymbalta) are both serotonin and norepinephrine reuptake inhibitors. Which of the following possible advantages does duloxetine have over other SSRIs and other antidepressants in general?

(A) In addition to antidepressant activity, it is anxiolytic.
(B) It is, in addition, an antipsychotic drug.
(C) It possesses analgesic properties.
(D) It possesses nonselective beta-blocking properties.
(E) It has antidiabetic properties.

17 A 48-year-old depressed patient, during an interview by his family doctor, reveals that his mood has been precipitated by his interpretation of his situation at work. He assumes that an impending change in his job description is a sign of his failure in his sales ability. Thus, he feels he has hopelessly lost out in his chosen field and feels it impossible to start over in a new direction at his age. Since finding out about the coming change, he has had difficulty in falling to sleep and is prone to frequent awakening; he is ultimately unable to complete a night's sleep. The physician engages him in a realistic discussion of the company's changing fortunes and helps him to conclude that, if anything, the change in job description within the company may be a vote of confidence in him, because he has not been asked to resign; that, in fact, the patient's interpretation of events has given rise to a negative value judgment. Which of the following therapeutic methods is being brought into play?

(A) Cognitive therapy
(B) Deep psychoanalytic therapy
(C) Reiki therapy
(D) Supportive therapy
(E) Corporate engagement therapy

Examination Answers

1. The answer is E. Depressed mood worse as the day progresses is the incorrect statement. Generally, in depression, if there is a diurnal variation, it is that symptoms *improve* as the day plays out. Diagnosis of major depression requires at least four of the following symptoms for a period of 2 weeks: impaired sleep; lack of interest (anhedonia); guilt; low energy; difficulty concentrating; poor appetite; psychomotor retardation; and suicidality. With psychotic depression, there may be prolonged grief and unreasonably perceived failure to meet self-defined or parental expectations; feelings of the body rotting away due to cancer or the like. Suicidality is to be taken more seriously the more specific the ideation, for example, consideration of method (firearms is the choice of 67% in both males and females) and absence of envisioning future plan. Suicide risk may be overlooked if the depression is masked by overt anxiety – especially when it attaches to unreasonable obsession with perceived faults, physical appearance, or job issues.

2. The answer is A. Bupropion is not an antidepressant, although it is employed as an adjuvant agent in conjunction with antidepressants. Zoloft and Prozac, as SSRIs, are highly popular because of their relatively high therapeutic to side effect ratio. Nortriptyline, as a TCA, is used less often due to its high rate of anticholinergic annoying side effects, some of which are life-threatening such as dysrhythmias in susceptible patients.

3. The answer is D. Organic hypoglycemia is *not* a side effect of lithium treatment. Polydipsia occurs due to a decreased renal responsiveness to anti-diuretic hormone. Hypothyroidism occurs in 10% of cases as well as euthyroid goiter in 3%. Upon discontinuance of the drug, manic symptoms will recur within an average of 2.7 months while depression returns as long as 14 months after cessation of lithium. Sodium loss makes diuretics relatively contraindicated. Lithium prevents both manic and depressive symptoms in about 70% of cases, more likely successfully in those whose attacks have been less frequent than once or twice per year.

4. The answer is C. A period of 25 to 34 years. However, depression remains a common diagnosis at all ages. Note that the peak age group for suicide (white boys or men, predominantly) and suicide attempts (white girls or women, predominately) is 15 to 24 years (see chapter 45).

5. The answer is E. Adjustment disorder with depressed mood or bereavement. Although this patient has some symptoms of a major depressive episode, they are temporally related to the recent loss of a loved one. Note also that she is basically functioning well and without impairment. She has had no manic or euphoric episodes to suggest a mixed disorder. Dysrhythmic and cyclothymic disorders are both characterized by a long term (>2 years) with mild mood alterations but without sustained remissions. In the former, patients have a chronically depressed mood of varying but milder intensity. In the latter, episodes of elevated mood alternate with periods of depression.

6. The answer is C. Alcoholism should be treated first if the two diagnoses exist, if one assumes that the suicide risk is assessed and accounted for. In many cases, the depression will abate after the patient has abstained from alcohol for a significant period. However, the depression is also treated if it persists after 1 month of alcohol abstinence. When the two diagnoses coexist, there is an increase in the incidence of attempted and successful suicides. Both alcoholic men and women have an increased incidence of depression.

7. The answer is C. About one-third of patients with chronic disease suffer from depression in roughly direct proportion to the length of time with the disease. The cause of this is not known, but contributing factors might include catecholamine depletion from chronic stress. It may be situational, based on a philosophically reasonable sense of defeat or discouragement (i.e., an adjustment disorder with depressed mood). Some diseases are better known than others for depression and suicide. These include AIDS prominently, renal failure under dialysis, chronic lung disease, multiple myeloma (often severely painful), other cancer, and coronary heart disease.

8. The answer is B. Each of the drugs mentioned is an SSRI, albeit less well known than fluoxetine, sertraline, paroxetine, and fluvoxamine.

9. The answer is B. SSRIs are known to cause headache, nausea, tinnitus, insomnia, and akathisia. Paroxetine (Paxil) also causes dry mouth. The greatest advantages of this class are the relative rapidity of onset and, the foregoing notwithstanding, the relative paucity of side effects.

10. The answer is A. TCAs are well known to cause anticholinergic effects, including cardiac dyrhythmias, sedation, and orthostatic hypotension. In regard to significant side effects that can lead to necessarily discontinuing the drug, this class has a narrow therapeutic window in comparison with the SSRIs.

11. The answer is D. MAOIs can precipitate hypertensive crises if the wrong dietary elements have been ingested. The management of MAOIs is complicated, and most primary care doctors (including the author) avoid them because of severe dietary restrictions that include most cheeses, fermented aged meats, broad bean pods, meat and yeast extracts, red wine and many other alcoholic beverages, soy sauce, and sauerkraut. These foods contain tyramine, which, when MAO has been exhausted, may result in a hypertensive crisis. The latter occurs not only through effects of the MAO inhibiting medications but also especially when much MAO has been depleted by prior exposure to phenylpropanolamine, phenylephrine, and the other drugs listed in the question. Thus, MAOIs are third-line drugs but nevertheless applicable for refractory panic disorder and depression.

12. The answer is E. Postpartum depression is sometimes considered an adjustment disorder with depressed mood. Postpartum depression tends to be milder with a shorter time period for spontaneous remission and less likely to be characterized by suicidal attempts. It affects about 10% of new mothers, although a less severe form, sometimes called the "postpartum blues," occurs in as many as 80% of new mothers. The foregoing is at odds with the sensational image given the illness by the mainstream media.

13. The answer is D. Bupropion is associated with seizures in approximately 0.4% of doses up to 450 mg/day. The usual starting dosage for adults is 300 mg/day in three divided doses. The risk of seizures is approximately 4 times that of any other antidepressant medication and therefore is contraindicated in patients with seizure disorder.

14. The answer is A. Trazodone, a heterocyclic antidepressant, has priapism among its side effects, according to its literature. Nefazodone might be a better heterocyclic alternative, especially in a male patient. Furthermore, it does not tend to produce the orthostatic hypotension as does trazodone, but both are sedating. Among the others, escitalopram (Lexapro), an SSRI, carries no similar caveat and has no other sexual side effects. Sertraline (the SSRI trade named Zoloft) may cause ejaculation failure; fluoxetine (the SSRI Prozac) may cause decreased libido.

15. The answer is C. The patient fulfills criteria for a major depressive episode. Patients with a major depression are more likely to commit suicide than those with more moderate depressions or other related diagnoses such as dysrhythmic disorder or adjustment disorder with depressed mood. The criteria for diagnosis of major depression are, aside from depressed mood, as follows: social withdrawal; anhedonia (inability to enjoy formerly enjoyable activities); and feelings of guilt. One aspect of suicidality not adequately emphasized in training of nonpsychiatrists is a state of frantic, catastrophizing agitation, with obsessive preoccupation with issues seemingly beyond reason. Asking the patient about suicidal ideation and plans is important to determine risk and does not increase the patient's rate of suicide.

16. The answer is C. It possesses analgesic properties. This new antidepressant agent is being touted as having analgesic properties, a possible advantage when pain is part of the cognitive aspects of a depressive affect. The latter often occurs in association with diabetes when the complication of painful neuropathy occurs and, for example, in chronic musculoskeletal pain in which the patient has developed circular thinking.

17. The answer is A. Cognitive therapy is based on an Ellis and Harper model, developed further by Tosi. It is predicated on the fact that every emotional impulse is preceded by an interpretation of an event. Thus, event A is followed by an interpretation B, which may add an unnecessarily negative value to the process and is thus followed by an emotion or affect that may be anxiety or depression, for example. In many cases, counseling may relatively easily unearth an irrationally negative thought and thus reverse the negative effect.

References

Bauman KA. Depression. In: Rudy DR, Kurowski K, eds. *Family Medicine: House Officer Series.* Baltimore: Williams & Wilkins; 1997:791–810.

Family Medicine Review. Kansas City, Missouri; May 3–10; 2009.

McPhee SJ, Papadakis MA. *Current Medical Diagnosis and Treatment.* 49th ed. New York/Chicago: Lange, McGraw-Hill; 2010.

Osipow SH, Walsh WB, Tosi DJ. *A Survey of Counseling Method.* Homewood, Illinois: Dorsey Press; 1984.

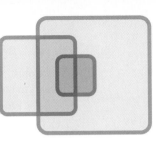

chapter **51**

Anxiety and Phobias

Examination questions: *Unless instructed otherwise, choose the ONE lettered answer or completion that is BEST in each case.*

1 Each of the following items is a side effect of withdrawal from benzodiazepines after modest to moderate usage except for which one?

(A) Insomnia
(B) Irritability
(C) Visual hallucinations
(D) Poor coordination
(E) Tremor

2 Selective serotonin reuptake inhibitors (SSRIs) are a mainstay of treatment of obsessive compulsive disorder (OCD). Which of the following is true regarding their use for OCD?

(A) Response time for SSRIs in OCD is shorter than that for depression.
(B) SSRIs may be used in dosages lower than those employed in treatment of depression.
(C) SSRIs are virtually always successful in treatment of OCD.
(D) Buspirone, although useful as an adjunct to SSRIs in treatment of depression, is not helpful as an adjunct to SSRIs in OCD
(E) Antipsychotic medications may be helpful adjuncts to SSRIs in treatment of SSRIs.

3 A 35-year-old female patient comes to your office complaining of bouts of palpitations, pounding heart, shortness of breath, and diaphoresis, along with feelings of impending doom. During an attack witnessed in the physician's office, the patient's blood pressure (BP) was 160/70 and her heart rate was 120 beats per minute and regular. The patient's face was flushed during the attack. After the attack passed over a period of 15 minutes, the BP had subsided to 110/75 and the heart rate to 80 beats per minute and regular. Which of the following would least resemble the clinical picture presented?

(A) Thyrotoxicosis
(B) Depression
(C) Carcinoid syndrome

(D) Pheochromocytoma
(E) Panic disorder

4 The patient in Question 3 is interviewed further. The onset of the first attack surprised her and led quickly to catastrophizing about possible situations that had never entered her mind before. She then began to dread the attacks and such ideations that accompanied them. She is stably married with three children, is college educated, and stays at home to care for her children. During the attacks, she feels that she is "losing (her) mind." Her affect is appropriate to the situation. Her vital signs, repeated, show BP is 115/75 and heart rate is 84 and regular. Along with counseling, which of the following would be the most appropriate for her acute attacks?

(A) Propranolol 20 mg by mouth (po)
(B) Diazepam 5 mg po
(C) Buspirone 10 mg po
(D) Lorazepam 0.5 mg, given sublingually
(E) Rebreathing exhaled air

5 In treating uncomplicated panic attacks with some success, which of the following pharmacologic approaches would be most helpful as maintenance therapy?

(A) Sertraline (Zoloft) 25 to 50 mg daily
(B) Propranolol (Inderal) 20 to 40 mg daily
(C) Trazodone (Desyrel) 50 mg daily
(D) Divalproex (Depakote) 250 mg daily
(E) Chlorpromazine (Thorazine) 25 mg daily

6 A 25-year-old woman with panic attacks has begun to structure her day around her attacks and collecting an increasing number of situations, which she avoids. She stays away from crowds and fears visits to a supermarket to shop for food for her family. Concluding that she now suffers from phobic disorder, which of the following would be the least reasonable therapeutic maintenance agent for this patient?

(A) Sertraline (Zoloft)
(B) Diazepam (Valium)
(C) Gabapentin (Neurontin)

(D) D-cycloserine (DCS, an antituberculous drug)

(E) Atenolol (Tenormin)

7 Which of the following statements regarding anxiety and depression is true?

(A) They usually (i.e., in the majority of cases) occur as clearly defined entities, easily separated from each other.

(B) Anxiety disorders are seldom confounded with medical conditions.

(C) Mixed anxiety and depression is less disabling than pure cases of anxiety or depression.

(D) One important aid in managing mixed anxiety and depression is to delay diagnostic closure and disposition while observing the patient through several visits.

(E) Clear diagnosis of anxiety or depression usually obviates the need to further evaluate for organic disease.

8 A 52-year-old woman complains to her family physician of bouts of anxiety and depression, the latter often very deep but short lived (i.e., lasting <24 hours). Between such bouts, she often feels "like I'm going to jump out of my skin." Her periods have changed within the past 6 months, becoming much less frequent but often heavy when they do occur. She denies suicidal ideation. She has difficulty sleeping through the night. Which of the following would be the most reasonable initial approach to this patient?

(A) Refer the patient to a psychiatrist

(B) Start a SSRI for panic disorder

(C) Start a tricyclic antidepressant (TCA)

(D) Draw a follicle-stimulating hormone level and start an estrogenic agent

(E) Perform thyroid function studies

9 A 30-year-old woman complains of irritability, apprehension, anxiety, difficulty concentrating, and various somatic complaints that differ with each visit to the doctor. She has had difficulty falling off to sleep for the past 8 months, although once she is asleep she generally remains so for the night. Vital signs are within normal limits; menstrual periods are regular and unchanged for the past 10 years. Although she has between 1 and 3 "good days" per week, she notes the foregoing more often than not. She has not changed her patterns of living, remaining in her stable marriage and her job as a receptionist for a small business, neither of which appears to be a focus of difficulty. Which of the following is the presumptive diagnosis?

(A) Panic disorder

(B) Phobic reaction

(C) Chronic depression

(D) Generalized anxiety

(E) Adjustment disorder

10 Which of the following could logically constitute the mainstay for therapy for the patient described in Question 8?

(A) Paroxetine (Paxil)

(B) Chloral hydrate (Noctec)

(C) Zolpidem (Ambien)

(D) Temazepam (Restoril)

(E) Diazepam (Valium)

11 A returning American soldier has recurring memories of scenes of his fellow soldiers being killed. He exhibits extreme reactions to sudden sounds, as well as insomnia, irritability, and avoidance of sights and sounds reminiscent of the precipitating event(s). Which of the following treatments have been shown to be of benefit to this condition?

(A) Antipsychotic agents

(B) Sedative–hypnotics

(C) SSRIs

(D) TCAs

(E) Major tranquilizers

12 What is the mean duration of posttraumatic stress disorder (PTSD) symptoms without treatment?

(A) Lifelong

(B) 10 years

(C) 64 months

(D) 32 months

(E) 24 months

13 Of the following benzodiazepine medications, which has the shortest half-life?

(A) Chlordiazepoxide (Librium)

(B) Diazepam (Valium)

(C) Clonazepam (Klonopin)

(D) Alprazolam (Xanax)

(E) Triazolam

Examination Answers

1. The answer is C. Visual hallucinations. They do not result from withdrawal from moderate long-term use of benzodiazepines. Withdrawal effects in that circumstance include insomnia, irritability, poor coordination, and tremor as well as nausea, muscle aches, poor concentration, mild depression, mild paranoia, and mild confusion. Abrupt withdrawal from chronic *excessive use* of these drugs can result in serious to fatal reaction including convulsions, psychosis, delirium, and autonomic dysfunction.

2. The answer is E. Antipsychotic medications may be helpful adjuncts to SSRIs in treatment of SSRIs. Response time for remediation of OCD in SSRI treatment is actually longer than for depression and requires larger dosages than for depression; buspirone is useful as an adjunct to SSRIs in treatment of OCD as it is in treatment of depression. SSRIs are about 60% successful in treatment of OCD.

3. The answer is A. Thyrotoxicosis is unlikely because the cardiac rate between attacks was normal. The typical BP and rate and rhythm in thyrotoxicosis are sinus tachycardia with systolic BP elevation. These persist until the condition is treated. Statistically, based on relative prevalence and incidence of attacks, panic disorder is the most likely basis for the picture portrayed, but the significant and threatening organic causes must first be ruled out. Furthermore, a significant portion of those individuals with panic disorder will prove to have an underlying depression. Carcinoid syndrome presents with attacks similar to that which is portrayed except that the BP is more likely to show a widened pulse pressure (systolic without diastolic elevation), as in the persistent pattern with thyrotoxicosis. Nearly all patients who present in the manner shown will be investigated for pheochromocytoma (and very few will prove out to have that syndrome). Pulmonary embolism presents in many ways, but acutely often with a picture similar to that in the vignette. However, such an acute attack would be unlikely to subside in such a short time. Acute angina may manifest the clinical picture shown, without chest pain, especially in a female patient; a similar situation may occur in the case of myocardial infarction.

4. The answer is D. Lorazepam, 0.5 mg (0.5 to 1 mg), given sublingually acts rapidly enough to make a difference, even in such short-lived bouts of anxiety as occurs with panic attacks, from which the patient in the vignette suffers. The other three medications mentioned do not act swiftly enough. Rebreathing exhaled air (e.g., breathing into a paper bag) may be beneficial if acute hyperventilation is a major manifestation of the panic attacks. In

fact, often the first few attacks are accompanied by hyperventilation, which compounds the somatic manifestations of panic. Panic disorder may lead to phobic responses. Panic disorder is more prevalent among female individuals (2:1 over male individuals), and the tendency is not entirely acquired, as there is a 50% concordance among twins and 18% among relatives.

5. The answer is A. Sertraline (Zoloft, an SSRI), 25 to 50 mg daily, is effective in suppressing panic attacks in a majority of cases. Trazodone, a TCA, may be equally effective but has the disadvantage of all TCAs, which is that of a higher incidence of side effects than SSRIs. Propranolol, the nonselective beta-adrenergic blocking agent, has not been satisfactory in panic disorder, except for specific phobias, such as stage fright, in which it suppresses the visceral response to panic while not impeding motor responsiveness. Divalproex is an anticonvulsant. Chlorpromazine is a previously developed antipsychotic agent, seldom any longer in use.

6. The answer is B. Valium, as a benzodiazepine with a long half-life, is not a practical agent for maintenance in phobic disorder, symptoms consisting of spasmodic panic attacks in response to the object(s) of the phobias. Sertraline as an SSRI is a valid treatment as are gabapentin (an anticonvulsant with anxiolytic properties) and the beta-adrenergic blocker. Perhaps surprising is the fact that the antituberculous drug, DCS, is an augmenting agent in advance of anticipated exposure to the objects of phobia. Panic attacks may lead to phobic reactions. Such progression in panic disorder can be prevented by proactive counseling of the patient not to change his/her lifestyle because of the panic attacks. Patients are fortified by the injunction to forge gamely ahead in staying the course of an organized life. If phobias develop early in life, intervention is obviously more difficult.

7. The answer is D. An important aid in managing mixed anxiety and depression is maintenance of "evenly hovering attention" and delay of diagnostic closure (assuming no evidence of suicidality). Mixed anxiety and depression is more common than either anxiety or depression alone. Anxiety is often confounded with medical conditions such as pheochromocytoma and thyrotoxicosis, and furthermore, it often occurs in conjunction with such conditions.

8. The answer is D. Draw a follicle-stimulating hormone level and start an estrogenic agent. If the hormone level is elevated, then the estrogen should be continued for a suitable period and the patient's psychological state observed.

Of such patients, 70% will complain of paroxysmal hot flashes, making the diagnosis more readily apparent. The acute menopause syndrome is a great imitator of other organic diseases. Only after the acute symptoms of estrogen withdrawal have been addressed and treated should the elements of depression and anxiety be addressed, if symptoms have not dissipated during the empiric therapeutic trial.

9. The answer is D. Generalized anxiety disorder is defined as the situation in which a person has symptoms of irritability, apprehension, anxiety, difficulty concentrating, somatic complaints, and insomnia on more days than he or she does not have them, over a period lasting at least 6 months. Panic attacks do not last all day, not to mention several days running. This patient has not changed her pattern of living to avoid symptoms; therefore, she does not have a phobic disorder. Her sleep patterns are not those usually encountered in depression (i.e., early and frequent awakening). Adjustment disorder does not fit the situation because nothing has changed materially in her life.

10. The answer is E. Diazepam (Valium), an intermediately long-acting benzodiazepine, is appropriate for generalized anxiety disorder. Not mentioned but quite acceptable and perhaps safer is buspirone for generalized anxiety. Paroxetine is an antidepressant (and in some cases, psychiatrists are not beyond mixing an anxiolytic and an antidepressant). Chloral hydrate, zolpidem, and temazepam are all sedatives for facilitation of sleep. On occasion, one of the latter group can be used adjunctively in generalized anxiety but is not the main aspect of therapy.

11. The answer is C. SSRIs have shown a 54% to 62% improvement in patients in 12-week trials, as opposed to 37% improvement in those who received placebo for PTSD. The diagnostic criteria for this entity are as follows: (a) the traumatizing event; (b) the recurrent reexperiencing of the event; (c) persistent avoidance of stimuli that remind the patient of the precipitating event; (d) persistent symptoms of increased arousal (e.g., the insomnia, irritability, and temper flare-ups); (e) duration of the symptoms for more than 1 month; and (f) significant resultant stress in social life.

12. The answer is C. A period of 64 months. With treatment, the average duration of symptoms is reduced to 32 months. These data come from research and call for a skeptical eye in dealing with patients who promote PTSD as a way of life.

13. The answer is E. Triazolam has no active metabolites to prolong its pharmacologic effects and partly as a result of this has a half-life of 1 to 3 hours. For this reason, it is promoted as a sleep-facilitating drug without significant morning "hangover." Its popular trade name is Halcion. All of the other drugs mentioned are employed as anxiolytic drugs, of which alprazolam has the shortest half-life (i.e., <24 hours); the remaining three benzodiazepines (chlordiazepoxide, diazepam, and clonazepam) each have a half-life of >24 hours. Clonazepam is used as an anticonvulsant. Drugs with short half-lives, when used as anxiolytics, may give rise to rebound anxiety within a dosage cycle. Those with half-lives of >24 hours should be used with caution in the aged population.

References

Eisendracht SJ, Lichtbacher JE. Psychiatric disorders. In: Tierney LM, McPhee SJ, Papadakis MA, eds. *Current Medical Diagnosis and Treatment*. 45th ed. New York: McGraw-Hill/Appleton & Lange; 2006:1038–1099.

Ronning GF. Anxiety, phobias, and the undifferentiated primary care syndrome. In: Rudy DR, Kurowski K, eds. *Family Medicine: House Officer Series*. Baltimore: Williams & Wilkins; 1997:811–828.

chapter 52

Somatic Symptoms without Organic Basis

Examination questions: Unless instructed otherwise, choose the ONE lettered answer or completion that is BEST in each case.

1 A 45-year-old woman university faculty person was referred to a family physician because of her chairman's and her husband's concerns for her light weight. Her body mass index is calculated as 21. Examination also reveals swelling of the parotid glands, erosions on the lingual surfaces of her teeth, and linear abrasions on the dorsal surfaces of her right hand, most prominently over the proximal phalanges. Which of the following is the most likely diagnosis?

(A) Chronic gastritis
(B) Generalized sialoadenitis
(C) Bulimia nervosa
(D) Chronic pancreatitis
(E) Regional enteritis

2 Which of the following constellations of symptoms is most likely to be psychologically based dizziness?

(A) Imbalance when standing or walking
(B) Motion sickness, visual vertigo, nausea
(C) Light-headedness, tunnel vision, or "graying out"
(D) Chronic floating, rocking, or fatigue
(E) Spinning, turning, or toppling sensation

3 A family doctor has been evaluating a 15-year-old boy for several weeks for nausea and vomiting. Which of the following would tend to allow a diagnosis of psychologically based nausea and vomiting?

(A) Nausea worst in the morning
(B) Nausea and vomiting associated with early satiety
(C) Nausea and vomiting over many weeks in the absence of weight loss
(D) Nausea and vomiting associated with vertigo
(E) Nausea and vomiting associated with epigastric pain

4 A family physician sees 30 patients a day, 5 days per week. Included in his practice are both sexes and all age groups. What percentage of the symptoms given by these patients will have no biomedical basis of explanation?

(A) 5% to 10%
(B) 10% to 20%
(C) 20% to 40%
(D) 40% to 60%
(E) 60% to 80%

5 A 22-year-old woman has been brought home from a private college on a medical basis because of the occurrence of seizures that often occurred in her room in a women's dormitory and, as described, would seem to be grand mal seizures. She is hospitalized and her family doctor visits her at her hospital bed. He witnesses a seizure and suspects that they are not organically based; that is, they are "hysterical" or pseudoseizures. Each of the following would be evidence of a pseudoseizure, except for which one?

(A) The patient is found to be urine incontinent.
(B) Her limbs flail in an asynchronous manner.
(C) She resists when her nose and mouth are held closed.
(D) She remains conscious as evidenced by her directional gaze.
(E) She began to manifest the seizure as soon as the doctor entered her hospital room for the first time since her admission.

6 Which of the following somatoform disturbances is present in the patient featured in Question 2?

(A) Conversion disorder
(B) Somatization disorder
(C) Pain disorder
(D) Hypochondriasis
(E) Malingering

7 In evaluating seizures as to true versus pseudoseizures, which of the following laboratory studies drawn during the seizure or shortly thereafter would be most helpful in making that determination?

(A) White blood cell count
(B) Blood sugar
(C) Lactic acid dehydrogenase
(D) Prolactin
(E) Alkaline phosphatase

8 A 28-year-old female complains of vague left chest pain, occasional feelings of shortness of breath, and fatigue. At other times, she has complained of right flank and lower quadrant abdominal pain. Two months ago, she complained of left upper quadrant abdominal pains that were intermittent and "nondescript." Over the past year, she has complained of urinary frequency; chest pains unassociated with exertion, light-headedness, or diaphoresis. At other times, this patient has cramping abdominal pain, constipation, and diarrhea as well as vague difficulty in swallowing. Today, the abdominal examination is negative for deep or rebound tenderness except for a probable exaggerated guarding response to deep palpation in the right lower quadrant. From which of the following somatoform disorders does this patient most likely suffer?

(A) Conversion disorder
(B) Somatization disorder
(C) Pain disorder
(D) Hypochondriasis
(E) Depression

9 A 45-year-old Caucasian man has sustained a cervical strain that prevents him from being able to manage the steering wheel to drive a truck as required on his job. Over a period of 6 months, he has remained off work because his employer won't entertain the concept of "light duty." He has returned regularly looking haggard, complaining of ongoing pain in both the neck and the lumbar spine regions. There are no radicular signs in either the cervical or the sciatic sectors of the physical examination. Electrical studies have returned negative results. Physical therapy modalities have failed to yield results satisfactory to the patient. From which of the following somatoform disorders does he suffer?

(A) Conversion disorder
(B) Somatization disorder
(C) Pain disorder
(D) Hypochondriasis
(E) Anxiety

10 A 35-year-old woman complains of vague abdominal sensations attributed to a hepatic cyst that has been diagnosed on a previous abdominal computed tomography scan. She has been followed for several years for "gastrointestinal dysautonomia." When she comes to the doctor's office, she invariably invokes a sensation with an anatomic attachment, not usually involving pain. In addition to the hepatic cyst, she has also cited a posterior lung field "cyst" attached to an otherwise vague right thoracic sensation. Which of the following somatoform syndromes does she display?

(A) Conversion disorder
(B) Somatization disorder
(C) Pain disorder
(D) Hypochondriasis
(E) Malingering

11 A 26-year-old man comes to the doctor with a complaint of low back pain radiating down the posterior left thigh to the midcalf. Deep tendon reflexes are difficult to evaluate and on occasion seem to anticipate the tap of the hammer. The straight-leg raising test is positive in that it results in a complaint of radiating pain in the same pattern as described in the chief complaint at 45 degrees. The doctor then has the patient sit up on the examining table and extends the knee to horizontal without resulting in a complaint or facial register of pain. Which of the following is the underlying condition?

(A) Herniated nucleus pulposus at L5 to S1
(B) Lumbosacral strain
(C) Pain disorder
(D) Hypochondriasis
(E) Malingering

12 Regarding the patient in Question 11, if instead of *worrying* that she has cancer of the stomach, suppose she insists she has cancer despite the definitive negative studies. Which of the following fits the clinical picture best among the choices?

(A) Somatization disorder
(B) Factitious disorder
(C) Depression
(D) Hypochondriasis
(E) Body dysmorphic disorder

13 A 42-year-old lawyer makes an appointment for chest pains approximately 1 week after a 52-year-old associate suffered a myocardial infarction. His pain is intermittent, not severe, not associated with exertion, and more likely to occur while he is sitting and watching television in the evening. A resting electrocardiogram

(EKG) is normal, as is a subsequent EKG treadmill stress test. One week after the stress test, the physician explains the results and the patient says the symptoms have disappeared. Which of the following is the best diagnosis?

(A) Somatization disorder
(B) Conversion disorder
(C) Depression
(D) Hypochondriasis
(E) Anxiety

14 A 34-year-old male complains of vague chest pain, more or less constant, although not severe, for the past 2 to 3 weeks. He cannot remember the date or time of onset and appears less than concerned about the pain, while appearing sadly disturbed. He indicates the location of the pain with two fingers and a soft pressure over the left precordium. An EKG stress test showed a normal response. Which of the following is the diagnosis?

(A) Somatization disorder
(B) Conversion disorder
(C) Depression
(D) Hypochondriasis
(E) Angina pectoris

Examination Answers

1. The answer is C. Bulimia nervosa anoxia nervosa negative, low erythrocyte sedimentation rate (ESR); later increased blood urea nitrogen (BUN) (dehydration), leukopenia, normal or low follicle-stimulating hormone (FSH), LH, T3, and T4. Bulimia nervosa conveys a risk of sudden death; the most common basis and precursor is prolonged QT and cardiac dysrhythmia. Signs include eroded teeth from vomiting and manual abrasions from self-induction of vomiting through application of fingers into the teeth. Parotitis is associated with the condition.

2. The answer is D. Chronic floating, rocking, or fatigue is characteristic of psychiatric dizziness. Imbalance when standing or walking describes disequilibrium without vertigo. Motion sickness, visual vertigo, and nausea describes physiologic dizziness or true vertigo, based on motion or a disconnect between position and messages from the vestibular apparatus. Light-headedness, tunnel vision, or "graying out" are typical of presyncope, associated with orthostatic hypotension. Spinning, turning, toppling sensation, and a free falling sensation are also symptoms of true vertigo that may be caused by medical conditions such as Meniere disease, benign positional vertigo, and vestibular neuronitis.

3. The answer is C. Nausea and vomiting over many weeks in the absence of weight loss is characteristic of psychological nausea and vomiting because only small amounts of food are vomited. Nausea worst in the morning, sometimes called matutinal nausea, may indicate increased intracranial pressure and, of course, pregnancy. Nausea and vomiting associated with early satiety may indicate gastric neoplasm. Nausea and vomiting associated with epigastric pain would tend to point toward gastric or duodenal pathology.

4. The answer is D. 40% to 60% of symptoms given by patients in a primary care setting have no biomedical basis of explanation. Reasons for presenting with such symptoms vary from straightforward desire for information and alleviation of fears to somatization of anxiety, depression, and hysterical conversion as well as other defined somatization syndromes discussed in this unit.

5. The answer is A. If a patient who is having a seizure is found to be incontinent of urine, almost certainly, the event is a genuine convulsion. Patients do not maintain consciousness as they enter into a grand mal seizure. In such a seizure, tonic–clonic movements tend to be symmetrical. The occurrence of a seizure just as soon as the doctor entered the room, taken from a real case, would be too coincidental to have happened by chance.

6. The answer is A. Conversion disorder. This picture, taken from a real case, is fairly typical of that condition. The student had learned early that she could escape certain responsibilities by deflecting attention to herself in a sympathetic manner. She was treated in a manner that walked the tightrope between reinforcement of neurosis and cure by allowing her self-respect and suggesting, without being direct, that she knew what to do to get herself reinstated at the college.

7. The answer is D. The prolactin level rises abruptly in the postictal state after a grand mal seizure and not so during or after a pseudoseizure. An electroencephalogram tracing available during the seizure is, of course, a crucial tool in determining the credibility of a seizure.

8. The answer is B. Somatization disorder. This patient satisfies the criteria of four symptoms, other than pain, in unrelated systems as well as four symptoms related to the gastrointestinal system, all of which have yielded no findings on clinical or ancillary evaluation. This disorder is most likely to have its onset before the time the individual reaches the age of 30 years, usually as early as adolescence, and occurs 10 times as frequently in female individuals as in male individuals. It has been referred to as Briquet syndrome.

9. The answer is C. Pain disorder. The criteria for this classification are that there is pain out of proportion to any anatomic evidence and that it coincides with certain psychological needs. In the present vignette, the patient was probably obtaining an escape from the responsibilities of his job and the necessity of supporting his family. His management consisted of allowing the medical evaluation phase to run to completion; then suggesting that he would have no more or less pain by returning to his job than by staying home; and finally supporting him in prescriptions of noncontrolled analgesics so as to allow preservation of self-respect.

10. The answer is D. Hypochondriasis. That which differentiates hypochondriasis from other somatoform syndromes, in particular, the chronic pain syndrome, is the patient's focus on a diagnosis rather than the pain itself. The patient may have her own "theory" of the pathophysiology, usually with an air of certainty, quaint although it may be.

11. The answer is E. Malingering. This is a conscious effort by the patient to feign a positive straight-leg test, which, if genuine, would have been matched by a positive Lesegue test, extending the knee on the ostensibly symptomatic side while the patient was in the sitting position.

12. The answer is C. Depression. There is a subtle but definite line between persistent worry and insistence in the patient who resists reasonable evidence against her having the serious organic disease, cancer of the stomach in this case. In the case of insistence, especially when associated with agitation, there may be depression, bordering on psychotic depression or other psychotic illness. Such agitation, especially when attached to fixation on body image or an unreasonable life issue such as employment, may signal a suicide risk.

13. The answer is E. Anxiety. One might well refer to this constellation as an anxiety somatic equivalent. As opposed to a patient with hypochondriasis, somatization disorder, conversion reaction, or depression, this patient has fears that are closely related to reality, amenable to reason, and subject to reassurance after presentation of the proof of testing and explanation.

14. The answer is C. Depression. Some psychiatrists would refer to this syndrome as somatic depressive equivalent. Whereas most patients with chest pain are anxious about the possibility of coronary disease, this patient lacks that symbolism. In fact, the two-finger mild touch analogy is more symbolic of "pressure" – that is, depression.

References

Margo KL: Psychological interventions for noncardiac chest pain (cochrane for clinicians). *Am Fam Physician.* 2005;72:1701.

Post DM, Rudy DR. Somatic symptoms without organic basis. In: Rudy DR, Kurowski K, eds. *Family Medicine: House Officer Series.* Baltimore: Williams & Wilkins; 1997:829–842.

Rakel RE, Bope EP: *Conn's Current Therapy.* Philadelphia: WB Saunders; 2009.

Miscellaneous Areas of Clinical Practice

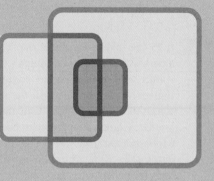

chapter **53**

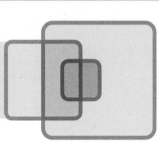

Dermatology

Examination questions: Unless instructed otherwise, choose the ONE lettered answer or completion that is BEST in each case.

1 Each of the following is true regarding scarlatina except which one?

(A) The rash may be described as "sandpapery."
(B) A desquamating "strawberry tongue" is a classical presentation.
(C) The rash spreads to the palms.
(D) Nausea and vomiting are features of a typical course.
(E) The disease has become increasingly benign.

2 Each of the following is true of hot tub folliculitis except for which statement?

(A) The proximal cause is *Pseudomonas aeruginosa*.
(B) The infection raises the pH of the external ear.
(C) Topical gentamicin is effective.
(D) Systemic symptoms such as fatigue, fever, and malaise are common.
(E) Culture of *Pseudomonas* from the water is unreliable.

3 In rocky mountain spotted fever (RMSF), which of the following laboratory values is most likely to be elevated?

(A) Serum sodium
(B) Hepatocellular functions tests
(C) Hematocrit
(D) Platelet count
(E) CSF glucose concentration

4 A young mother comes to you with her 8-month-old formula-fed baby. She is concerned about a rash involving the facial cheeks and the tops of folds of skin over various parts of the body. On occasion, the patches weep and form crusts. The baby does not seem to be bothered greatly by the rash. Both the parents are healthy and without especially apparent inherited diseases, except that the mother has allergic rhinitis in the autumn months and the father had asthma as a child. Which of the following is the most likely diagnosis of the rash?

(A) Psoriasis
(B) Eczema
(C) Chafing caused by lip licking
(D) Candidiasis
(E) Cellulitis

5 A 25-year-old male complains of severe sore throat for 3 days with no coryza or cough. Upon examination, he speaks with a "hot potato voice" and manifests an impressive membrane about the fauces and his intact tonsils plus cervical adenopathy that is not particularly tender. A quick streptococcus flocculation test and a Monospot test are negative. The doctor treats the patient empirically with ampicillin–clavulanate, and 3 days later, the patient complains that he is not improved and now has a morbilliform rash that includes pruritus in certain areas. Which of the following is the diagnosis?

(A) Streptococcal pharyngitis
(B) Viral pharyngitis
(C) Infectious mononucleosis
(D) Measles
(E) Urticaria

6 Which of the following would be the approach most fundamental toward addressing the causation of infantile eczema?

(A) Triamcinolone ointment applied twice daily for 1 month and a follow-up visit at that time
(B) Systemic glucocorticoid course over a 2-week period
(C) Admission to the hospital for intravenous antibiotics
(D) Trial of change in formula from patient's cow milk-based preparation to a soybean-based formula
(E) Application of topical antibiotic ointment

7 A 12-year-old complains of pruritic patches of dry, scaly skin at the antecubital fossae, the medial aspects of the ankles above the malleoli and the popliteal spaces. Which of the following therapeutic modalities would be most appropriate and effective?

(A) Applications of lotion containing 1% hydrocortisone 2 to 3 times daily
(B) Ten-day course of tapering prednisone, beginning with 40 mg daily
(C) Prescription of hydroxyzine, 25 mg per os, every 4 hours as needed for pruritus
(D) Prescription of 2% hydrocortisone ointment to be applied 4 times daily to the pruritic patches as needed for itching
(E) Prescription of a food-elimination diet

8 A 35-year-old male type 2 diabetic patient comes to you with severe contact dermatitis caused by poison ivy, 2 days after he worked in his garden with short sleeves, for the first time in several years. The dorsal aspects of his forearms manifest weeping areas involving about two-thirds of the surfaces distributed in the midportions where there had been blebs that rup-

tured yesterday. The fluid has a serous appearance, and there is no purulence and no red streaking. There is no extraordinary degree of pain in the affected areas. Which of the following treatments is the most rational approach to this condition at this time?

(A) Prednisone per os 40 mg/day, tapering over a 10-day period
(B) Hydrocortisone ointment applied 2 to 3 times daily under an occlusive dressing twice daily for the next 3 days, and a revisit at that time
(C) Application of 1% hydrocortisone in a lotion, applied under loose gauze until the dressing dries, repeated 2 to 3 times daily; revisit in 3 days
(D) Ten-day course of an antibiotic effective against both beta-hemolytic streptococci and staphylococci
(E) Desensitization with poison ivy antigen

9 A 28-year-old man notes the onset over the past few months of intensely pruritic vesicles distributed over the lateral aspects of the shoulders, buttocks, elbows, and knees. The axillae and interdigital web spaces are spared. The condition has not abated during this time, and the patient has had to rely on systemic anti-pruritic prescriptions to get to sleep. You have put the patient on standard food-elimination diets with no alleviation of the symptoms. Topical ointments containing hydrocortisone have not been effective in controlling the itching. At the time of onset, the patient had been on no prescription or nonprescription drugs. On examination, you see excoriations but no patch thickening. Which of the following diagnoses is most likely?

(A) Psoriasis
(B) Discoid lupus erythematosus
(C) Scabies
(D) Food allergy
(E) Dermatitis herpetiformis

10 A 55-year-old white female patient draws your attention to a pigmented 15-mm raised lesion on the posterolateral aspect of her left arm. Because she does not often see that part of her body, she is not certain how long it has been present and denies sensory irritation of any kind. She is concerned about the possibility of melanoma. On examination, you find the lesion to be well demarcated both at the base and at the circumference of its shallowly raised (i.e., raised with a flat rather than a domed top) and flat surface that extends to a diameter that is slightly broader than the base. In addition, you find three other similar lesions that are located on the back of the torso that range from 5 mm to 1.5 cm in diameter, none of which shows signs of inflammation or breakdown of the surface. Which of the following is the most likely diagnosis?

(A) Squamous cell carcinoma
(B) Malignant melanoma
(C) Basal cell carcinoma
(D) Seborrheic keratosis
(E) Actinic keratosis

11 A 28-year-old white male former college basketball player complains of intermittent arthralgias over the past 3 months, which involve the left ring finger proximal interphalangeal joint (PIP) and right index and middle finger distal interphalangeal (DIP) joints. He admits to morning stiffness. On examination, you note dysplasia of the right index nail with some pitting. The remainder of the integument is within normal limits. Which of the following is the most likely diagnosis?

(A) Rheumatoid arthritis
(B) Psoriatic arthritis
(C) Osteoarthritis
(D) Gouty arthritis
(E) Traumatic arthritis

12 A 35-year-old man comes to you with the complaint of a rash virtually covering the anterior chest and abdomen to well below the beltline and the upper half of his posterior trunk. The patient has taken neither prescription nor over-the-counter medications. Since onset, the course has been steady, without waxing or waning in intensity. The lesions are papulosquamous and ovoid with their long axes oriented more or less horizontally, tilting downward and laterally. He has had the rash for about 1 week and remembers a period of mild malaise and slight nausea 3 weeks ago. On closer examination, you find neither vesiculation nor bulla formation. The patient says he has not changed soaps and wears cotton T-shirts that are tucked outside of his underwear that is made of a synthetic fiber. You look for a larger patch that may have preceded the rash and find none. The patient is monogamous and shows neither oral nor palmar lesions. Which of the following is the most likely diagnosis?

(A) Pityriasis rosea
(B) Secondary syphilis
(C) Contact dermatitis
(D) Nummular eczema (neuro eczema)
(E) Food allergy

13 A blond mother of a red-headed daughter seeks information to fortify her in counseling her teenaged daughter not to pursue suntans during the summer months. Which of the following is the least protective of skin against skin cancer and aging?

(A) Avoidance of sun exposure between the hours of 10 AM and 2 PM
(B) Daily low-grade exposure to sunlight (e.g., experienced by people in outdoor occupations)

(C) Use of sunscreens that block ultraviolet B (UVB)
(D) Use of sunscreens that block UVB and ultraviolet A (UVA)
(E) Sunlight exposure to normally unexposed areas of the body only during special occasions such as trips to the beaches and winter vacations in tropical or semitropical latitudes

14 A 45-year-old black woman complains to you of hyperpigmented spotty areas on her lower legs, especially prominent just above the medial malleoli. She reminds you that, last month, you treated her successfully for itching patches in those areas that had been present for several weeks. She is concerned from the cosmetic point of view and worries as to the cause. You notice no fasciculations. Which of the following is the diagnosis of the condition?

(A) Hyperpigmentation caused by Addison disease
(B) Melanoma
(C) Acanthosis nigricans
(D) Hyperpigmentation secondary to inflammation
(E) Pigmented seborrheic keratosis

15 Your patient, a 45-year-old white woman, complains to you of having irregular menses, being overweight, and having hair on her upper lip. On examination, in addition to the foregoing, you notice a pigmented velvety thickening of the skin in 3- to 4-cm patches on her dorsal neck surface and deep in the axillae. Her palms and sublingual areas are unremarkable. Which of the following is the likely diagnosis?

(A) Addison disease
(B) Seborrheic keratoses
(C) Nummular eczema
(D) Epidermoid cysts
(E) Acanthosis nigricans

16 Regarding the patient in Question 12, to which of the following endocrine conditions should you be alert?

(A) Polycystic ovary syndrome (PCOS)
(B) Autoimmune thyroiditis
(C) Addison disease
(D) Graves disease
(E) Pregnancy

17 A 35-year-old woman complains that, for about a year, she has had a mysterious rash involving her face that is nonpruritic. She stopped using topical facial make-up preparations 6 months ago. In the past 2 months, she has noticed muscle weakness of the neck, trunk, and limbs. You see on inspection that her eyes manifest a purple discoloration and discernible periorbital edema. Which of the following is the correct diagnosis?

(A) Lupus erythematosus
(B) Dermatomyositis
(C) Polymyositis
(D) Charcot–Marie–Tooth disease
(E) Contact dermatitis

18 A 55-year-old man complains of stinging pain for 3 days in the facial area involving the right forehead from beneath the scalp anteriorly and as low as the level of the right eye, seemingly out of proportion to a red rash he notes that is appearing today. The area of erythema involves a band that matches the area of pain reported by the patient. Examination reveals 1- to 3-mm vesicles on the right cheek against the erythematous background. Which of the following is the most likely diagnosis?

(A) Herpes simplex (HS)
(B) Dermatitis herpetiformis
(C) Contact dermatitis
(D) Herpes zoster
(E) Nummular eczema

Examination Answers

1. The answer is C. The incorrect statement regarding scarlatina is that the rash spreads to the palms. Each of the other statements is true. The sandpaper rash has sometimes been called pampiniform. The strawberry tongue is classic; as a form of beta-hemolytic streptococcal pharyngitis, it may manifest symptoms of systemic illness such as nausea and vomiting. That said, the disease is much less frequent and more benign than it was two generations ago.

2. The answer is E. *Culture of Pseudomonas from the water is unreliable* is the incorrect statement. In fact, all reports on water exposure folliculitis, *P. aeruginosa*, has been isolated. Although the infection in healthy people is self-limited, systemic symptoms occur in the majority of cases as well as external otitis. Each of the other statements is correct. Successful treatments include polymyxin B spray and oral cipromycin.

3. The answer is B. In RMSF, hepatocellular functions tests may be elevated. Serum sodium, hematocrit, platelet count, and CSF glucose may each be lower than normal, the latter (hypoglycorrhachia) signaling meningitis in this disease, caused by *Rickettsia ricketsii*, carried by the dog tick in the east and the wood tick in the west. The petechial rash begins on the legs before spreading to the hands. Immunofluorescence titers do not rise until the 2nd week of symptoms. Treatment in children under 9 years is chloramphenicol, otherwise doxycycline. Untreated cases have a high risk of dying due to pulmonary hemorrhage.

4. The answer is B. Infantile eczema. Psoriasis rarely occurs on the face, and the mean age at onset is between 20 and 30 years. Compulsive licking followed by chafing the lips usually occurs during the juvenile years, and the lesions in this case are farther from the mouth than the reach of the tongue. Candidiasis affects the intertriginous areas, opposite from the rash in this case, which involves the tops of the folds of skin. Cellulitis is a serious bacterial infection that occurs in a focal area, not in separate distinct patches, and it would not manifest chronicity as the patient's illness would bring the affair to an early crisis. Finally, statistically, not only the greater prevalence of infantile eczema but also the fact that this disorder is a manifestation of the heavily familial-inherited group of atopic diseases mark this as eczema. The other members of the group are allergic rhinitis and conjunctivitis ("hay fever") and asthma.

5. The answer is C. Infectious mononucleosis is noted for an associated morbilliform rash when the patient has been treated with ampicillin, the famous ampicillin rash. The mononucleosis test is not reliable until the illness has been present for 5 to 7 days. Streptococcal pharyngitis nearly always manifests *tender* adenopathy if the nodes are enlarged. Rubeola causes indeed a morbilliform eruption, but the exudative pharynx is not part of the picture. Urticaria may be mixed with the rash of mononucleosis, which may account for the occasional pruritic aspect of the rash on the vignette but that would not account for the remainder of the presentation.

6. The answer is D. Infantile eczema, although genetically determined, is often precipitated by a food allergy in the first year of life. For a baby on a common formula (e.g., as opposed to breast feeding), the most likely causation is allergy to cow's milk. Later, after advancement of the feeding schedule beyond liquid formula, common offenders are egg whites and wheat. Often, a simple empiric change of formula to one based on soy will result in total clearing of the eczema within 1 week. Systemic glucocorticoids would be a radical step for an infant who is not critically ill. Although topical glucocorticoids may be employed for infantile eczema, preparations such as triamcinolone are too potent and carry a high rate of complications of atrophy and scarring striae at the areas of application, particularly on infantile skin. Antibiotics, either systemic or topical, have no place in a noninfectious inflammatory process such as infantile eczema.

7. The answer is D. The patient has what is variously called *neuro eczema, nummular eczema,* and *neurodermatitis.* There is a predisposition for atopic diseases in these patients. The skin is more sensitive and has a lowered threshold for itching. In the accessible areas referred to in the vignette, scratching and rubbing causes a thickening, called, by dermatologists, *lichenification.* Paradoxically, lichenification causes the threshold for pruritus to be further lowered and leads to further rubbing and the vicious circle of itching and scratching. This cycle is effectively interrupted in the vast majority of cases by topical glucocorticoids. Systemic glucosteroids are not effective, and systemic antipruritics such as hydroxyzine (e.g., Vistaril) are usually not needed. Although some allergists may try food elimination in intractable cases, food allergy is rarely a factor and usually the elimination diet is ineffective.

8. The answer is C. The most significant part of the treatment of a weeping lesion is to apply a drying agent. The most drying are the wettest upon application, such as saline or Burrow solution, and the most moistening are occlusive agents such as petrolatum (Vaseline). Creams are positioned toward the moistening end of the spectrum and lotions toward the drying end. When the etiology is a noninfectious inflammatory process as in contact dermatitis, not as a part of a chronic connective tissue disease, glucocorticoids are a legitimate therapeutic modality. Systemic glucocorticoids are not as effective on the thicker parts of the dermal organ (as opposed to being more effective on the glabrous skin, e.g., volar forearm, face, and genitalia). In this case, the presence of diabetes is relatively contraindicated because of predictable certain rocketing levels of blood sugar during their use. In the latter cases, topical glucocorticoids are not only more effective but are also fraught with complications involving skin atrophy and local striae formation if the preparation is too potent or used for too long a period. Thus, in this instance, the mild agent hydrocortisone at the low concentration of 1% is chosen rather than a potent preparation such as a fluorinated ointment.

9. The answer is E. Dermatitis herpetiformis is a vesiculating disease of the skin that makes its onset during the 3rd and 4th decades and then is generally lifelong. The vesicles are approximately the size of those found in varicella and occur on the extensor surfaces of the body referred to in the vignette. The vesicles are often not present on examination because of the excoriations (which are due to the intense itching and scratching) that obliterate them. However, most patients readily describe the vesicles that recur and lead to scratching. The disease is genetically transmitted, with a strong prevalence in people with human leukocyte antigen types HLA-B8 and HLA-DR3. Diagnosis requires an index of suspicion suggesting skin biopsy that shows immunoflourescently visible immunoglobulin A deposits at the tips of dermal papillae. Therapy with oral dapsone, given as 25 to 50 mg daily, is dramatically effective. An alternative, sulfapyridine, for those with allergy or intolerance to the foregoing, or colchicine, in usual dosages has been found to be effective. Neither psoriasis nor discoid lupus is pruritic. Discoid lupus occurs in isolated, usually single, plaques. Scabies, although pruritic to a degree rivaling dermatitis herpetiformis, does not produce vesicles and tends to affect the axillae and web spaces. Food allergy typically causes urticaria and virtually never vesicles.

10. The answer is D. Seborrheic keratosis is typically well demarcated, often pigmented and rough on the surface without inflammatory signs. It has been described by dermatologists as waxy and "stuck on" in appearance as if it could be peeled off. Squamous cell carcinoma nearly always displays an inflammatory appearance and an irregular buildup of keratin. Squamous cell carcinoma may be pigmented but occurs on sun-exposed parts of the body. Actinic keratosis occurs in the regions where squamous cell carcinoma is found, is less inflammatory, and is less likely to be pigmented. Melanoma also is likely to be irregular at the edges or early manifesting inflammatory foci centrally. Basal cell carcinoma displays a very slow progression, often pearly appearance, and sometimes central ulceration. In any of the foregoing situations, a biopsy is necessary for confirmation.

11. The answer is B. Psoriatic arthritis occurs in about 45% of patients with psoriasis and may precede the onset of dermal manifestations of psoriasis by varying amounts of time. As an inflammatory arthritis (psoriasis is an autoimmune disease), this arthritis exhibits morning stiffness and gelling after periods of inactivity. What differentiates psoriatic arthritis from rheumatoid arthritis is its asymmetrical involvement of hands and feet and that it includes the DIP as well as PIP joints and occasionally knees and hips. The pinpoint-type pitting of fingernails is a hallmark of psoriasis, occurring in 30% of patients. The DIP joints of the hands are involved in osteoarthritis in people in their 6th and 7th decades (Heberden nodes). Traumatic arthritis is mentioned as a red herring, given the patient's history of basketball activity and presumed history of numerous stoving injuries. Traumatic arthritis is a form of osteoarthritis and thus is noninflammatory, manifesting no significant stiffness. Gout would not be seriously considered in this age group without more classic presentations such as great toe metatarsophalangeal joint involvement.

12. The answer is A. Pityriasis rosea occurs without a discernible herald patch in about 50% of cases. Secondary syphilis should be considered in all cases of pityriasis rosea but is unlikely in a monogamous man. (Nevertheless, the standard of care dictates a serologic test for syphilis in all cases.) Contact dermatitis is unlikely in a situation in which the affected areas of the skin are in contact with different fabrics. Nummular eczema will not occur in unreachable areas such as the upper back; classically, it affects the antecubital and popliteal fossae among other places. Food allergies follow a waxing–waning course, depending on meals and their times of ingestion.

13. The answer is E. Intermittent intense sun exposure constitutes a greater skin cancer risk than daily less intense exposure over a period of years. This is apparent to people who have experienced sunburns to the trunk and legs on numerous occasions during their youth and young adult years and daily but less intense exposure to the head, neck, and forearms. In the late middle years, actinic changes are found to a much greater degree on the thighs and lower legs than in the head, neck, and forearms, the latter areas having received many more hours of sun exposure than the intermittently and more intensely exposed areas. The best prevention is total blockade and shade. Next would be sunscreens that block both UVA and UVB; next would be sunscreens that block UVB. Avoidance of the most direct hours of sunlight (10 AM to 4 PM, according to the U.S. Preventive Services Task Force) is advisable but does not confer secure protection against skin aging and cancer.

14. The answer is D. Dark-skinned people, be they of African, Southeast Asian, or other ethnic origin, manifest, as a result of the subacute phase of an inflammatory process, a muddy-looking hyperpigmentation locally. Inflammation that lasts much longer causes the opposite, that is, a loss of pigmentation. Both conditions will reverse after subsidence of the inflammatory process. Hyperpigmentation will reverse itself sooner than hypopigmentation.

15. The answer is E. Acanthosis nigricans. This patient probably has PCOS and thus stands a strong chance of being insulin resistant, hence prediabetic type 2 or clinically diabetic. Acanthosis nigricans accompanies such conditions in a minority but significant proportion of cases. The pigmentation of Addison disease tends to involve the creases of the palms, soles, axillae (as opposed to the concavities), extensor joint surfaces, tongue, nails, and belt or bra lines. Seborrheic keratoses may be pigmented, but they occur as "stuck on" 1-cm^2 lesions on the open areas of the skin. Nummular eczema is pruritic and pigmented only in dark-skinned people. Epidermoid cysts are not noted for dark coloration except at the punctum, where the sebaceous comedone is found.

16. The answer is A. PCOS is associated with irregular menses, obesity, hirsutism, and insulin resistance. Acanthosis nigricans is connected with the insulin resistance of type 2 diabetes, both type A (PCO) and type B (autoimmune). Addison disease does not fit the pattern of pigmentation (see discussion of Question 12). Thyroid diseases have no particular association with pigment abnormalities in humans. Pregnancy often manifests the "mask of pregnancy," involving the face. In the age group of the 40s and 50s, acanthosis nigricans is associated also with the following cancers: non-small cell lung, breast, gastrointestinal, prostate, and myeloproliferative disease as well as carcinoid.

17. The answer is B. Dermatomyositis in its classic presentation involves the purple discoloration of the eyelids and periorbital edema ("heliotrope eyes") and proximal muscle weakness. In 10% of patients, the rash precedes myositis by up to 2 years. Lupus erythematosus causes a classic facial rash (seldom seen in primary care practice); polymyositis is generally assumed to be dermatomyositis without dermatitis. Charcot–Marie–Tooth disease is a demyelinating disease of the central nervous system involving the distal extremities, leading to the stork-leg deformity. Contact dermatitis seldom occurs on the face except in reaction to cosmetics and virtually always is pruritic.

18. The answer is D. Herpes zoster (HZ, "shingles") is characterized by a searing superficial type pain associated with a varicelliform vesicular rash. The vesicles occur on an erythematous background. The rash occurs simultaneously or within 2 to 3 days after the onset of the pain and last about 10 days through phases of subsequent crusting, dark colored eschar, and resolution, sometimes with scar formation. Shingles is seldom confused with HS because the vesicles of HS are distributed within an area of only a few centimeters, whereas HZ usually covers the majority of a complete dermatome or as this case, a cranial nerve, that is, the ophthalmic branch of cranial n. V. Dermatitis herpetiformis, contact dermatitis, and eczema are all pruritic while HZ is not, unless late in the healing phase. There is a close correlation, when the ophthalmic branch of the trigeminal nerve is involved in herpes zoster, between involvement of the tip of the nose and involvement of the cornea.

References

Fitzgerald PA. Endocrinology. In: Tierney LM, McPhee SJ, Papadakis MA, eds. *Current Medical Diagnosis and Treatment.* 43rd ed. New York: McGraw-Hill/Appleton & Lange; 2004:1062–1145.

Fitzpatrick TB, Eisen AZ, Wolff L, Freedberg IM, Austen KF, eds. *Dermatology in General Medicine.* 3rd ed. New York/St. Louis/San Francisco:McGraw-Hill; 1971.

Habif TP. *Clinical Dermatology.* St. Louis: Mosby; 2004.

Jemal A, Tiwari RC, Murray T, et al. Cancer statistics 2004. *CA Cancer J Clin.* 2004; 54:8–29.

McPhee SJ, Papadakis MA. *Current Medical Diagnosis and Treatment.* 49th ed. New York/Chicago: Lange, McGraw-Hill; 2010.

Schwayder T. Common skin problems in children. *Patient Care.* 2004; July:32–36.

U.S. Preventive Services Task Force. Recommendations and rationale. *Am Fam Physician.* 1996; 69:903–904.

chapter 54

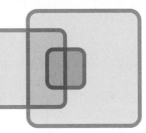

Geriatrics

Examination questions: Unless instructed otherwise, choose the ONE lettered answer or completion that is BEST in each case.

1 Which of the following is the most effective regimen, besides pre-procedure generous hydration, to protect against acute renal failure before injection of radiographic contrast medium?

(A) IV mannitol
(B) IV furosemide
(C) IV prednisone
(D) N-acetylcysteine
(E) IV diphenhydramine

2 Which of the following most simply differentiates the pain of pedal fat pad atrophy (FPA) from plantar fasciitis (PF)?

(A) Time of day when pain is the worst *PF ↑ am*
(B) Location of the pain *FPA↑ as day goes on*
(C) Drugs to which the pain responds
(D) Response specifically to glucocorticoids
(E) Response to footwear

3 A 67-year-old woman with abdominal pain enters the office of a family physician. Which of the following statements regarding the diagnosis of the pain in this patient is true?

(A) A surgical cause is ruled out by lack of fever and leukocytosis.
(B) Acute cholecystitis is likely to present with radiating flank and back pain.
(C) The patient's chances of having ascending cholangitis are greater than those for a younger person.
(D) One can expect appendicitis to be accompanied by a temperature of 100°F (37.7°C).
(E) Elevated alkaline phosphatase levels will not be helpful in diagnosing ascending cholangitis.

4 Which of the following is the most significant difference between "old–old" patients (>75 years) and younger patients in the diagnosis of perforated peptic ulcer?

(A) The >75 group has devastating pain heralding perforation.
(B) Patients older than 75 years are more likely to demonstrate free air under the diaphragm.
(C) Serum amylase is less helpful in the diagnosis of perforation of these patients than it is in patients younger than 75 years.
(D) Symptoms and signs of perforated viscus are more likely to occur without prior symptoms in patients older than 75 years.
(E) Leukocytosis is more likely to be present in the older patient than in the younger one.

5 A 70-year-old man complains of abdominal pain that is steady and building. Abdominal examination reveals a widened abdominal aortic palpable pulsation; otherwise, it is remarkable only for vague deep tenderness (i.e., showing no rebound tenderness). Abdominal ultrasound discloses an aneurysm 5 cm in diameter below the origin of the renal arteries. Which of the following is nearly certainly true regarding atherosclerotic risk factors present in this patient?

(A) Dyslipidemia
(B) Smoking
(C) Hypertension
(D) Psychological stress
(E) Diabetes type 2

6 An 80-year-old previously well and self-sufficient great-grandfather who lives alone is brought to the family doctor because of newly occurring falls, urinary incontinence, and confusion over the past 4 days. His temperature and blood pressure are normal for him. Which of the following is the least likely cause of this change?

(A) Acute pneumonia
(B) Urinary tract infection
(C) Acute myocardial infarction
(D) Stroke
(E) Alzheimer disease (AD)

7 A 78-year-old white man is brought to his family doctor for confusion. He is visiting his daughter, son-in-law, and their college-age children. His vital signs, including orthostatic pressures, are within normal limits. The patient's confusion had its onset after he had been at the family's home for 2 days. There had been a recent change of medications for the gentleman, who has established diagnoses of diabetes, hypertension, and depression. Although other factors may cause confusion, which of the following medications is the most likely cause of confusion in this patient?

(A) Hydrochlorothiazide/triamterene (Dyazide)
(B) Verapamil
(C) Lisinopril
(D) Amitriptyline
(E) Metformin

8 A 65-year-old man has persistent blood pressure levels averaging 150/78, although his diastolic pressure has never been above 90 mm Hg. Which of the following drugs would have the best chance of controlling the blood pressure as a single medication in reasonable dosages?

(A) Lisinopril (an angiotensin-converting enzyme inhibitor)
(B) Propranolol (a nonselective beta-adrenergic blocker)
(C) Irbesartan (an angiotensin II receptor inhibitor)
(D) Hydrochlorothiazide/triamterene (a combination thiazide diuretic and potassium-saving diuretic)

9 A family doctor began seeing patients in a nursing home and assumed care of several dozen patients. One 85-year-old female patient sat impassively during the 3 days required for the family doctor to make initial rounds, familiarizing himself with each patient while still pursuing his office practice. While exchanging a joke with the rounding nurse, the patient suddenly laughed out loud. The doctor found that she fed herself, albeit laboriously. Except for the humorous response, her face remained flat and expressionless. The doctor checked the medication list on the woman's chart and discovered that it included 5 mg of diazepam 4 times a day. This medication was discontinued forthwith. Within 1 to 2 days, she became talkative and began exploiting her keen sense of humor. Which of the following was the diagnosis if this woman's problem was relevant to the described findings?

(A) AD
(B) Parkinson disease
(C) Supranuclear palsy
(D) Depression
(E) Delirium

10 A 75-year-old woman is brought in by her family because of failure to adequately take care of herself alone in her apartment. Problems include errors and neglect in her private financial records; life-threatening errors concerning her kitchen stove; and a decreasing ability to dress herself. The possibility of AD is considered. Each of the following is a criterion to be fulfilled for diagnosis of AD, except for which one?

(A) Disturbance of consciousness
(B) Progressive impairment of memory and at least one other cognitive function (e.g., language)
(C) Onset between 40 and 90 years of age
(D) Dementia documented by examination and confirmed by testing
(E) Absence of another brain disorder or systemic disease that could cause dementia

11 An 81-year-old father of a 47-year-old female patient of a family physician is brought to the doctor because of urinary retention. Recently, he made a trip to a local emergency department and had to be catheterized. In culling the list of medications on which the patient has been placed, you note that each of the following may cause urinary retention, except for which one?

(A) Trihexyphenidyl for Parkinsonian rigidity
(B) Amitriptyline for facilitation of sleep
(C) Amlodipine for hypertension
(D) Terazosin (Hytrin) for benign prostatic hyperplasia
(E) Hydrocodone (Vicodin) for severe pain

Examination Answers

1. The answer is D. N-acetylcysteine, the agent used to protect the liver after a toxic dose of acetaminophen, is nephroprotective after intravenous radiocontrast dye. Mannitol and furosemide do not work for that purpose. Prednisone and diphenhydramine are indicated in allergic reactions, including those in response to contrast dyes but will not protect the kidneys against acute failure due to such dyes.

2. The answer is A. Time of day when pain is the worst. PF causes pain in the morning that remits with activity while plantar fat atrophy, a condition common to "old-old" people (see Question 4), hurts more as the day progresses.

3. The answer is C. Her chances of having ascending cholangitis are greater than those for a younger person. This complication of acute cholecystitis is rare before a person reaches the age of 40; half of all patients older than 65 years of age who have cholecystitis suffer complications including ascending cholangitis, perforated gallbladder, emphysematous gallbladder, bile peritonitis, and gallstone ileus. Older patients are less likely to present with radiating flank and back pain than are younger patients. The majority of people with ascending cholangitis manifest elevated alkaline phosphatase levels. Acute surgical abdomen in patients older than 65 years of age is less likely to present with fever or leukocytosis.

4. The answer is D. Symptoms and signs of perforated viscus are more likely to occur without prior symptoms. The first symptom of ulcer disease is more likely to be that of perforated viscus. Leukocytosis is blunted in old–old individuals in situations that, in younger patients, result in white cell elevation. Amylase levels rise after perforation, the same in the older group as in younger patients. Older patients are equally likely as younger ones to demonstrate free air under the diaphragm.

5. The answer is B. Smoking is the strongest risk factor for abdominal aortic aneurysm, and 90% of patients with abdominal aortic aneurysm are smokers. The U.S. Preventive Services Task Force has advocated aortic aneurysm screening for all men who are between 65 and 75 years of age and have a history of smoking.

6. The answer is E. AD is unlikely in a previously independent octogenarian. AD would not have such a rapid onset. The point of the vignette is that the old–old (>75 years) frequently develop a set of nonspecific symptoms of mental dysfunction in response to any of the conditions mentioned. Other precipitants of such a change include gastrointestinal bleeding, starting a new sedating medication, or simply moving the venue of the patient's living conditions. Virtually all of the conditions not related to AD that are mentioned in this unit are amenable to treatment of the underlying cause, and for variable periods, the dementia is thus reversible.

7. The answer is D. Amitriptyline, a tricyclic antidepressant, has a marked anticholinergic action, well known to cause confusion in older people. None of the other drugs' literature, among the other choices, mentions this side effect. Anticholergics are relatively contraindicated in the "old–old," those 75 years or older, for that reason.

8. The answer is D. Hydrochlorothiazide/triamterene, a combination of thiazide diuretic and potassium-saving diuretic (trade name of Dyazide, among others), may be effective for isolated systolic hypertension, the form of hypertension seen most often in elderly people. The pathophysiology of isolated systolic hypertension leans toward that of salt or water retention (volume load increased) as opposed to increased peripheral vascular resistance. The former is associated with lower renin levels for a given salt balance than normal. As the blood pressure tends to be more or less dependent on blood volume, it responds, in a majority of cases, to a simple diuretic. Angiotensin-converting enzyme inhibitors, angiotensin II receptor inhibitors, alpha-1 adrenergic blockers, and beta-blockers each function to relieve increased peripheral resistance, which is not as likely to be a mechanism of hypertension in the elderly population.

9. The answer is D. Depression. There are two messages from this true-life experience. First, true sedatives should be used very judiciously in elderly people and for the most part avoided. Second, treating with a sedative, any "nervous" or somewhat agitated state in elderly individuals can aggravate or even precipitate depression. The patient did not demonstrate Parkinsonian or supranuclear palsy-like symptoms except for the facial flatness. AD was ruled out by the patient's rapid intellectual recovery when she stopped taking the diazepam. Delirium is acute organic brain syndrome, whose symptoms she did not manifest.

10. The answer is A. Disturbance of consciousness is the one criterion among those listed that does not fit AD. In addition, supporting evidence (but lacking specificity) includes loss of motor skills, family history of AD, and cerebral atrophy on a computed tomography scan. The latter, however, is found frequently in ages even as young as the 70s while the subject may continue to function and grow intellectually. That said, all reversible causes of dementia must be ruled out. In addition to those conditions discussed in Question 4, these conditions include chronic anemia, hypothyroidism, vitamin deficiencies, electrolyte imbalance, disease related to acquired immunodeficiency syndrome and human immunodeficiency virus, congestive heart failure, and seizure disorders.

11. The answer is D. Terazosin (Hytrin), when used to combat benign prostatic hyperplasia or as an antihypertensive, may cause urinary incontinence, especially in women. Each of the other choices has anticholinergic activity as a significant part of their pharmacologic effectiveness or as a significant side effect. Thus, urinary retention is a logical sequela. Each of the choices has legitimate applications in the aged population but must be utilized prudently. Other drugs with anticholinergic side effects include vincristine (anticancer drug); all the other calcium channel blockers; all antihistamines; thioridazine (antipsychotic drug) and many other antipsychotic agents; and opiates, including hydrocodone, benztropine, and many others.

References

Dickman R. Care of the elderly. In: Rakel RE, ed. *Textbook of Family Practice.* 6th ed. Philadelphia: WB Saunders; 2002:88–130.

Family Medicine Review. Kansas City, Missouri; May 3–10; 2009.

Johnston B, Harper GM, Landefeld S. Geriatric medicine. In: Tierney LM, McPhee SJ, Papadakis MA, eds. *Current Medical Diagnosis and Treatment.* 45th ed. New York: McGraw-Hill/Appleton & Lange; 2006:49–66.

Lyon C, Clark DC. Diagnosis of acute abdominal pain in older patients. *Am Fam Physician.* 2006; 74:1537–1544.

The Guide to Preventive Services 2009. Recommendations of the U.S. Preventive Services Task Force. Agency for Healthcare Research and Quality.

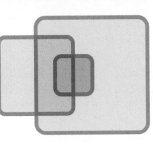

chapter 55

Hematology

Examination questions: *Unless instructed otherwise, choose the ONE lettered answer or completion that is BEST in each case.*

1 Each of the following, when presenting with abnormal mean cell volume (MCV), manifests microcytic anemia except for which one?

(A) Thalassemia
(B) Lead intoxication
(C) Sideroblastic anemia
(D) Iron deficiency
(E) Anemia of chronic disease

2 Iron storage is notably elevated in each of the following conditions except for which one?

(A) Hemochromatosis
(B) Lead poisoning
(C) α-Thalassemia
(D) Sickle cell disease (SCD)
(E) Sideroblastic anemia

3 A 45-year-old woman with four healthy grown children has undergone subtotal hysterectomy for refractory menorrhagia, which had caused an iron deficiency anemia. Two months after the operation, she still has a hemoglobin of 10 g/dL despite adequate dosage of oral iron, and the reticulocyte count has not risen significantly during the treatment. A decision is made to institute a course of parenteral iron. Each of the following situations may result in failure of oral iron except for which one?

(A) Patient has not taken the oral iron because of distaste for the prescription.
(B) Refractoriness to oral iron
(C) Heavy alcohol intake
(D) Allergy to oral iron
(E) Inflammatory bowel disease

4 A 55-year-old woman complains of attacks of painful hands and fingertips that are not pruritic and are relieved by cold applications. As a manifestation of a systemic condition, which of the following diseases would she most likely have?

(A) Essential thrombocytosis
(B) Raynaud disease
(C) Secondary syphilis
(D) Dyshidrotic eczema
(E) Myelodysplasia

5 A newborn has a relative polycythemia with a hemoglobin range of 16.5 to 21.5 g/dL that declines to levels whose range is roughly 10 to 16 g/dL before slowly correcting to a more narrow range in the preteen years. At what age does the infant's hemoglobin range reach the nadir?

(A) 15 to 30 days
(B) 1 to 2 months
(C) 3 to 5 months
(D) 6 to 11 months
(E) 4 to 7 years

6 Which of the following is true regarding iron deficiency anemia?

(A) MCV is higher than normal.
(B) Mean cell hemoglobin is elevated.
(C) Variability of red blood cell distribution width (RDW; range of red blood cell diameter) is increased.
(D) The ratio between the red blood cell count in millions and the hemoglobin is increased.
(E) Serum ferritin is elevated.

7 A 24-year-old woman has been suffering from prolonged and frequent menses (i.e., menometrorrhagia) for 7 months. She now complains of light-headedness when she stands erect from sitting. She weighs 120 lb (54.4 kg) at a height of 5 ft, 4 in. (1.63 m). Her blood pressure sitting is 110/80 with a regular heart rate at 80 beats per minute, and she exhibits orthostatic hypotension with 95/60 after 30 seconds. Her blood hemoglobin level is 10 g/dL. Which of the following laboratory test results is most likely those of this patient?

(A) Serum iron level of 100 μg/dL, total iron-binding capacity (TIBC) of 300 μg/dL
(B) Serum iron level of 200 μg/dL, TIBC of 300 μg/dL

317

(C) Serum iron level of 40 μg/dL, TIBC of 120 μg/dL
(D) Serum iron level of 40 μg/dL, TIBC of 400 μg/dL
(E) Serum ferritin level of 200 ng/mL

8 Each of the following is true regarding hemochromatosis except for which statement?

(A) It is diagnosed by finding an elevated transferrin saturation.
(B) It is a cause of impotence and fatigue.
(C) It is most common in people of Asian descent.
(D) The staging of the disease is measured by serum ferritin content.
(E) Onset of symptoms occurs at an earlier age in men as opposed to women.

9 An 83-year-old woman who has had late-onset rheumatoid arthritis for the past 10 years arrives for a routine periodic examination. She has had negative stool examinations for occult blood and has had no gastrointestinal (GI) symptoms. Her complete blood count (CBC) showed anemia of chronic disease. Which of the following findings is compatible with that diagnosis?

(A) Decreased mean red cell hemoglobin content
(B) Increased mean red cell volume
(C) Serum iron level of 20 μg/dL, TIBC of 60 μg/dL
(D) Increased reticulocyte count
(E) Serum ferritin level of 1,000 ng/mL

10 A 55-year-old man enters the health care system in the office of a family doctor, complaining of problems of maintaining balance. The CBC shows a hemoglobin of 6 g/dL (14 to 16); MCV 110 μmm^3 (80 to 96), 3,000 to 5,800, and platelet count 1,00,000/mm^3 (1,50,000 to 3,00,000). He takes no medications. He has also complained of lessening of his appetite and some diarrhea. Which of the following most likely explains his symptoms?

(A) Aplastic anemia
(B) Malnutrition
(C) Malabsorption syndrome
(D) Blood dyscrasia
(E) Pernicious anemia

11 A 34-year-old woman has had four bouts of deep vein thrombosis, one of which resulted in pulmonary embolism. None was associated with trauma nor occurred after a surgical procedure. Routine CBC result was unremarkable, including a platelet count of 50,000. A thorough evaluation for occult malignancy has turned up none. There is therefore a strong possibility of an inherited coagulopathy. Which of the following is the most likely cause?

(A) Protein C deficiency
(B) Resistance to protein C activation
(C) Deficiency of protein S
(D) Antithrombin III deficiency
(E) Prothrombin nucleotide mutation

12 A 45-year-old man suffered a pulmonary embolus during his second bout of deep vein thrombosis. During the therapeutic phase, it was noted that heparinization was not quite successful in bringing the partial thromboplastin time into the therapeutic range and that anticoagulation was not achieved until the 5th day through normal oral warfarin anticoagulation. Which of the following was the cause of the hypercoagulability?

(A) Protein C deficiency
(B) Resistance to protein C activation
(C) Deficiency of protein S
(D) Antithrombin III deficiency
(E) Prothrombin nucleotide mutation

13 A 45-year-old man of Greek descent reports to his primary care physician with complaint of fatigue. Examination of the skin reveals telangiectasias about the face and upper chest. His weight is 195 lb (88 kg) at a height of 5 ft, 6 in. (1.68 m). Neurological review and examination are grossly normal, including proprioception by the Romberg test. Routine laboratory studies show a blood urea nitrogen (BUN) level of 10 mg/dL, a creatinine level of 0.8, an alanine aminotransferase level of 110 U/L (1 to 45), and an aspartate aminotransferase level of 76 U/L (1 to 36). The hemoglobin level is 10 g/dL. Hematocrit is 29, MCV is 120 fL (80 to 96), and the mean corpuscular hemoglobin concentration is 34 g/dL (32 to 26). Which of the following accounts for this patient's hematologic findings?

(A) Pernicious anemia
(B) Iron deficiency anemia
(C) Hemolytic anemia
(D) Folic acid deficiency
(E) Beta-thalassemia

14 A 16-year-old male African-American patient has been seriously ill all his life with SCD. He displays sickled red cells with hemoglobin SS and generally runs a hemoglobin level of 8 g/dL. Each of the following is a potential cause of crisis in this patient, except for which one?

(A) Splenic sequestration
(B) Vaso-occlusive events
(C) Acute chest syndrome
(D) Hemolytic crisis
(E) Infarctions caused by polycythemic crises

15 A 45-year-old busy male attorney complains of headaches and generalized pruritus. He flew into an eastern American city from Denver, Colorado, to attend a high-level legal conference. He smokes 1 pack of cigarettes per day. He denies recent upper respiratory tract infection, foci of specific pain, and urinary and GI symptoms. On examination, he manifests a blood pressure of 160/105, a temperature of 98.6°F, a ruddy complexion, and splenomegaly and hepatomegaly. Blood gases are not immediately available. His CBC showed the hemoglobin level to be 18 g/dL, the white blood cell count to be 14,000, and the platelet count to be 7,00,000. Red blood cells are normochromic and normocytic. The BUN level is 18 mg/dL and the creatinine level is 1.1 mg/dL. Urinalysis is within normal limits with a specific gravity of 1.015. Which of the following is the diagnosis?

(A) Polycythemia vera
(B) Secondary polycythemia from altitude accommodation
(C) Secondary polycythemia caused by chronic obstructive pulmonary disease
(D) Spurious polycythemia from dehydration caused by air travel
(E) Secondary polycythemia compensating for carboxyhemoglobin in a heavy smoker

16 A 65-year-old woman complains of pain in the back and chest with localized tenderness at the spine of T8 and ribcage pain with tenderness at the right seventh rib. The patient appears to be quite pale and admits to fatigue. These symptoms have come on gradually over a period of several weeks, with the back pain becoming the reason for consulting the physician. A dip urinalysis shows proteinuria. Screening CBC reveals a normochromic, normocytic anemia with 8 g/dL of hemoglobin and marked rouleau formation with normal platelets and white cell counts and morphology. Serum chemistry results include calcium elevation to 12.2 mg/dL with normal alkaline phosphatase. Plain x-rays show a fracture of the right seventh rib, compression of the eighth vertebra. Of the following, which is the most likely diagnosis?

(A) Alcoholism
(B) Metastatic carcinoma
(C) Multiple myeloma
(D) Waldenström macroglobulinemia
(E) Severe osteoporosis

17 A 26-year-old man has noted painless swelling in the left side of his neck. Furthermore, he has noted afternoon chills and night sweats for several weeks. He has stopped smoking because inhaling tobacco smoke makes him ill. Although he seldom drinks alcohol, during the past week, he took a glass of wine and only then noted pain in the swelling about the neck. Examination is unremarkable except for the neck, which exhibits a firm irregular mass measuring approximately 3 cm × 5 cm located in the left anterior cervical region. The CBC and laboratory chemical battery are within normal limits. Which of the following is the most likely significant cause of these symptoms?

(A) Hodgkin disease
(B) Sialoadenitis
(C) Viral respiratory tract infection
(D) Streptococcal pharyngitis
(E) Carotid artery aneurysm

Examination Answers

1. The answer is C. Sideroblastic anemia is the one choice that is not normally an example of microcytic anemia. This disorder results from inability to incorporate iron into the protoporphyrin in the erythropoiesis process. A prominent characteristic is accumulation of iron as iron absorption is accelerated in response to low hemoglobin, resulting in elevated serum iron and transferrin saturation, although not to the level found in hemochromatosis; usually this produces a macrocytic or normocytic situation. A classic cause is a generalized marrow disorder and may culminate in myelodysplasia. Cases that may be secondary to lead poisoning account for some of the few instances in which sideroblastic anemia manifests microcytosis. Each of the other conditions presented is characterized by microcytic anemia, that is, thalassemia, iron deficiency, and anemia of chronic disease. The latter is either normocytic or microcytic.

2. The answer is B. Lead poisoning harms by neurological and GI symptoms and pathology. Only 25% are anemic and the anemia tends to be mild, so that iron storage is not a great part of the clinical picture. Hemochromatosis is defined by pathological storage of iron. Thalassemia is a multivariate disease but when clinically expressed the hemoglobin runs 6 to 10 gm/dL due to hemolysis, and the tendency for overabsorption of dietary iron is inversely related to the hemoglobin level. SCD is of course also intensely hemolytic, and iron storage is a characteristic for the same reason. Sideroblastic anemia has several causes, but the pathophysiology of each of them features blocked erythropoiesis, and the resultant low hemoglobin has the same effect on iron absorption as do the hemolytic anemias. The measure of elevation of the process of iron storage is transferrin saturation (occupation of greater proportion of the transferrin molecule, the vehicle of transport), and the measure of total body storage is serum ferritin. These parameters are not very prominent in the non-iron deficiency anemias as they are in hemochromatosis.

3. The answer is C. Heavy alcohol intake, unless complicated by GI bleeding, does not impede oral iron absorption. In fact, regular ingestion of alcohol increases GI absorption as does large dosages of ascorbic acid and inflammatory hepatic disease. Each of the other factors mentioned may be a cause of failure of iron deficiency to respond to oral iron.

4. The answer is A. Essential thrombocytosis often features erythromelalgia, described in the vignette. The condition is characterized by platelet counts for up to 2 million/dL without significant other abnormalities of formed peripheral blood elements. It occurs predominantly in the 50 to 60 years age group, and incidental discovery of the elevated platelet count is the most frequent presentation. Other cases are found because of the occurrence of frequent thromboses in unusual sites such as mesenteric, hepatic, and portal veins. Treatment with hydroxyurea to keep the platelet count at 5,00,000 or below is the therapeutic approach. Raynaud disease features the Raynaud phenomenon wherein the finger tips exhibit pain and color changes, usually demarcated at the proximal interphalangeal joints (PIP). The attacks are *precipitated* by exposure to cold, the opposite in that regard to erythromelalgia. Secondary syphilis manifests generalized macular non-pruritic lesions that the palmar and solar areas. Dyshidrotic eczema occurs on the palms and soles as pruritic lesions with mild tendency to desquamation. Myelodysplasia is a group of diseases that feature cytopenias with hypercellular marrows and morphologic abnormalities in two or more hematopoietic cell lines. Sometimes, the collective diseases are classified as "preleukemias" because many cases evolve into myeloid leukemia. Usually, symptomatic presentation is based on clinical marrow failure with fatigue, infection, or bleeding. There is no particular acral dermatologic manifestation with this group of diseases.

5. The answer is B. One to two months is the low point of hemoglobin and the level at which it remains until the child reaches about the age of 8 years. In a comparison of the analogous hematocrit level, the months of 3 to 11 reveal a relative hypochromia (hemoglobin-to-hematocrit ratio of <1:3). This begins to be corrected after the growth rate slows markedly after the child's first birthday. If we assume these data apply to the population at large and all socioeconomic groups, then the reason for the lag in correction to the teen levels is quite likely due to iron deficiency, which reflects the rapid growth in the 1st year that outruns the dietary iron. The latter reveals that too often the hemoglobin of the growing infant is still not checked frequently enough or that iron-fortified formula is not being prescribed as a routine in the majority of well baby care practice. Either is acceptable, as some practitioners prefer to forego iron-fortified formula because of frequent GI side effects, usually hard stools. *In lieu* of fortified formula, hemoglobin should be checked by about 9 months; in many cases, iron should be prescribed separately when needed.

6. The answer is C. Variability of red cell width (range of RDW) is increased in iron deficiency. MCV is lower than normal in iron deficiency (i.e., the anemia is microcytic).

Mean cell hemoglobin is lower than normal (i.e., hypochromic). The ratio between the red cell count in millions and the hemoglobin is lower than normal, which is another indication of hypochromia. The serum ferritin level is low, reflecting low total body iron stores, a condition that exists before the hemoglobin begins to fall in iron deficiency.

7. The answer is D. A serum iron level of 40 μg/dL and a TIBC of 400 μg/dL would be an expected relationship between serum iron and TIBC, given the probability of iron deficiency anemia in a woman with prolonged menometrorrhagia. A serum iron level of 100 μg/dL and a TIBC of 300 μg/dL (Choice A) represents virtually the median normal values for iron and TIBC, and the ratio of 1:3 is expected (i.e., the transferrin saturation of 33% is the median point of normal). In iron deficiency, as the serum iron falls, the iron-binding capacity rises in a homeostatic response. A serum ferritin level of 200 ng/mL, an indirect measure of total body iron, represents 2 g, where normal is 1 to 4 g of total body iron. In iron deficiency, the total body iron level will have fallen to well less than 1 g by the time the serum iron level begins to fall.

8. The answer is C. The incorrect statement is that hemochromatosis is most common in people of Asian descent. The ethnic group in whom the disease is virtually always found is white Anglo-Saxon, particularly northern Europeans, North Americans, Australians, and New Zealanders. Transferrin saturation is elevated from the first year of life, over 60% as compared to the normal of 30%. It is a cause of impotence, fatigue arthritis in the DIPs and PIPs as well as, in the advanced stages, cirrhosis and risk of hepatocellular carcinoma. Total body iron is accumulated with the passage of time, and in men, usually this causes organ damage and symptoms at the age of 50 or later, at least 10 years before women due to their monthly iron loss in otherwise normal women. The staging of the disease is measured indirectly by serum ferritin content. Approximately 85% of cases are conveyed by the *C282Y* gene, recessive but partially penetrant. About 7% of susceptible groups carry the mutation, resulting in a 0.5% frequency of homozygotes. Of those, 8% of males and 1% of females will develop clinical symptoms. Treatment is by phlebotomy.

9. The answer is C. Serum iron level of 20 μg/dL and TIBC of 60 μg/dL, as characteristic of anemia of chronic disease. Note that the serum iron level (normal is 100 μg/dL) and the TIBC (250 to 410 μg/dL) are each decreased by the same proportions so that the transferrin saturation remains at about 33%. This is seen most often in aged individuals but may occur as well in younger people who are chronically ill. Mean cell hemoglobin and MCV should be normal. Ferritin level should also be normal, reflecting

normal iron stores. The ferritin example given is abnormally high, in the range of hemochromatosis. The reticulocyte count increases in recovery from reversible anemias, such as iron deficiency, and in other conditions calling for increased erythropoiesis, such as hemolytic anemias.

10. The answer is E. Pernicious anemia manifests a macrocytic peripheral picture and may reach strikingly low hemoglobins. Furthermore, late in the course, one finds a neutropenia with hypersegmented cells and thrombocytopenia. The proximate cause is vitamin B$_{12}$ (cobalamin) deficiency, which in pernicious anemia comes about as the result of a lack of intrinsic factor, needed for dietary B$_{12}$ absorption. Cobalamin is also a cofactor in the conversion of folate to its active form; thus, folic acid therapy may go a long way in redressing the macrocytic anemia in pernicious anemia but does not prevent the neurological sequelae, to be described. Cobalamin deficiency may occur in dietary deficiency and malabsorption (e.g., in sprue), but these two conditions are comparatively rare. The red cell aberrations are identical in the three diseases. Marrow aplasia, which may be expressed as aplastic anemia or as pure red cell aplasia, is characterized by normochromic, normocytic red cells. The neurologic complications of pernicious anemia are peripheral neuropathy (stocking/glove hypesthesia) followed later by posterior column degeneration, accounting for balance problems (subacute combined degeneration). Atrophic gastritis is a heralding condition, is associated with other GI symptoms, and conveys an increased risk of gastric carcinoma. Low B$_{12}$ level is present in the absence of dietary or GI cause. Differentiation from nutritional B$_{12}$ deficiency is effected by the finding of elevated methylmalonic acid, the product of the metabolic arrest in the development of cobalamin. Treatment of pernicious anemia is vitamin B$_{12}$ 1 mg daily IM for 8 weeks followed by monthly dosing as maintenance therapy. Preceding the failure of B$_{12}$ production in the gastric mucosa, it has undergone atrophic change on an autoimmune basis.

11. The answer is B. Resistance to protein C activation (resistance to anaphase-promoting complex activation) is the cause of 50% of cases of venous thrombosis not accounted for by another explicable cause. This abnormality is a mutation in Leiden factor V and thus produces a functional deficiency of protein C, which normally works in part by inactivating Leiden factor V. Protein C thus prevents hypercoagulability by inactivating coagulation factors V and VIII. Inherited deficiency of protein C accounts for 5% of otherwise unexplained deep vein thrombosis. Protein S functions with and depends on vitamin K as an endogenous anticoagulant factor. Inherited deficiency of protein S is a less common form of constitutional hypercoagulability. Prothrombin nucleotide mutation occurs in the prothrombin gene, wherein adenine is substituted for guanine at position 20210. The result is excessive levels of prothrombin and hypercoagulability, the second most common cause of otherwise unexplained venous thrombosis.

12. The answer is D. Antithrombin III deficiency is associated with a relative resistance to heparin because heparin is a cofactor in the physiologic function of antithrombin III. Thus, heparin needs antithrombin III presence for its effectiveness. In cases in which heparin resistance is encountered, fresh-frozen plasma should be given along with heparin.

13. The answer is D. Folic acid deficiency explains a macrocytic anemia in an alcoholic who displays no signs of posterior column abnormalities or peripheral neuropathy. Alcoholism is nearly certain, given the macrocytic anemia, lower than expected BUN and creatinine levels (insufficient protein intake), mild hepatocellular enzyme elevations with alanine aminotransferase more strikingly so, and the physical stigmata of telangiectasias. (These are the form fruste of spider angiomata.) The discussion of Question 7 covers most of the reasoning for this unit. Pernicious anemia manifests a macrocytosis but with eventual neurologic involvement. Iron deficiency shows a microcytosis and hypochromia; hemolytic anemias manifest increase in urine urobilinogen and elevated unconjugated serum bilirubin levels; beta-thalassemia is a hemolytic anemia that happens to manifest microcytosis and normochromia. Both beta- and alpha-thalassemias tend to occur in Mediterranean ethnic groups. The presentation of the patient as being of Greek descent was a red herring.

14. The answer is E. Infarctions that are due to polycythemic crises do not occur as sequelae of SCD. On the contrary, SCD is, of course, a condition of anemia, not polycythemia. The African-American infant with SCD is typically well until 6 to 8 months of age while his predominantly fetal hemoglobin is gradually replaced by hemoglobin S (SS), in a homozygous sickle cell sufferer. After that age, he may begin suffering from bouts of severe pain caused by splenic red cell sequestration, and he manifests splenomegaly. In addition, the patient often suffers from dactylitis. By the time the infant reaches the age of 2, the spleen has infarcted to the point of atrophy and functional asplenia. Most of the critical events attendant to SCD are directly or indirectly related to sludging of red cells and concomitant vaso-occlusive phenomena. Microinfarctions of various tissues, such as mesentery and bone, are results of sludging. Bone infarctions cause aseptic necrosis of the humerus and femoral heads. There is also an acute chest syndrome that carries a 10% mortality rate and is thought to be based on microvascular pulmonary infarctions, occasionally leading to pulmonary embolism.

Unrelated directly to vaso-occlusive disease is the hemolytic crisis that may occur in SCD and, if not recognized, may lead to acute heart failure within a few hours.

15. The answer is A. Polycythemia vera involves increased levels of all the formed blood elements. The only other problem choice that fits that picture would be Choice D, spurious polycythemia caused by dehydration and hemoconcentration. The latter is ruled out by the relatively dilute urine. Secondary polycythemia caused by altitude, chronic lung disease, or smoking should involve only the erythroid elements. Polycythemia vera is a myeloproliferative disorder that is characterized by hypervolemia (hence hypertension), plethora, splenomegaly, and generalized pruritus. There is a significant chance of evolution into myeloid leukemia. Thrombotic disease is a frequent complication caused by the increased viscosity of the blood. Treatment historically has been phlebotomy, and this is still used. Also in the past, more definitive therapy included (radioactive) ^{32}P. Presently, hydroxyurea or anagrelide is used for myelosuppression. Low-dose aspirin is employed for prevention of thromboses.

16. The answer is C. Multiple myeloma. The most common presentations are complaint of bone pain, pathologic fractures, pallor, and symptoms of fatigue; and laboratory findings of normocytic, normochromic anemia and hypercalcemia. Metastatic carcinoma to bone usually is characterized by elevated alkaline phosphatase. Multiple myeloma features lytic but not blastic bone lesions; hence, alkaline phosphatase is not elevated, and such pathologic fractures will not show on radionuclide bone scan. Plain x-rays may demonstrate the typical lytic "punched out" metastatic lesions. Although proteinuria is not always present, as multiple myeloma proteins are light chain and not often found in the urine, proteinuria may be present early. Waldenström macroglobulinemia does not involve the bones and features heavy chain (hence the term *macroglobulin*) paraprotein. Although osteoporosis results in pathologic fractures, it would not explain the other findings in the vignette. (Occasionally, osteoporosis may be the sole skeletal finding in multiple myeloma.) Serum protein electrophoresis readily demonstrates the monoclonal spikes. These occur in the beta- or (gamma)-globulin region in multiple myeloma, with 60% being immunoglobulin (Ig)G, 25% IgA paraprotein, and 15% light chain only. The spike occurs in the IgM region in Waldenström macroglobulinemia. The latter, because of the large chain protein, is characterized especially by hyperviscosity and problems attendant thereto. Bone marrow examination shows infiltration by plasma cells in multiple myeloma, comprising 5% to 100% of the content; in Waldenström macroglobulinemia, abnormal-appearing plasmacytic lymphocytes are seen in the marrow and in small numbers in the peripheral smear, whereas in multiple myeloma plasma cells are only rarely seen peripherally. One percent of all adults and three percent of people over the age of 70 years have monoclonal gammopathy of unknown significance, most commonly an IgG spike with less than 2.5 g/dL. In 25% of cases, this progresses over a period of many years to overt malignancy. Nearly all patients with IgG spikes >3.5 g/dL prove to have multiple myeloma.

17. The answer is A. Hodgkin disease presents as a painless mass, often in the cervical lymph nodes or with constitutional symptoms suggesting low-grade fever. Nearly specific is pain in the lymphoid mass with alcohol ingestion and often intolerance to tobacco.

References

Blinker CA. Blood. In: Tierney LM, McPhee SJ, Papadakis MA, eds. *Current Medical Diagnosis and Treatment.* 45th ed. New York/Chicago/San Francisco: Lange, McGraw-Hill; 2006.

Family Medicine Review. Kansas City, Missouri; May 3–10; 2009.

Fitzpatrick TB, Eisen AZ, Wolff L, Freedbuerg IM, Austen KF, eds. *Dermatology in General Medicine,* 3rd ed. New York/St. Louis/San Francisco: McGraw-Hill; 1987.

Lee GR, Bithell TC, Foerstel J, Athens JW, Lukens JN, eds. *Clinical Hematology.* Philadelphia; London: Lea and Febiger; 1993.

McKnight JT, Eklund EA. Hematology. In: Rakel RE, ed. *Textbook of Family Practice.* 6th ed. Philadelphia: WB Saunders; 2002.

McPhee SJ, Papadakis MA, eds. *Current Medical Diagnosis and Treatment,* 49th ed. New York/Chicago: Lange, McGraw-Hill; 2010.

Mengel MB, Schiebert LP, eds. *Family Medicine Ambulatory Care & Prevention,* 5th ed. New York: Lange, McGraw-Hill; 2009.

chapter 56

Drug Interactions, Caveats, and Primary Care

Examination questions: Unless instructed otherwise, choose the ONE lettered answer or completion that is BEST in each case.

1 A 25-year-old male complains of a mildly pruritic rash that appears on the trunk as evenly distributed ovoid papulosquamous lesions. Besides pityriasis rosea, each of the following drugs may precipitate this rash as an expression of allergy except for which one?

(A) Captopril
(B) Barbiturates
(C) Sulfonamides
(D) Metronidazole
(E) Metoprolol

2 A middle-aged male has been diagnosed with onychomycosis and wishes to be rid of the troublesome bilateral great toe subungual accumulations of sloughed squamous material. The patient takes several medications. Each of the following drugs or categories of drugs should be considered for lowering their current dosages except which one?

(A) Tricyclic antidepressants
(B) Beta-adrenergic blocking agents
(C) Selective serotonin reuptake inhibitors (SSRIs)
(D) Ethinyl estradiol
(E) Class C antidysrhythmia drugs

3 A 55-year-old male patient with treated hypertension has been referred to a psychiatrist for bipolar disorder. He returns within a few weeks for his routine follow-up visit, having been placed on lithium carbonate. Each of the following drugs is relatively contraindicated in this patient due to the danger of precipitating toxicity of lithium except for which one?

(A) Acetazolamide
(B) Hydrochlorothiazide
(C) Carbamazepine
(D) Lisinopril
(E) Metronidazole

4 Symmetrel (amantadine) is indicated in two quite different types of conditions: prophylaxis against and treatment of influenza A and extrapyamidal central nervous system (CNS) disease and extrapyramidal drug side effects. Which of the following drugs or preparations given simultaneously with amantadine has been shown to worsen the tremor of Parkinson disease?

(A) Hydrochlorothiazide/triampterene
(B) Amitriptyline
(C) Benztropine
(D) Thioridazine
(E) Trihexyphenidyl

5 A 34-year-old woman has been diagnosed with type 2 diabetes, with a 2-hour postprandial blood sugar level of 160 mg/dL. Her glycohemoglobin is 8% of the total. She has had no operations, and her health is unremarkable except for her moderate obesity. The family doctor plans to start metformin. Which of the following must be measured before commencing with this plan?

(A) Complete blood cell count
(B) Liver function battery
(C) Lipid screen
(D) Serum creatinine
(E) Chest x-ray

6 Regarding the patient in Question 5, she has been started on metformin 500 mg twice daily. The family doctor considers placing her on an angiotensin-converting enzyme inhibitor (ACEI) to maximize preservation of renal function in a diabetic. The patient says that she is attempting to achieve pregnancy. Which of the following is a strict contraindication to this drug?

(A) Chronic renal failure
(B) Chronic obstructive lung disease
(C) Pregnancy in the second trimester
(D) Asthma
(E) Pregnancy in the first trimester

7 A 45-year-old man has been treated for hypertension with clonidine (e.g., Catapres), titrated to 0.2 mg daily. However, he has begun to complain of fatigue, and the primary care doctor makes a decision to change the antihypertensive medication to the beta-1 selective blocking agent, atenolol. Which of the following is the wisest method for making the change?

(A) Start the atenolol as 50 mg daily 2 days before discontinuation of the clonidine.

(B) Start atenolol 4 days before the discontinuance of clonidine as 25 mg daily and increase it to 50 mg daily 2 days before the change.

(C) Start the atenolol at the maintenance dosage of 50 mg on the day after the last dose of clonidine.

(D) Discontinue clonidine and wait 2 days before starting atenolol at a prudent beginning dosage.

(E) Taper the clonidine off as the atenolol is started low and accelerates, with the two drugs overlapping in their subtherapeutic levels over a 4-day period.

8 Besides the manifestations of Cushing syndrome, which of the following may be a complication of systemic glucocorticoid administration over several weeks?

(A) Decreased insulin requirements in diabetics

(B) Lymphoproliferative disorder

(C) Atrophic gastritis

(D) Premature closure of epiphyses in growing children

(E) Glaucoma

9 A 33-year-old woman is brought to an emergency department in stupor with a history of attempting suicide with a prescribed benzodiazepine. Which of the following is the specifically indicated drug for this emergency?

(A) Naloxone

(B) Buprenorphine

(C) Flumazenil

(D) Dextroamphetamine

(E) Phenobarbital

10 Fluoxetine (Prozac, an SSRI antidepressant) has been prescribed for a 35-year-old woman with depression. Which of the following side effects would be more likely, given this combination, if she is to be given tolterodine (Detrol) for her recurrent trigonitis that is causing urinary frequency (Detrol, urinary antispasmodic agent)?

(A) Bradycardia

(B) Gastritis

(C) Gastroesophageal reflux disease (GERD)

(D) Dry mouth

(E) Decreased near point of visual focus

11 A 34-year-old male patient is seen by a physician for the first time; he presents himself as depressed and taking tranylcypromine (Parnate) prescribed by a doctor in another city for the past 4 months. The patient expressed doubt, insecurity, and frustration with the current regimen because of the necessity to avoid aged cheeses, wines, and other foods to avoid the risk of serious behavioral and neurological side effects. The adopting physician conducts her own interview and is satisfied that the man is indeed depressed and still in need of completing a 1-year course of medication. The new doctor is considering a change to fluoxetine (Prozac, an SSRI) for the patient's depression. Which of the following is the best technique for effecting the transition from tranylcypromine to fluoxetine?

(A) Continue tranylcypromine and start fluoxetine. Discontinue tranylcypromine after 2 days.

(B) Continue tranylcypromine and start fluoxetine. Discontinue tranylcypromine after 2 weeks.

(C) Discontinue tranylcypromine and start fluoxetine the next day.

(D) Discontinue tranylcypromine and wait 2 weeks before starting fluoxetine.

(E) Discontinue tranylcypromine and wait 4 weeks before starting fluoxetine.

12 Risperidone (Risperdal), an antipsychotic agent, is contraindicated in which of the following groups of people?

(A) Teenaged patients

(B) Elderly patients

(C) Schizophrenic patients

(D) Patients with pneumonia

(E) Patients with urinary tract infections

13 A 37-year-old male patient with schizophrenia has been treated with pimozide (Orap) with satisfactory control. He now has developed a community-acquired pneumonia. Which of the following antibiotics is contraindicated?

(A) Clarithromycin

(B) Ampicillin

(C) Amoxicillin

(D) Sulfamethoxazole

(E) Doxycycline

14 The high-potency topical glucocorticoid, betamethasone, is indicated for certain inflammatory skin conditions on a temporary basis. Each of the following side effects is known to be caused by prolonged application of this preparation, except for which one?

(A) Cushing syndrome

(B) Adrenocorticotropin suppression

(C) Systemic effects passed through breast milk

(D) Atrophy of the treated area of the skin

(E) Precipitation of diabetes

15 If a pregnant woman has been treated for dyslipidemia, which of the following drugs would be safe to continue throughout the period of gestation?

(A) Cholestyramine

(B) Gemfibrozil

(C) Simvastatin

(D) Atorvastatin

(E) Fenofibrate

16 Atorvastatin (Lipitor) will have its blood levels increased when given in combination with each of the following, except for which drug?

(A) Ketoconazole

(B) Diltiazem

(C) Gemfibrozil

(D) Grapefruit juice

(E) Beta-adrenergic blocking agents

17 The anticoagulant warfarin interacts with many medications to increase its blood level, risking bleeding complications. Which of the following drugs in combination with warfarin acts to decrease warfarin blood levels?

(A) Dextrophenydate

(B) Rifampin

(C) Amiodarone

(D) Fluconazole

(E) Metronidazole

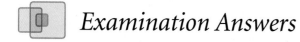

Examination Answers

1. The answer is C. Sulfonamides is the group or drug mentioned that is not included among those that may precipitate a pityriasis-like rash. Other agents that may do so besides those mentioned (captopril, barbiturates, metronidazole, and metoprolol) include bismuth, clonidine, gold salts, methopromazine, and tripelennamine.

2. The answer is D. Ethinyl estradiol is not metabolized in the 2D6 system. Lamisil (terbutaline) inhibits 2D6 metabolism, and the other drugs presented in the vignette are metabolized in that system; hence, their dosages might need to be lowered due to their enhanced metabolism when terbutaline is administered at the same time. In addition to tricyclics, beta-blockers, SSRIs, and class C antidysrhythmics (e.g., flecainide and propafenone), other CYP 450 2D6 metabolized drugs that would fall under this alert include monoamine oxidase inhibitors (MAOIs).

3. The answer is A. Acetazolamide increases renal excretion, thus reducing the chance of lithium toxicity. All other diuretics, that is, thiazides and loop diuretics like furosemide, as well as any clinical dehydration states and conditions that result in dehydration including diarrhea and vomiting enhance the tendency to reduce serum sodium manifesting lithium toxicity. ACEIs increase the risk of lithium intoxication. Carbamazepine enhances the risk of neurotoxicity of lithium. Metronidazole may provoke lithium toxicity due to reduced renal clearance as do urea, xanthines, and alkalinizing agents. Lithium toxicity encompasses a large spectrum of physiological systems including cardiovascular (e.g., dysrhythmias), gastrointestinal, dermatologic (including alopecia, anesthesia, acne, xerosis cutis, and psoriasis).

4. The answer is D. Thioridazine has been reported to worsen the tremor of Parkinson disease when given along with amantadine (Symmetrel). It is not known whether other phenothiazines have the same effect. Hydrochlorothiazide/triampterene (Dyazide, Maxzide) has been shown to increase the blood level of amantadine when the two are taken during the same period. Amitriptyline (Elavil), trihexyphenidyl (Artane), and benztropine (Cogentin) each potentiates the anticholinergic effects of amantadine.

5. The answer is D. The serum creatinine level must be checked before metformin is started. Lactic acidosis, albeit rare, has been reported with the usage of metformin in the presence of renal failure. The pharmaceutical guidelines state that metformin should not be prescribed if the serum creatinine level is above 1.5 mg/dL in male patients or 1.4 in female patients. Metformin should be held for 48 hours before general anesthesia. The foregoing is emphasized more in diabetics, the very group for whom it is prescribed.

6. The answer is C. Pregnancy in the second or third trimester is a firm contraindication for ACEIs and for angiotensin-converting enzyme receptor blocking agents (e.g., valsartan). These drugs may cause fetal injury or death. Although dry cough may be a side effect of ACEIs (not angiotensin-converting enzyme receptor blocking agents) and this may be a subclinical expression of asthma or reactive airway disease, a history of these conditions is not a contraindication to the use of ACEIs.

7. The answer is D. Discontinue clonidine and wait 2 days before starting atenolol at a prudent beginning dosage. Beta-blockers may exacerbate rebound hypertension following discontinuance of clonidine. Thus, if the beta-blocking agent is present when discontinuance of clonidine is contemplated, then the beta-blocker should be stopped 2 days before the clonidine. If the beta-blocker is to replace clonidine, then it should wait for 2 days after discontinuance of clonidine before being started.

8. The answer is E. Glaucoma as a complication of prolonged usage of glucocorticoids is perhaps not appreciated; it is less well known than side effects such as precipitation of diabetes, elevation of blood pressure, Cushing syndrome, aggravation of certain viral infections (varicella, herpes zoster keratitis), and osteoporosis. The other choices have no relationship to glucocorticoids and are true distracters.

9. The answer is C. Flumazenil is a benzodiazepine receptor blocker and is specific for overdose of this family of drugs. Naloxone and buprenorphine are virtually complete and partial opioid antagonists respectively. Phenobarbital, one of the most ancient sedatives, would, of course, aggravate the sedative effects of the benzodiazepine. Dextroamphetamine, although a sympathomimetic medication, is not employed in sedative overdose management. However, dextroamphetamine inhibits gastrointestinal absorption of the sedative phenobarbital.

10. The answer is D. Dry mouth. Fluoxetine (Prozac), being CYP2D6 system metabolized, increases blood level of tolterodine, an anticholinergic antispasmodic and as such would be expected, even normally to result in a high percentage of incidence of dry mouth. This would be compounded and enhanced by any drug that increases its blood level. Each of the other "side effects" mentioned as distracters is actually a condition that would be ameliorated by the anticholinergic effects of the medications presented. Thus, tachycardia, not bradycardia; reduction of acid production, salutary for both gastritis and GERD; *increase* in near focal distance, concurrent with pupillary mydriasis and paralysis of accommodation.

11. The answer is D. Discontinue tranylcypromine; wait 2 weeks before starting fluoxetine. Under threat of hypertensive crisis, behavioral emergencies, hyperthermia, and other problems, these two medications should not be given together and should not overlap in time. Parnate is an MAOI, and several other drugs are strictly contraindicated when given in conjunction with MAOIs. These include dextroamphetamine; all other SSRIs; any drug with anticholinergic effects including tricyclic antidepressants; any sympathomimetic such as the amphetamines; meperidine within 3 weeks of MAOI on board; dextromethorphan. Also, foods that contain significant amounts of tyramines such as cheeses must be avoided.

12. The answer is B. Elderly patients with dementia should seldom be treated with risperidone. In field studies, elderly individuals were 1.4 to 1.6 times as likely as placebo-taking subjects to die while under treatment. The deaths were most often due to cardiovascular and cerebrovascular events as well as infection. Therefore, if the drug is used in elderly people, those conditions as underlying or symptomatic should be ruled out before deciding in favor of starting the medication. None of the other conditions appears as definite or relative contraindications.

13. The answer is A. Clarithromycin in conjunction with pimozide (and with astemizole, cisapride, and terfenadine) may result in life-threatening ventricular dysrhythmias, including ventricular tachycardia, ventricular fibrillation, and torsade de pointes. This is assumed to be related to inhibition of metabolism of these drugs by clarithromycin. The phenomenon occurs with erythromycin as well.

14. The answer is C. Systemic effects passed through breast milk have not been shown with topical applications of glucocorticoids on nursing mothers. All of the other effects mentioned, well known in association with oral or injected glucocorticoids, are possible as a result of the topical route.

15. The answer is A. Cholestyramine, colesevelam, and colestipol are known to be safe for pregnancy and the fetus. Gemfibrozil, fenofibrate, and especially all HMG-CoA reductase inhibitors place the fetus at risk.

16. The answer is E. Beta-adrenergic blocking agents do not appear on the lengthy list of medications that increase the blood levels of atorvastatin. That list, however, includes not only ketoconazole, diltiazem, gemfibrozil, and grapefruit juice but also bosentan, clarithromycin, cyclosporine, erythromycin, fluconazole, and itraconazole. The presence of fenofibrate with atorvastatin increases the chances of rhabdomyolysis.

17. The answer is B. Rifampin is among the few drugs that interact with warfarin to decrease its blood level, risking hypercoagulability, and compromise of the therapeutic goal of the anticoagulant regimen. Other examples are tabulated in Table 56–1. Far longer is the list of drugs that increase warfarin levels and exaggerate the anticoagulant effect (see Table 56–1).

TABLE 56–1 Tabulation of Drugs by Effect on Warfarin Levels or Risk of Hemorrhage

Raise Level	Lower Level or Otherwise Risk Bleeding
Barbiturates	Amiodarone dextrophenydate
Bosentan	Cefamandole
Capecitabine	Cefmetazole
Mercaptopurine	Cefoperazone
Phenytoin (chronic)	Cefotetan
Rifampin	Chloramphenicol
Carbamazepine	Fluconazole
	Fluvoxamine
	Itraconazole
	Ketoconazole
	Metronidazole
	Phenytoin (acute)
	Salicylates (specifically enhance bleeding chances)
	Sulfamethoxazole
	Ticlopidine
	Voriconazole
	Zafirlukast

References

Green GB, Harris IS, Lin GA, et al. *The Washington Manual of Medical Therapeutics*, 31st ed. Philadelphia: Williams & Wilkins; 2004.

McPhee SJ, Papadakis MA. *Current Medical Diagnosis and Treatment*, 49th ed. New York/Chicago: Lange, McGraw-Hill; 2010.

Suarez RA, Fleming MF. Abuse of controlled substances. In: Rakel RR, ed. *Textbook of Family Practice*. 6th ed. Philadelphia: WB Saunders; 2002:1539–1547.